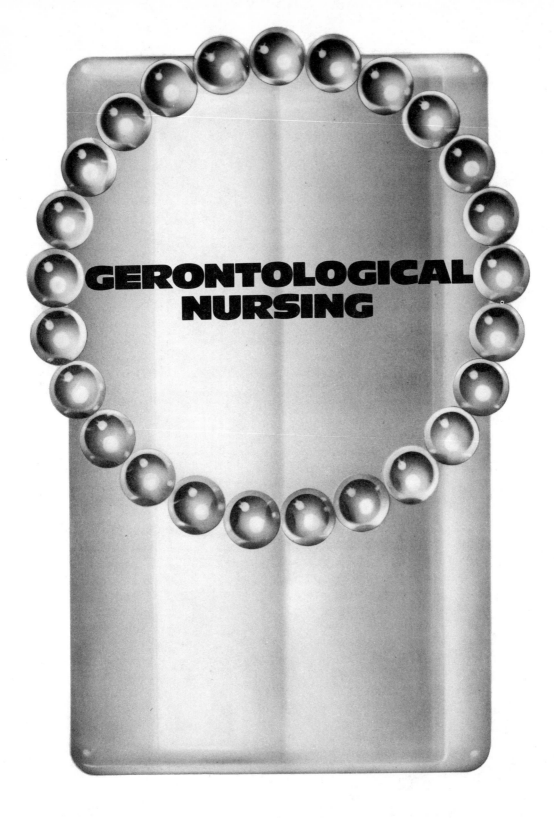

GERONTOLOGICAL NURSING

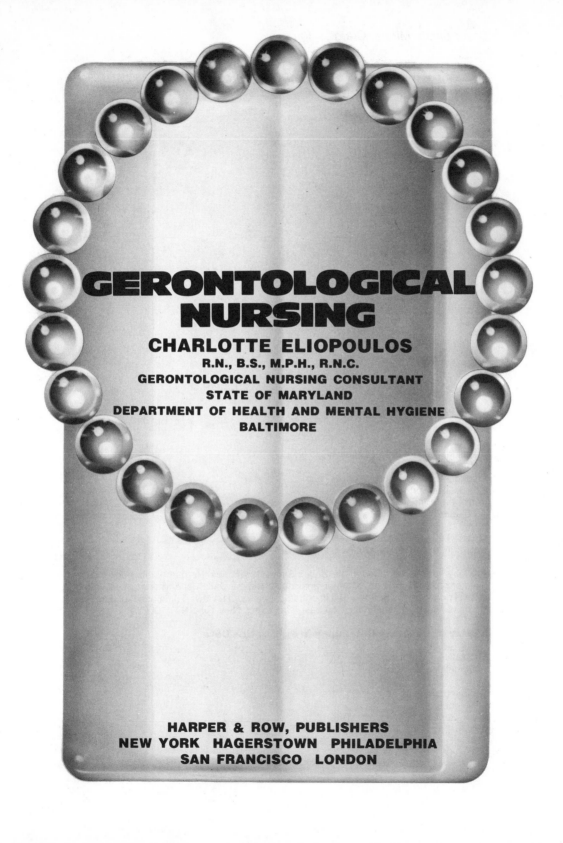

GERONTOLOGICAL NURSING

CHARLOTTE ELIOPOULOS

R.N., B.S., M.P.H., R.N.C.
GERONTOLOGICAL NURSING CONSULTANT
STATE OF MARYLAND
DEPARTMENT OF HEALTH AND MENTAL HYGIENE
BALTIMORE

HARPER & ROW, PUBLISHERS
NEW YORK HAGERSTOWN PHILADELPHIA
SAN FRANCISCO LONDON

Cover photo: Michel Craig

Photographs on pages 4, 41, 75, 95, 201, 219, 245, 263, 287, 327, 335, and 351: Robert Goldstein.

Sponsoring Editor: Bonnie Binkert
Designer: Michel Craig
Production Supervisor: Marion A. Palen
Compositor: Port City Press
Printer and Binder: The Murray Printing Company
Art Studio: J & R Technical Services, Inc.

GERONTOLOGICAL NURSING

Library of Congress Cataloging in Publication Data

Eliopoulos, Charlotte.
  Gerontological nursing.

  Bibliography: p.
  Includes index.
  1. Geriatric nursing. I. Title.
[DNLM: 1. Geriatric nursing. WY152 E42g]
RC954.E44   610.73'65   78-25587
ISBN 0-06-043754-5

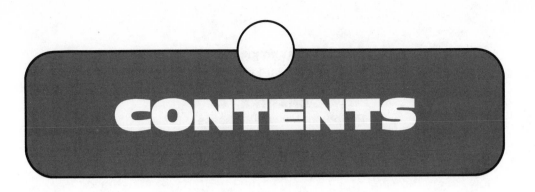

CONTENTS

CONTENTS

CONTENTS

vii

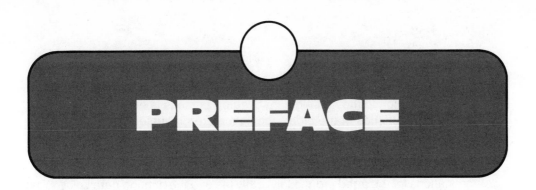

PREFACE

The growing number of elderly persons in the population, and the more active role they are assuming, have increased society's awareness of the qualities, rights, and needs of its older members. Popular literature that dispels myths concerning the aging process, proliferates. Government is demonstrating greater sensitivity to the problems of old age, as evidenced by legislation promoting increased security and care for the aged. The media exposes the public to the often overlooked pleasures and problems of growing old in America. Society thus has a new concern for the aging population.

The increased numbers of the aged have influenced the helping professions to become more closely involved in the fields of gerontology and geriatrics. During the past few decades alone, tremendous strides have been made in conducting research, preparing specialists, developing educational programs, increasing literature, and providing clinical services in gerontology and geriatrics. Because of the complexities and challenges of working with the aged, greater numbers of professionals are entering this area of specialization.

The nursing profession is experiencing an outstanding attitudinal shift in its view of caring for the aged. Once viewed as the bottom rung of the nursing ladder—a stepchild speciality—gerontological nursing has blossomed into one of the most popular and expanding fields of practice. The sophisticated blend of knowledge and skill required to deliver appropriate gerontological care supports the fact that gerontological nurses must have special cognitive and clinical capabilities.

An introduction to the nursing care of aging persons is offered in this book. Characteristics of the older population are presented to help the reader differentiate myths from realities. There is a review of aging theories, emphasizing their strengths and weaknesses. Characteristics of the normal aging process will be identified and transferred into implications for the aged individual's daily life and the nursing care he or she may require. The unique knowledge and skill utilized in applying the nursing process to the aged will be discussed.

In addition to information pertaining to normal aging and health promotion in old age, it is important for gerontological nurse to understand the special features of the aged's illnesses. A portion of this book reviews major problems that affect each body system, and outlines differences in symptomatology, diagnosis, management, and related nursing care.

Currently popular issues in aging and geriatric care have special chapters devoted to them. Included among these topics are: geriatric pharmacology, sexuality, the dying process, surgical care, sensory deficits, services for the aged, and mental health and illness.

This book is designed as an introduction to gerontology, geriatrics, and nursing care of the aged. It provides a basic framework upon which gerontological nursing practice can be developed. Rather than being all inclusive, this book is a stepping-stone to assist the reader into a deeper exploration of gerontology literature.

The reader should note that the words *old, aged,* and *geriatric* are used throughout the text to describe older persons. Although a negative connotation is often associated with these words, it is the author's belief that the attitudes and behaviors demonstrated to older persons are far more significant than the labels they are given.

C. E.

ACKNOWLEDGMENTS

No author writes a book alone; the ideas, support, and efforts of persons too numerous to mention go into the birth of a book.

There are many persons to whom I'd like to express my gratitude. From Jim Kopelke and Sandy Orem I received the encouragement and support that only very special friends can provide as I experienced the many peaks and valleys in the process of writing this book. Praise must go to Gladys Spiller who performed the vital task of transferring hundreds of handwritten pages into typewritten form.

Last, but not least, I am deeply indebted to the many older persons who taught me the wisdom, strength, and beauty of old age.

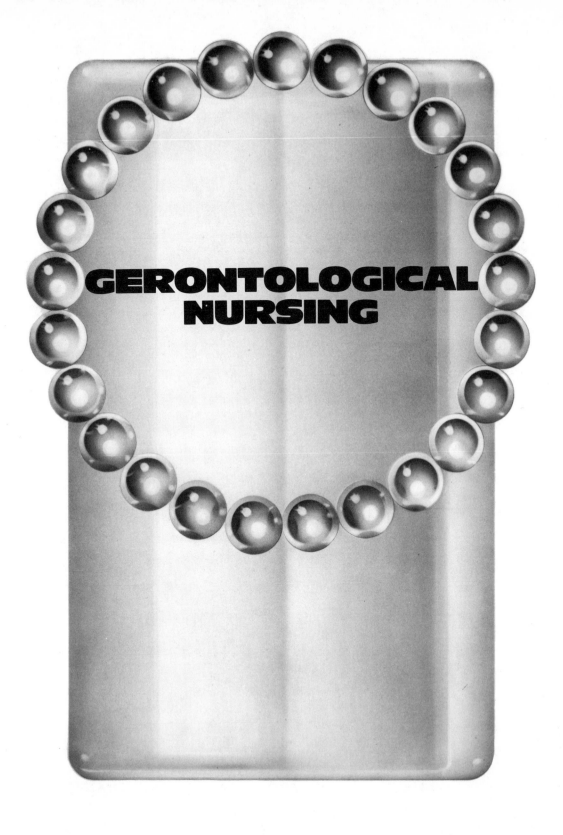

GERONTOLOGICAL NURSING

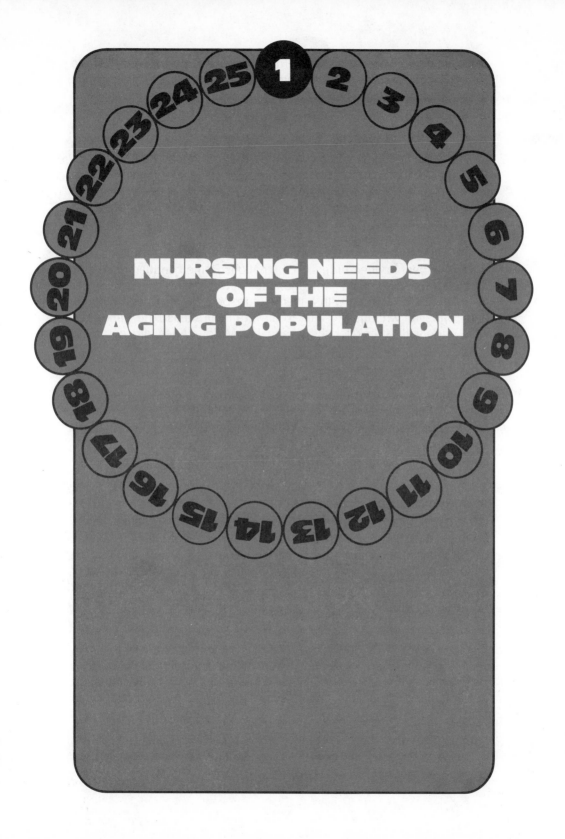

NURSING NEEDS OF THE AGING POPULATION

Older members of a society have always received some degree of attention, and many historical writings depict both the positive and the negative attributes of growing old. Confucius' time expressed a direct correlation between one's age and the respect to which one was entitled. Taoism viewed old age as the epitomy of life, and the ancient Chinese believed that attaining old age was an accomplishment deserving the greatest honor. The early Egyptians, on the other hand, dreaded old age and experimented with a variety of potions and schemes to avoid that end. Greek views were divided—the myths portraying many struggles between old and young and quests for immortality and fountains of youth, Plato promoting the aged as society's best leaders, and Aristotle denying them any role in government matters. Ancient Romans, according to descriptions, had limited respect for their elders; in the nations Rome conquered the sick and the aged were customarily the first killed.

The Bible is laced with a theme of respect for the aged, although early Christian writings did little to elevate their status. The Dark Ages were especially bleak for them, and the Middle Ages did not bring considerable improvement. A strong feeling for the superiority of youth occurred during medieval times, with uprisings of sons against fathers. The art of this period also portrayed an uncomplimentary image of the aged, Father Time for example. The aged were also among the first to be hurt by famine and poverty and the last to benefit during better times. Many gains made during the eighteenth and nineteenth centuries were lost because of the cruelties of the industrial revolution. While child labor laws were developed to guard the frail lives of minors, the frail lives of the aged were left unprotected, and those unable to meet industrial demands were placed at the mercy of their offspring or forced to beg on the streets for sustenance.

Although Dr. I. L. Nascher, known as the father of geriatrics, wrote the first geriatric textbook in 1914, American literature during the first half of the twentieth century reflects little improvement in the status of the aged. Most significant was the passage under the Social Security Act of the Federal Old Age Insurance Law in 1935, which provided some financial security for older persons. Only recent literature has viewed the age with positivism rather than prejudice, intelligence rather than myth, and concern rather than neglect. The past few decades have brought a profound awakening of interest in older people as their numbers in society have grown. A generally more humanistic attitude toward all people has affected the aged also, and improvements in health care and general living conditions ensure more people of the opportunity to achieve old age.

There has been a growing recognition that the unique needs and problems of older persons require separate attention, evidenced by the development of the American Geriatrics Society in 1942, the beginning of the Gerontological Society in 1944, the first National Conference on Aging in 1950, the founding of the Senior Citizens of America in 1954 and the American Society for the Aged in 1955, and the establishment of a Federal Council on Aging in 1956. Concurrent efforts have been made to expand research, develop educational programs, and provide comprehensive services pertaining to aging individuals.

Before continuing, we should define some of the terms we will encounter throughout this book.

Aged: used as an adjective to mean old, as a noun to mean old people.
Aging: continuous process of maturation beginning at conception and terminating at death.
Geriatrics: concerned with diseases of old age.
Gerontology: study of the normal aging process.
Incidence: number of new cases of a condition occurring during a specific period of time.
Life expectancy: average number of years that an organism will probably live.
Life span: full extent of years that an organism is capable of living.
Old age: conventionally accepted as being the period of life past age 65, although realistically, chronological age alone does not determine if one is young or old. May be subcategorized into younger old for those 60–75 years of age, and older old for those over 75.
Prevalence: number of cases of a condition existing at a given time.
Senescence: period of life in which changes related to the aging process are evident; not related to senility, which implies a deterioration of function.

STANDARDS FOR NURSING THE AGED

Nurses, long interested in the care of the aged, seem to have assumed more responsibility than any other profession for people in this group. In 1904 the *American Journal of Nursing* printed the first nursing article on the care of the aged, presenting many principles that still guide gerontological nursing practice today (Bishop, 1904):

> You must not treat a young child as you would a grown person, nor must you treat an old person as you would one in the prime of life.

Interestingly, in that same year the same journal featured an article entitled "The Old Nurse," which emphasized the value of the aging nurse's years of experience (DeWitt, 1904).

After the passage of the Federal Old Age Insurance Law in 1935, many older persons had an alternative to alms houses and could

3

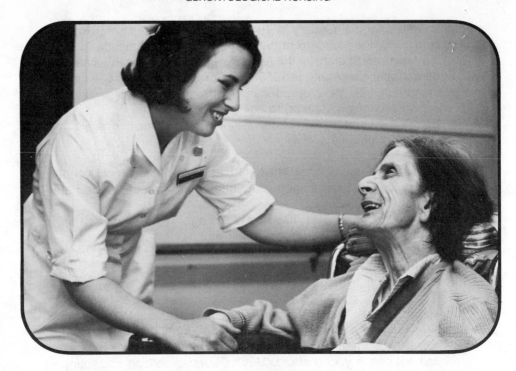

independently pay for their room and board. Because many homes for the aged were opened by women who called themselves nurses, it is not coincidental that such residences later became known as nursing homes. For many years care of the aged was an unpopular branch of nursing practice. A stigma was attached to geriatric nurses, implying that they were somewhat inferior in capabilities or not good enough for acute settings or ready to go to pasture. Geriatric facilities may have further discouraged many competent nurses from working in these settings by paying low salaries, and little was found to counterbalance the negativism in educational programs, where experiences with older persons were inadequate in quantity and quality and focused on the sick rather than the well, who were actually more representative of the older population. While nurses were among the few groups who were exposed to experiences with the aged, gerontology was nonexistent in most nursing curriculums until recently.

Frustration over the lack of value of geriatric nursing led to an appeal to the American Nurses' Association for assistance in promoting the status of geriatric nursing. After years of study, the American Nurses' Association recommended in 1961 that a specialty group for geriatric nurses be formed. In 1962 the American Nurses' Association's Conference Group on Geriatric Nursing Practice held its first national meeting. This group became the Division on Geriatric Nursing in 1966, gaining full recognition as a nursing specialty. An important contribution by this group was the development in 1969 of Standards for Geriatric Nursing Practice, first published in 1970. Certification of nurses for excellence in geriatric nursing practice followed, with the first 74 nurses achieving this recognition in 1975. Another significant event in 1975 was the birth of the *Journal of Gerontological Nursing,* the first professional journal to meet the specific needs and interests of gerontological nurses.

Interest grew in changing the name from Geriatric to Gerontological Nursing since geriatrics is concerned with the diseases of old age and nurses working with the aged in addition to caring for illnesses have the broader goal of helping individuals maximize their capacities throughout the aging process. In 1976 the Geriatric Nursing Division became the Gerontological Nursing Division. This landmark and others in the growth of gerontological nursing appear in the chronological listing here.

> 1904—First nursing article on care of the aged published in *American Journal of Nursing*
> 1961—American Nurses' Association recommendation for formation of specialty group for geriatric nurses
> 1962—First national meeting of American Nurses' Association's Conference Group on Geriatric Nursing Practice in Detroit, Michigan
> 1966—Formation of Geriatric Nursing Division of American Nurses' Association
> 1969—Development of Standards for Geriatric Nursing Practice
> 1970—First publication of Standards for Geriatric Nursing Practice
> 1975—First nurses certified in Geriatric Nursing
> 1975—*Journal of Gerontological Nursing* first published
> 1976—Geriatric Nursing Division changes title to Gerontological Nursing Division

Standards have been developed to guide nurses who work with the aged in achieving a high quality of practice, and to guarantee quality service to the public. With the change in the name of the Division came a change in the title of its standards. These Standards of Gerontological Nursing Practice are presented below. It is essential for the gerontological nurse to be knowledgeable about them and to use them as a framework for practice.

STANDARDS OF GERONTOLOGICAL NURSING PRACTICE

Standard I
Data are systematically and continuously collected about the

health status of the older adult. The data are accessible, communicated, and recorded.

Rationale: In order to provide comprehensive nursing care of the older adult, the data are collected from a framework that includes the scientific findings and knowledge derived from the fields of gerontology and nursing.

Assessment Factors
1. Health status data includes the older adult.
   Normal responses to the aging process
   Physiological, psychological, sociological, and ecological status
   Modes of communication
   Individual's patterns of coping
   Prior life-style
   Independent performance of activities of everyday living
   Perception of and satisfaction with current health status
   Health goals
   Human and material resources available and accessible
2. Health status data are collected from:
   The older adult, significant others, health care personnel
   Other individuals in the immediate environment who are involved in the care of the older adult
   Interviews, examination, observation, records, and reports
3. The data are:
   Accessible on the older adult's records
   Retrievable from record-keeping system
   Communicated to those responsible for the older adult's care
   Accurate
   Confidential

Source: The American Nurses' Association, Washington, D.C., 1976.

Standard II
Nursing diagnoses are derived from the identified normal responses of the individual to aging and the data collected about the health status of the older adult.

Rationale: Each person ages in an individual way. The individual's normal response to aging must be identified before deviations in response requiring nursing actions can be identified.

Assessment Factors:
1. The older adult's health status is compared to the norm, and a determination is made regarding deviations from the norm.

2. The older adult's prior life-style, responses to the aging process, and personal goals and objectives are identified.
3. The older adult's strengths and limitations are identified.
4. The nursing diagnosis is related to and congruent with the diagnosis and plan of all other professionals caring for the older adult.

Standard III
A plan of nursing care is developed in conjunction with the older adult and/or significant others that includes goals derived from the nursing diagnosis.

Rationale: Goals are a determination of the results to be achieved and are an essential part of planning care. All goals are ultimately directed toward maximizing achievable independence in everyday living.

Assessment Factors:
1. Goals are congruent with other planned therapies, are stated in realistic and measurable terms, and are assigned a time period for achievement.
2. Goals determine specific nursing approaches that will promote, maintain, and restore health.
3. Goals are measured by the eventual outcomes of nursing care.
4. The established goals incorporate
   Normal developmental processes of aging
   Individuality of the older adult
   Needs for intimacy and sexual expression
   Slowing down
   Losses
   Adaptability

Standard IV
The plan of nursing care includes the priorities and the prescribed nursing approaches and measures to achieve the goals derived from the nursing diagnosis.

Rationale: Priorities and approaches are an integral part of the planning process and are necessary to the successful achievement of the goals.

Assessment Factors:
1. Physical and psychosocial measures are planned to prevent, ameliorate, or control specific problems of the older adult and

7

are related to the nursing diagnosis and goals of care.
2. Environmental hazards, which may include high-frequency sounds, glaring surfaces, and overproduction of stimuli that cause confusion are eliminated.
3. Methods of adaptation using concepts of wellness are taught to the older adult.
4. Specific approaches are identified to orient the older adult to new roles and relationships, to any new surroundings, and to relevant health resources.
5. Specific approaches are identified to promote social interactions and effective communication.

Standard V
The plan of care is implemented, using appropriate nursing actions.

Rationale: Appropriate nursing actions are purposefully directed toward the stated goals.

Assessment Factors:
Nursing actions are:
Consistent with plan of care developed in collaboration with the older adult and with appropriate input from other health disciplines
Based on scientific principles
Individualized to the specific situation
Modified to allow for alternative approaches
Used to provide a safe and therapeutic environment
Compatible with the physiological, psychological, and social data acquired
Task-delegated as deemed appropriate
Planned to meet specific criteria as described in protocols

Standard VI
The older adult and/or significant others participate in determining the progress attained in the achievement of established goals.

Rationale: The older adult and/or significant others are essential components in the determination of nursing's impact upon the individual's health status.

Assessment Factors:
1. Current data are used to measure progress toward goal achievement.
2. Nursing actions are analyzed for effectiveness in goal achievement.
3. The older adult and/or significant others evaluate nursing actions and goal achievement.
4. Plans for the nursing follow-up of the older adult are made to permit the ongoing assessment of the effects of nursing care.

Standard VII
The older adult and/or significant others participate in the ongoing process of assessment, the setting of new goals, the reordering of priorities, the revision of plans for nursing care, and the initiation of new nursing actions.

Rationale: Comprehensive nursing care is dependent upon actively involving the older adult and/or significant others in a continuing dynamic process.

Assessment Factors:
1. Assessment is based on the level of progress of the older adult in goal achievement.
2. The older adult and/or significant others assist in the identification of new goals and the reordering of priorities.
3. Plans are updated and revised.
4. New nursing actions are appropriately initated.

Some requisites of the gerontological nurse testify to the uniqueness and validity of this nursing specialty. Gerontological nurses must understand the normal aging process and recognize deviations from normal. They must be aware that aging is a highly individualized process with different outcomes in each individual. The atypical pattern of disease frequently displayed in the aged, and the differences in disease diagnosis and management in this group, must be realized. The gerontological nurse should be acquainted with the psychosocial factors associated with aging and must be able to work with professionals in other

9

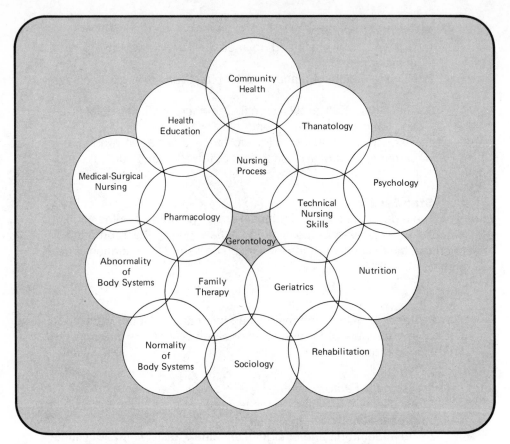

Figure 1-1. Information system of the gerontological nurse.

disciplines to achieve effective outcomes. Empathy, sensitivity, sincerity, and patience are particularly important attributes of the gerontological nurse. It is also helpful for gerontological nurses to understand and accept their own aging process, recognizing their own mortality.

Today a growing number of nurses are recognizing the complexities and challenges of gerontological nursing. Few other specialties provide an opportunity for nurses to blend the knowledge and skills from so many disciplines. (See Figure 1-1.) The broad scope of gerontological nursing allows nurses to contribute to the care of the aged in settings for community, chronic, and acute conditions through direct clinical practice, research, education, and administrative or advocacy activities. Entering the field of gerontological nursing ensures a career that is unique, challenging, and rewarding to its practitioners.

TABLE 1-1: POPULATION 65 YEARS OF AGE AND OVER

Year and Population Group	Number of People (× 1000)	Percentage of Total Population
1960		
Total	16,560	9.2
Male	7,503	
Female	9,056	
White	15,304	
Male	6,908	
Female	8,396	
Black	1,176	
Male	547	
Female	629	
1970		
Total	19,972	9.9
Male	8,367	
Female	11,605	
White	18,272	
Male	7,615	
Female	10,657	
Black	1,544	
Male	669	
Female	876	
1974		
Total	21,815	10.3
Male	8,966	8.7
Female	12,849	11.8
White	19,883	10.8
Male	8,129	
Female	11,755	
Black	1,732	7.2
Male	733	
Female	999	
Percent		
1960	9.2	
1970	9.9	
1974, total	10.3	
Male	8.7	
Female	11.8	
White	10.8	
Negro	7.2	

Source: U.S. Bureau of the Census, *U.S. Census of Population: 1960 and 1970*, Vol. 1; and *Current Population Reports*, series P-25, No. 529.

TABLE 1-2: EXPECTATION OF LIFE AT BIRTH, 1920 TO 1973

Year	U.S. Population			White Population			Black Population and Others		
	Total	Males	Females	Total	Males	Females	Total	Males	Females
1920	54.1	53.6	54.6	54.9	54.4	55.6	45.3	45.5	45.2
1930	59.7	58.1	61.6	61.4	59.7	63.5	48.1	47.3	49.2
1940	62.9	60.8	65.2	64.2	62.1	66.6	53.1	51.5	54.9
1950	68.2	65.6	71.1	69.1	66.5	72.2	60.8	59.1	62.9
1955	69.6	66.7	72.8	70.5	67.4	73.7	63.7	61.4	66.1
1960	69.7	66.6	73.1	70.6	67.4	74.1	63.6	61.1	66.3
1965	70.2	66.8	73.7	71.0	67.6	74.7	64.1	61.1	67.4
1970	70.9	67.1	74.8	71.7	68.0	75.6	65.3	61.3	69.4
1971	71.1	67.4	75.0	72.0	68.3	75.8	65.6	61.6	69.7
1972	71.1	67.4	75.1	72.0	68.3	75.9	65.6	61.5	66.9
1973	71.3	67.6	75.3	72.2	68.4	76.1	65.9	61.9	70.1

Source: U.S. National Center for Health Statistics, *Vital Statistics of the United States* (annual), in U.S. Bureau of the Census, *Statistical Abstract of the United States: 1975,* p. 59, No. 82.
Note: Prior to 1960, Alaska and Hawaii are excluded.

PROFILE OF THE AGED

Gerontological nurses must know the characteristics of the aged not only to deliver effective services to this population but also to clarify misconceptions among persons of all ages. Many people erroneously believe that families put their aged in nursing homes and forget them or that most old people are sick all the time or that social security provides a comfortable life-style in retirement or that most old people benefit from senior citizen centers while Medicare takes care of all their health care costs. Such ideas are an injustice not only to the aged but also to younger adults, who need accurate information to prepare realistically for their own old age.

In the United States there are more than 22 million people 65 years of age or older, representing over 10 percent of the population. As shown in Table 1-1, more are female than male, more white than nonwhite. Table 1-2 shows the increase in life expectancy since 1920. As shown, females enjoy a longer life expectancy than males in both white and nonwhite races: 76.1 years for white females, 70.1 years for nonwhite females, 68.4 years for white males, and 61.9 years for nonwhite males. Several factors have contributed to a longer life expectancy for Americans: advancements in disease control and health technologies; an increase in the number of people able to survive the previously hazardous period of infancy and other dangers throughout the lifespan (Table

TABLE 1-3: DEATH RATES

	Death Rate per 1000	
Year	Total Population	Infants
1910	14.7	NA
1915	13.2	99.9
1920	13.0	85.8
1925	11.7	71.7
1930	11.3	64.6
1935	10.9	55.7
1940	10.8	47.0
1945	10.6	38.3
1950	9.6	29.2
1955	9.3	26.4
1960	9.5	26.0
1965	9.4	24.7
1970	9.5	20.0
1971	9.3	19.1
1972	9.4	18.5
1973	9.4	17.7
1974	9.1	16.5

Source: U.S. National Center for Health Statistics, *Vital Statistics of the United States* (annual).

NA: Not available.

1-3); improved sanitation and general living conditions. As can be seen in Table 1-4, the ratio of older males to older females has steadily declined throughout this century, to 69.8 to 100. Over half the women 65 years of age and older are widowed, whereas a majority of older men are married (Table 1-5); and women in the older age group (75 and over) are the ones most affected by widowhood (Table 1-6). The customary practice of women marrying men older than themselves also contributes to this picture.

A recent survey by Louis Harris and Associates disproved the widespread belief that families forget their parents and grandparents, thus contributing to isolation of the aged. It was found that most older persons had seen their children and grandchildren within the past week; many had seen them within the past few days. Only a small percentage had not seen their families for several months. Interestingly, not only did older persons have contact with their family on a regular basis, but they were often found to provide meaningful services to the family, such as baby-sitting, giving gifts, and caring for the ill. Most older persons also have siblings with whom they have frequent contact. We should be

13

TABLE 1-4: SEX RATIO IN POPULATION 65 YEARS AND OLDER

Year	Number of Males per 100 Females
1910	101.1
1920	101.3
1930	100.5
1940	95.5
1950	89.6
1960	82.8
1970	72.1
1974	69.8

Source: U.S. Bureau of the Census, based on *U.S. Census of Population: 1950, 1960, and 1970,* part B; and *Current Population Reports,* series P-25, No. 529.

aware that families are an important support system to the aged (Harris, 1975a).

Figure 1-2 presents an overview of the distribution of the aged population among the states. Most of the aged live in urban settings, and many live in rural areas, but the suburbs have not attracted a large number of older persons because of limited public transportation, the prevalence of large homes for growing families, and the general cost of living. A majority of older persons are not employed, due primarily to retirement. Although only 12 percent are either fully or partially employed, the employment rates for persons 65 to 69 years of age are much higher than those for 70 years and over: 18 percent of those 65 to 69 years old are employed, 4 percent full time and 14 percent part time

TABLE 1-5: MARITAL STATUS
OF POPULATION 65 YEARS OLD AND OVER IN 1975

	Number of Males and Females (× 1000)	Number of Males (× 1000)	Number of Females (× 1000)
Number of people 65 and over	20,602	8,528	12,074
Single	1,155	389	766
Married	11,396	6.727	4,669
Widowed	7,556	1,224	6,332
Divorced	497	189	308

Source: U.S. Bureau of the Census, *Current Population Reports,* series P-20, No. 271, and series P-60, No. 93.

TABLE 1-6: MARITAL STATUS
OF OLDER POPULATION IN 1974 BY AGE AND SEX

	Number of Males (× 1000)		Number of Females (× 1000)	
	65–74 Years	75 Years and Over	65–74 Years	75 Years and Over
Total older population	5,680 (100%)	2,848 (100%)	7,412 (100%)	4,662 (100%)
Single	246 (4.3%)	143 (5.0%)	487 (6.6%)	279 (6.0%)
Married	4,790 (84.3%)	1,937 (68.0%)	3,531 (47.6%)	1,138 (24.4%)
Widowed	507 (8.9%)	717 (25.2%)	3,155 (42.6%)	3,177 (68.1%)
Divorced	137 (2.4%)	52 (1.8%)	239 (3.2%)	69 (1.5%)

Source: U.S. Bureau of the Census, *Current Population Reports,* series P-20, No. 271.

(Harris, 1975b). The older persons who are employed represent a small percentage of the total labor force (Table 1-7). The reasons given for not being in the labor force are shown below (U.S. Department of Labor, 1975). Of those not in the labor force who "would like to work" (31 percent of unemployed aged), the major obstacles to their employment are: poor health (57 percent) feeling "too old" (28 percent), and lack of opportunity or availability of jobs (15 percent) (Harris, 1975c). Concern over loss of pensions and other benefits accounts for only a small percentage of the reasons given for older persons not being employed. The median income in 1975 for people 65 years and older was $3809 for males and $2375 for females (U.S. Bureau of the Census, 1975a). With the rising cost of living, this amount can do little more than meet the essential expenses of a modest life-style. It is not surprising that over 15 percent of the aged have incomes at or below the poverty level—with many more surviving on slightly more than that amount (U.S. Bureau of the Census, 1975b).

The aged are among the less educated members of society. Less than half of today's older population graduated from high school, and of those who did, only 18 percent completed a college education (Table 1-8). The aged have a greater percentage of illiteracy than any other age

REASONS GIVEN BY MALES	PERCENT	REASONS GIVEN BY FEMALES	PERCENT
Retirement, old age	24.8	Home responsibilities	81.6
Ill health, disability	16.8	Retirement, old age	8.6
Home responsibilities	1.8	Ill health, disability	8.3
Other	6.5	Other	1.6

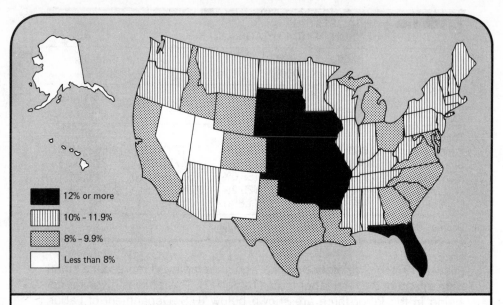

12% or more

10% – 11.9%

8% – 9.9%

Less than 8%

ESTIMATED POPULATION AGED 65+, BY STATE, 1975

State	Number (000's)	Percent of Total Population	Rank[1]	Percent Increase, 1970-75	State	Number (000's)	Percent of Total Population	Rank[1]	Percent Increase, 1970-75
Total	22,613	10.4	—	12.2	Montana	75	10.0	29[t]	9.5
Excluding Puerto Rico					Nebraska	194	12.5	6	6.2
and outlying					Nevada	44	7.4	49	42.9
areas	22,400	10.5	—	12.2	New Hampshire	87	10.6	22	11.4
Alabama	378	10.5	23[t]	16.6	New Jersey	767	10.5	23[t]	10.6
Alaska	9	2.6	54	32.4	New Mexico	90	7.8	47	28.2
Arizona	223	10.0	29[t]	38.6	New York	2,030	11.2	16[t]	4.0
Arkansas	271	12.8	2	14.5	North Carolina	492	9.0	38	19.5
California	2,056	9.7	34	14.8	North Dakota	73	11.5	13[t]	10.3
Colorado	210	8.3	44[t]	12.3	Ohio	1,066	9.9	32[t]	7.3
Connecticut	321	10.4	26	11.6	Oklahoma	334	12.3	8	11.8
Delaware	50	8.6	42	14.6	Oregon	259	11.3	15	14.7
District of Columbia	71	9.9	32[t]	1.0	Pennsylvania	1,377	11.6	12	8.7
Florida	1,347	16.1	1	36.7	Rhode Island	113	12.2	9	8.8
Georgia	430	8.7	41	17.7	South Carolina	229	8.1	46	20.6
Hawaii	57	6.6	50[t]	29.6	South Dakota	85	12.4	7	5.9
Idaho	79	9.6	35	17.2	Tennessee	441	10.5	23[t]	15.4
Illinois	1,153	10.3	27[t]	5.9	Texas	1,158	9.5	36	17.3
Indiana	531	10.0	29[t]	8.0	Utah	91	7.5	48	18.1
Iowa	364	12.7	3	4.2	Vermont	52	11.0	19	9.9
Kansas	285	12.6	4[t]	7.4	Virginia	424	8.5	43	16.4
Kentucky	368	10.8	20[t]	9.6	Washington	365	10.3	27[t]	13.9
Louisiana	346	9.1	37	13.4	West Virginia	211	11.7	11	8.9
Maine	125	11.8	10	9.5	Wisconsin	512	11.1	18	8.8
Maryland	340	8.3	44[t]	14.0	Wyoming	33	8.8	40	9.7
Massachusetts	672	11.5	13[t]	6.1	American Samoa	1	2.4	55	4.8
Michigan	815	8.9	39	8.8	Guam	2	1.8	56	21.6
Minnesota	440	11.2	16[t]	8.0	Puerto Rico	203	6.6	50[t]	14.6
Mississippi	253	10.8	20[t]	14.4	Trust Territories	4	3.5	53	27.9
Missouri	601	12.6	4[t]	7.6	Virgin Islands	4	3.8	52	52.8

[1] States are ranked in order of decreasing percentages (higher percentage is rank 1, lowest is 54).
[t] Tied in ranking. States with identical percentages receive identical rank number with following rank number(s) shipped to allow for number in tie.

TABLE 1-7: DISTRIBUTION OF LABOR FORCE IN 1974 BY AGE

Age in Years	Percent
16–19	9.9
20–24	15.0
25–34	23.4
35–44	18.2
45–54	18.4
55–64	12.0
65 and over	3.1

Source: U.S. Bureau of Labor Statistics, *Employment and Earnings* (monthly), in U.S. Bureau of the Census, *Statistical Abstract of the United States*, 1975, p. 344, No. 560.

group (U.S. Bureau of the Census, 1975c). Only 2 percent of those enrolled in educational institutions or taking courses are 65 years of age and older, and there is a direct relationship between the level of education achieved and the likelihood of enrolling in a course (Harris, 1975d). The reasons given by older persons for taking courses are primarily to expand their knowledge about a particular field or hobby and to use their spare time productively; few seek to acquire job skills by taking a course. Rather than lack of availability or expense, the main reason given by those older persons not enrolled in courses is that they are "not interested" (Harris, 1975c). Perhaps a higher quantity and quality of educational opportunities, specific to the interests of this group, can involve more aged persons in formal educational programs.

Most older persons view religion as a very important part of their lives and attend a church or synagogue regularly. As is true of the general population, most of the aged are Protestant (70 percent); less than one-fourth are Catholic (24 percent), and only a small proportion are either Jewish (2 percent) or some other religion (Harris, 1975f). In addition to their religious functions, religious organizations often provide many social services for the aged, such as senior citizen clubs, household assistance, and lunch programs. Although over 50 percent of the aged have convenient access to a senior citizen center, only a minority actually utilize such a service. These centers seem to appeal to

Figure 1-2. Geographic distribution of population over 65 years of age in 1975. (Source: U.S. Dept. of Health, Education, and Welfare, Office of Human Development, Administration on Aging, *Facts About Older Americans, 1976.*

TABLE 1-8: HIGH SCHOOL AND COLLEGE
GRADUATES, 1900 to 1975, AND PROJECTIONS
TO 1984, BY SEX, AND BY CONTROL OF HIGH SCHOOL

High School Graduates

Year of Graduation	Total Number (× 1000)	Percentage of Total 17-Year-Old Population[a]	Males (× 1000)	Females (× 1000)
1900	95	6.4	38	57
1920	311	16.8	124	188
1940	1,221	50.8	579	643
1950	1,200	59.0	571	629
1955	1,351	60.7	648	703
1960	1,864	65.1	898	966
1965	2,665	74.0	1,314	1,351
1966	2,632	75.8	1,308	1,325
1967	2,679	75.5	1,332	1,348
1968	2,702	74.5	1,341	1,360
1969	2,829	75.7	1,402	1,427
1970	2,896	75.7	1,433	1,463
1971	2,943	75.2	1,456	1,487
1972	3,006	74.4	1,490	1,516
1973	3,037	74.3	1,501	1,536
1974 Est	3,095	74.5	1,537	1,558
1975 Est	3,119	74.4	1,549	1,570
1980	3,043	74.6	1,511	1,532
1982	2,908	75.0	1,443	1,465
1983	2,783	75.4	1,381	1,402
1984	2,679	72.6	1,329	1,350

Source: U.S. National Center for Education Statistics, *Earned Degrees Conferred* (annual); *Digest of Educational Statistics* (annual); *Projections of Educational Statistics to 1983–84*; and unpublished data in U.S. Bureau of the Census: *Statistical Abstract of the United States: 1975*, p. 135, No. 222.
Note: Prior to 1960, excludes Alaska and Hawaii.
NA: Not available.
EST: Estimated.
[a] Beginning 1962, based on persons 18 years of age.
[b] Bachelor's or first professional degree. Data cover public and private institutions.

						College Graduates[b]

Control						

Public	Private (Est)	Total Number (× 1000)	Per 1000 Persons 23 Years Old	Per 100 High School Graduates 4 Years Earlier	Males (× 1000)	Females (× 1000)
NA	NA	27	19	36	22	5
NA	NA	49	26	19	32	17
NA	NA	187	81	18	110	77
NA	NA	432	182	40	329	103
1,208	143	286	151	24	183	103
1,633	231	392	182	27	254	138
2,366	298	530	203	27	316	214
2,334	298	551	186	29	329	222
2,381	298	590	212	30	353	237
2,402	300	667	243	29	391	276
2,529	300	764	282	29	444	320
2,596	300	827	223	31	484	343
2,643	300	878	255	33	511	367
2,706	300	927	269	34	538	389
2,737	300	1,005	293	36	580	425
2,795	300	1,031	290	36	583	448
2,819	300	1,029	NA	NA	575	454
2,743	300	1,091	NA	NA	588	502
2,608	300	1,106	NA	NA	596	510
2,483	300	1,094	NA	NA	588	506
2,379	300	1,086	NA	NA	584	503

women more than to men, and to lower income groups more than to higher income groups. There is no significant difference in the attendance of senior citizen centers based on race, in spite of the fact that these centers are least accessible to blacks (Harris, 1975g).

The voting record of the older segment of the population is quite impressive. Over 50 percent of the voting population 65 years of age and older vote, second only to the 45- to 64-year-old group. Although the

19

TABLE 1-9: ACTIVITY LIMITATIONS RESULTING
FROM SELECTED CHRONIC CONDITIONS IN PERSONS 65
AND OLDER, BASED ON NONINSTITUTIONALIZED PERSONS, 1972

	Persons 65 and Over		
Limitation Factor	Total Population	Males	Females
Persons with activity limitation per 1000	8613	3904	4709
Percentage limited by			
heart conditions	18.8	19.2	18.5
arthritis and rheumatism	16.9	11.6	21.3
visual impairments	3.0	3.2	2.8
hypertension without heart			
involvement	4.0	2.8	4.9
mental and nervous conditions	1.7	1.3	2.1
Percentage with			
no activity limitation	56.8	53.0	59.5
activity limitation	43.2	47.0	40.5
limitation in major activity	37.9	43.3	34.1

Source: U.S. National Center for Health Statistics, *Vital and Health Statistics,* series 10, No. 96.

aged represent 10 percent of the total population, they constitute 15 percent of the voting population (U.S. Bureau of the Census, 1975d). In general, older voters are well informed, write to their legislators more frequently, and are more highly represented in political organizations.

Health Problems

The maintenance of health becomes more difficult with age. A lifetime of poor health care practices may combine with age-related bodily changes to make the aged more susceptible to health problems. Once present, health problems are more troublesome for the aged, usually requiring a longer recovery period and often subjecting the individual to multiple complications. A simple health problem for the younger adult can be life threatening to the aged individual. A common cold in an older person can easily progress to pneumonia, which may be undiagnosed until it has reached an advanced stage due to differences in the aged person's symptomatology. The resulting weakness and discomfort associated with pneumonia may lead the older person to stay in bed, causing the many complications associated with immobilization, which are compounded by such age-related factors as fragile skin, less

TABLE 1-10: MORTALITY RATES FOR
LEADING CAUSES OF DEATH IN THE AGED IN 1973

Males		Females	
Cause	Rate per 100,000	Cause	Rate per 100,000
Heart disease	3214.6	Heart disease	2242.0
Cancer	1274.6	Stroke	829.9
Stroke	852.9	Cancer	716.4
Pneumonia	266.1	Pneumonia	171.1
Accidents	159.6	Diabetes	134.1
Emphysema	151.4	Accidents	105.3
Diabetes	115.2	Cirrhosis of liver	22.5
Cirrhosis of liver	59.9	Emphysema	22.3
Suicide	38.1	Suicide	7.8
Homicide	8.7	Homicide	3.0

Source: U.S. National Center for Health Statistics, *Vital Statistics of the United States* (annual).

active respiratory muscles, poorer circulation, and decreased peristalsis.

The aged have more health problems than other age groups and have more than twice the per capita health care expenditure of any other age group (U.S. Social Security Administration, 1975). Older persons have four times the incidence of chronic diseases of other age groups; and almost half of all aged persons have some limitation in their ability to meet their self-care demands as a result of chronic diseases (Table 1-9). Although the incidence of acute conditions in the aged is less than half of that of the general population, the aged have more days of hospitalization for acute conditions than younger persons (U.S. Bureau of the Census, 1975e). Table 1-10 shows the leading causes of death in the aged. Heart disease, cancer, and stroke are the three major threats to the lives of older people. Many of the major causes of death can be prevented or more successfully managed with regular checkups and early detection and treatment. The aged, however, are among the least likely to engage in preventive health care services. A lifetime of crisis-oriented health care practices and limited finances are some factors contributing to this situation. Less than one-third of the aged population have annual checkups, chest x-rays, breast examinations, and vision screening (U.S. Bureau of the Census, 1975f).

Only 5 percent of the aged population are institutionalized, mostly in nursing homes. The percentage of national health expenditures for nursing home care has increased at a greater rate than any other type of

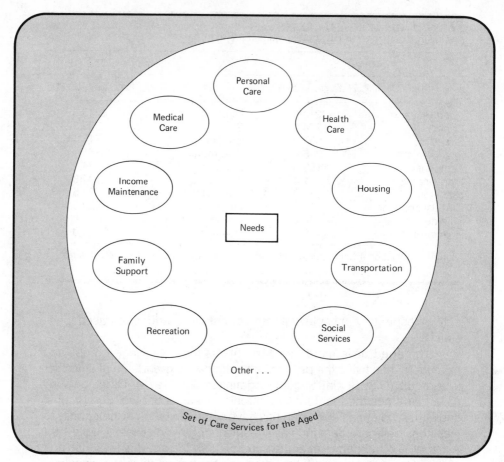

Set of Care Services for the Aged

Figure 1-3. Multidimensional care for the aged. Services must enter the circle of needs at appropriate times for optimal results.

health care service (U.S. Bureau of the Census, 1975g), and the nursing home industry is now a big business in this country. Many nursing homes provide excellent services for their residents; in others the limited quantity and quality of personnel, the physical facility, and fiscal constraints result in inadequate care for aged residents. The fact that the ratio of employees to residents in hospital settings is 2 to 1, whereas in nursing homes it is 1 to 5, gives some clue to the differences in services provided—especially since the need for personal care and therapeutic needs are often just as great. (U.S. Bureau of the Census, 1975h). Perhaps as the complexities of caring for older adults are realized there will be a change in the systems for delivering care in nursing homes.

The needs of the aged are in a dynamic state. As older persons move along the health-illness continuum, and as their capacities for functioning change both from normal aging and from abnormal conditions, the mix of services required to meet these needs will vary—not only among individuals but also at different times for any given individual. Although different services will predominate at various times, no single service or resource can function autonomously in the care of older persons. Effective gerontological nursing requires that the specialized talent of the nurse be used in concert with other disciplines to achieve multidimensional services for the aged (Figures 1-3).

REFERENCES

Bishop, L. F. "The Relation of Old Age to Disease, with Illustrative Cases." *American Journal of Nursing,* 4:679, 1904.

DeWitt, K. "The Old Nurse." *American Journal of Nursing,* 4:177–181, 1904.

Harris, L., and Associates. *The Myth and Reality of Aging in America.* National Council on Aging, Washington, D.C., 1975. (a) pp. 73–74, (b) p. 82, (c) pp. 89–90, (d) pp. 106–107, (e) pp. 108–109, (f) pp. 181–182, (g) pp. 182–183.

Nascher, Ignatz L. *Geriatrics.* Blakiston, Philadelphia, 1914.

U.S. Bureau of the Census. *Statistical Abstract of the United States, 1975.* (a) p. 287, No. 456; (b) p. 403, No. 658; (c) p. 120, No. 195; (d) p. 450, No. 728; (e) p. 85, No. 134; (f) p. 86, No. 137; (g) p. 70, No. 101; (h) p. 78, No. 121.

U.S. Department of Labor, Bureau of Labor Statistics. *Handbook of Labor Statistics, 1975.*

U.S. Social Security Administration. *Social Security Bulletin,* June 1975.

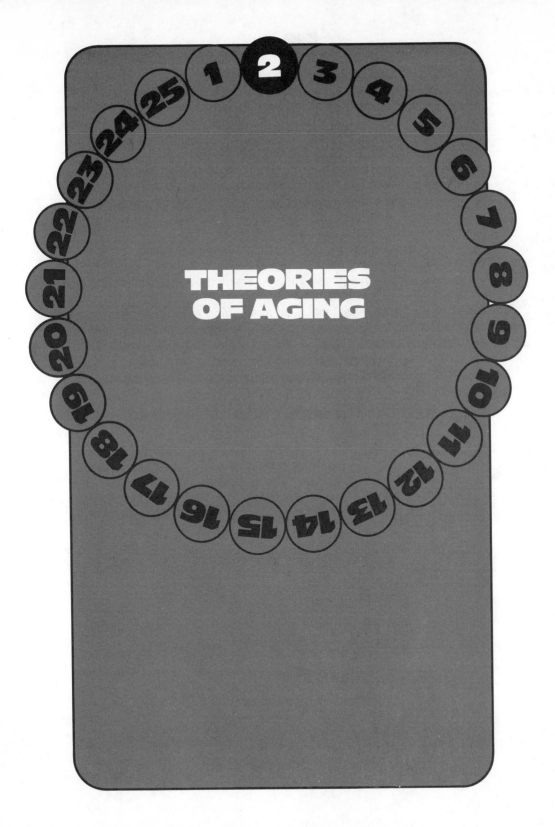

THEORIES
OF AGING

For centuries humanity has explored the mystery of aging, trying to discover a way to lengthen the lifespan and conducting numerous searches for a fountain of youth, the most famous being that of Ponce de Leon. Ancient Egyptian and Chinese relics show evidence of concoctions designed to prolong life or achieve immortality, and various other cultural practices throughout history include specific dietary regimens and the ingestion of herbal preparations. Ancient chemical life expanders prepared from the testicles of tigers may seem ludicrous until compared with modern day injections of embryonic tissue and novocaine, for example. Yoghurt, vitamins, cosmetic creams, and youth spas are some of the many items currently used to maintain youth and prolong the onset of old age.

There is no single factor which causes or prevents aging; the complexities of aging cannot be explained by one theory. Explorations into biological, psychological, and social aging continue, and although some activities focus on a "cure" for aging, most research efforts are aimed toward a better scientific understanding of this process. Aging theories, all in a formative stage and increasing in number, offer varying degrees of universality, validity, and reliability. Recognizing the limitations of these theories, the nurse may find a knowledge of them beneficial to understanding and caring for aging and aged individuals.

BIOLOGICAL THEORIES

The process of biological aging differs from species to species and also demonstrates much diversity in humans. Some general statements can be made about biological aging—for example, glomerular filtration rate at age 90 is one-half that at age 20, and the proportion of body fat is increased with age. However, no two individuals age identically, and you will find varying degrees of physiological changes, capacities, and limitations within a given age group. In addition, the rate of aging among various cells within one individual differs; one body system may show marked declines with advanced age while the others demonstrate no significant changes. Many theories have been espoused in an effort to explain biological aging according to intrinsic or extrinsic factors. Intrinsic factors include genetic programming, cellular mutation, autoimmune reactions and other inherent processes. Environmental influences, such as diet and radiation, are considered extrinsic factors.

Intrinsic Factors

Several theories assume that individuals inherit a genetic program that determines their specific life expectancy. In fact, various studies have shown a positive relationship between parental age and filial life span. Genetic mutations are also thought to be responsible for aging, a pattern depicted below; but laboratory experiments which have accelerated mutation rates have not produced proportionate increases in the rate of aging, thus reducing support of this theory. Some theorists believe that a growth substance fails to be produced causing the cessation of cell growth and reproduction, whereas others hypothesize that an aging factor responsible for development and cellular maturity throughout life is excessively produced. Cross-linkage of DNA strands may impair the cell's ability to function and divide, and the continued occurrence of this process may lead to the manifestations of aging. Although minimal research has been done to support this theory, aging may be a result of a decreased ability of RNA to synthesize and translate messages.

The accumulation of lipofuscin "age pigments" has been considered a biochemical basis for aging. Lipofuscin, a lipoprotein by-product of metabolism, can be seen under a fluorescent microscope. This insoluble, nonfunctional material is known to accumulate with age as a result of some unplanned, rare metabolic accident. The liver, heart, ovaries, and neurons are the sites in which lipofuscin tends to accumulate. Although the function and significance of this age pigment is not clear at this point, there is a positive relationship between the age of the individual and the number of lipofuscins (Strehler, 1962). Investigators have discovered the presence of lipofuscin in other species at amounts proportionate to the life span of the species, that is, an animal with one-tenth the life span of humans accumulates lipofuscin at a rate approximately ten times greater (Few and Getly, 1967). The existence of well-documented laboratory findings gives popularity to this theory.

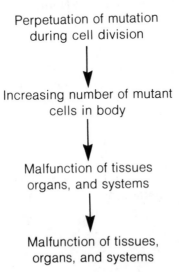

Mutation of DNA

Perpetuation of mutation
during cell division

Increasing number of mutant
cells in body

Malfunction of tissues
organs, and systems

Malfunction of tissues,
organs, and systems

27

Another fascinating group of theories postulates autoimmune reactions as being responsible for aging. Simply stated, the host attacks its own kind, either because of the presence of foreign cells or substances to which there has been no exposure, or because of a breakdown in the body's immunochemical memory, which makes it sensitive to its own constituents. This is shown diagramatically below. Diseases associated with normal aging and caused by autoimmune reactions, such as rheumatoid arthritis, could be explained by this theory.

One theory used to explain biological aging links collagen to the aging process. There is thought to be an increase in the amount of collagen and a loss of ground substance with age. Collagen may become cross-linked, rigid, and less permeable. The great density of the connective tissue may reduce the rate at which nutrients are deposited and wastes removed, leading to a deterioration of collagen and consequent slowing down of bodily processes. Excess collagen has been found in old tissue, but investigators are not able to determine if this is a causative factor or a result of the aging process.

Another theory attributes aging to the wear and tear of the cells of the body as they perform their highly specific functions over time. Insults and stresses to the body take their toll, and the result is less efficient functioning of the cells. Proponents of this theory point to the shortened life span caused by a life of overexertion and stress. Since each individual reacts differently to life's stresses, it is difficult for this theory to be universally valid.

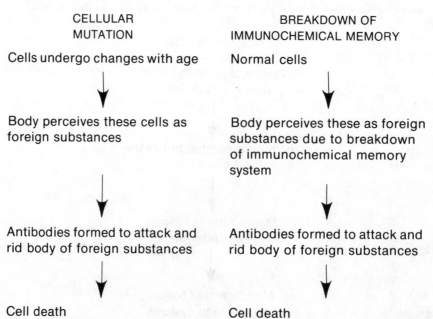

CELLULAR MUTATION	BREAKDOWN OF IMMUNOCHEMICAL MEMORY
Cells undergo changes with age	Normal cells
↓	↓
Body perceives these cells as foreign substances	Body perceives these as foreign substances due to breakdown of immunochemical memory system
↓	↓
Antibodies formed to attack and rid body of foreign substances	Antibodies formed to attack and rid body of foreign substances
↓	↓
Cell death	Cell death

Extrinsic Factors

Disease-producing organisms are often associated with biological aging. Bacteria, fungi, viruses, and other organisms are thought to be responsible for certain physiological changes during the aging process. Although no conclusive evidence presently exists to link these pathogens with the aging process, interest in this theory has been stimulated by the fact that humans and animals have been shown to live longer with the control or elimination of certain pathogens via immunization and the use of antimicrobial drugs.

The relationship of radiation and age changes has been, and continues to be, explored. Research in rats, mice, and dogs has shown a decreased life span resulting from exposures to nonlethal doses of radiation (Strehler, 1962). Repeated exposure to ultraviolet light is known to cause solar elastosis, "old age" type of skin wrinkling resulting from the replacement of collagen by elastin, and also to cause skin cancer in humans. There is some thought that radiation may induce cellular mutations which promote aging.

Nutrition is considered to have a significant influence on the aging process. Experiments with underfed fish have shown their growth rate to be retarded and their life span to be unusually longer (Hershey, 1974). Underfed rats have also proven to live longer than their overfed cohorts, who aged at a faster rate. Obesity in people is said to shorten life, a view supported by insurance statistics. Quality as well as quantity of diet is thought to influence aging. Deficiencies of vitamins and other nutrients and excesses of nutrients such as cholesterol may cause malfunction. Although the full relationship of diet and aging is not understood, there is enough confidence in what is known to suggest that certain dietary habits may minimize or eliminate some ill effects of the aging process.

Several environmental factors known to threaten health are often associated with the aging process. Ingested mercury, lead, arsenic, radioactive isotopes, certain pesticides, and other substances are known to produce pathological changes in the human organism. Smoking and breathing tobacco smoke and other air pollutants have known adverse effects. Emotional stress, crowded living conditions, excessive alcohol intake, and "coping" ability are among the factors thought to influence the aging process.

No single biological theory completely explains the multifarious phenomenon of aging. Some populations are known to have a high proportion of aged individuals, such as in the Caucasus in southern Russia, where there are 12,000 people over age 90 and almost 5,000 who are centenarians (Leaf, 1975). But even extensive investigations have not been able to attribute the longevity in such people to any one factor. Nursing practice can utilize these theories, however, by identifying the elements known to influence aging and then discouraging the exposure to adverse factors and encouraging those which promote health and proper function.

PSYCHOSOCIAL THEORIES

Psychological and social changes during the aging process are closely united, and they have a significant impact on each other. It is difficult to explain mental processes, behavior, and feelings without the perspective of social roles, positions, and norms. A theory of aging that is purely social or psychological would be most unusual, and it is more appropriate to approach these aging factors as *psychosocial* theories. Probably the most controversial and widely discussed is the *disengagement theory,* developed by Elaine Cumming and William Henry (Cumming and Henry, 1961; Cumming, 1964). This theory views aging as a process whereby society and the individual gradually withdraw, or disengage, from each other, to the mutual satisfaction and benefit of both. The benefit to individuals is that they can reflect and be centered on themselves, having been freed from societal roles. The value of disengagement for society is that some orderly means is established for the transfer of power from the old to the young, making it possible for society to continue functioning after its individual members have died.

The theory does not indicate whether it is society or the individual who is responsible for initating the disengagement process, but one may readily detect several difficulties with the premise. Many older persons are highly satisfied to remain engaged and do not want their primary satisfaction to be derived from reflection on younger years. Senators, supreme court judges, and college professors are among those who commonly derive satisfaction and provide a valuable service for society by not disengaging. Since the health of the individual, cultural practices, societal norms, and other factors influence the degree to which a person will participate in society during the later years, some critics of this theory claim that disengagement would not be necessary if society improved the health care and financial means of the aged and increased the acceptance, opportunities, and respect afforded them.

A careful examination of the population studied in the development of the disengagement theory indicates certain of its limitations. The disengagement pattern which Cumming and Henry described was based on a study of 172 middle-class persons between the ages of 48 and 68. This group was wealthier, better educated, and of higher occupational and residential prestige than the general aged population. No blacks or chronically ill persons were involved in the study. Caution is advisable in generalizing for the entire aged population findings based on less than 200 persons who are not representative of the average aged person. While nurses should appreciate that some older individuals may wish to disengage from the mainstream of society, this is not necessarily a process to be expected from all aged persons.

At the opposite pole from the disengagement theory, the *activity theory* (Havighurst, 1963) proclaims that an older person should continue a middle-aged life-style, denying the existence of old age as long as possible, and that society should apply the same norms to old age as it does to middle age and not advocate diminishing activity, interest, and involvement as its members grow old. This theory suggests ways of maintaining activity in the presence of multiple losses associated with the aging process—including substituting intellectual activities for physical activities when physical capacity is reduced, replacing the work role with other roles when retirement occurs, and establishing new friendships when old ones are lost. Declining health, loss of roles, reduced income, a shrinking circle of friends, and other obstacles to maintaining an active life are to be resisted and overcome instead of being accepted.

This theory is not without merit. Activity is generally assumed to be more desirable than inactivity as it facilitates physical, mental, and social well-being. Like a self-fulfilling prophecy, the expectation of a continued active state during old age may be realized. Because of society's currently negative view of inactivity and "acting old," it is probably best to encourage an active live-style among the aged, consistent with society's values. Also supportive of the activity theory is the reluctance of many older persons to accept themselves as old, although one of its problems is the assumption that most older people desire and are able to maintain a middle-aged life-style. Some want their world to shrink to accommodate their decreasing capacities or their preference for less active roles. Many lack the physical, emotional, social, or economic resources to continue active roles in society. Aged people who are expected to maintain an active middle-aged life-style on a retirement income of less than half that of middle-aged people may wonder if society isn't giving them conflicting messages. The results and consequences of multiple expectations to remain active that cannot be fulfilled by the aging individual still need to be researched.

The *developmental theory* of aging, also referred to as the *continuity theory,* (Neugarten, 1964) relates the factors of personality and predisposition toward certain actions in old age to similar factors during other phases of the life cycle. Personality and basic patterns of behavior are said to be unchanged as the individual ages. The activist at age 20 will most likely be an activist at age 70. On the other hand, the young recluse will probably not be active in the mainstream of society when he or she ages. Concepts and patterns developed over a lifetime will determine whether an individual remains engaged and active or becomes disengaged and inactive. The recognition that the unique features of each individual allow for multiple adaptations to aging and that

31

the potential exists for a variety of reactions gives this theory reality and support. Aging is a complex process, and the developmental theory considers these complexities to a greater extent than most other theories. While the implications and impact of this promising theory are uncertain, since it is in an early stage of research, it should be closely followed.

Several other theories, although less developed, need mentioning. One theory (Rose, 1965) views the aged as a subculture whose members are typically forced to interact primarily with each other, due to their negative treatment by society. One problem with this theory is that it is not valid for all social classes of aged people. A similar theory (Streib, 1965) views the aged as a minority group which, like the handicapped and certain racial groups, has visible characteristics that are discriminated against—the signs of being old. Aged persons who do not display such characteristics and are able to maintain a youthful appearance are less discriminated against. This is not valid in all circumstances, however, since older individuals possessing great wealth, status, or fame are often the subjects of admiration rather than discrimination.

To an extent, the biological, psychological, and social processes of aging are interrelated and interdependent. Frequently, loss of a social role alters an individual's drives and speeds physical decline, and poor health forces retirement from work, promoting social isolation and the development of a weakened self-concept. While certain changes occur independently, as separate events, most are closely associated with other age-related factors. It is impractical, therefore, to subscribe solely to one theory of aging. Wise nurses will be eclectic in choosing the aging theories they will utilize in the care of older adults; they will also be cognizant of the limitations of these theories.

REFERENCES

Cumming, Elaine. "New Thoughts on the Theory of Disengagement." In Kastenbaum, Robert, *New Thoughts on Old Age*. Springer, New York, 1964.
—— and Henry, William E. *Growing Old: The Process of Disengagement*. Basic Books, New York, 1961.
Few, A., and Getty, R. "Occurrence of Lipofuscin as Related to Aging in the Canine and Porcine Nervous System." *Journal of Gerontology*, 22:357–367, 1967.
Havighurst, Robert J. "Successful Aging." In Williams, Richard H., Tibbitts, Clark, and Donahue, Wilma (eds.), *Processes of Aging*, Vol. I. Atherton Press, New York, 1963, pp. 299–320.
Hershey, Daniel. *Lifespan: And Factors Affecting It*. Thomas, Springfield, Ill, 1974.
Leaf, Alexander. *Youth in Old Age*. McGraw-Hill, New York, 1975.
Neugarten, Bernice L. *Personality in Middle and Late Life*. Atherton Press, New York, 1964.

Rose, Arnold. "The Subculture of the Aging: A Framework for Research in Social Gerontology." In Rose, A., and Peterson, W. (eds.), *Older People and Their Social World.* Davis, Philadelphia, 1965, pp. 3–16.

Strehler, Bernard L. *Time, Cells, and Aging.* Academic Press, New York, 1962.

Streib, Gordon F. "Are the Aged a Minority Group?" In Gouldner, A. W., and Miller, S. M. (eds.), *Applied Sociology.* Free Press, New York, 1965.

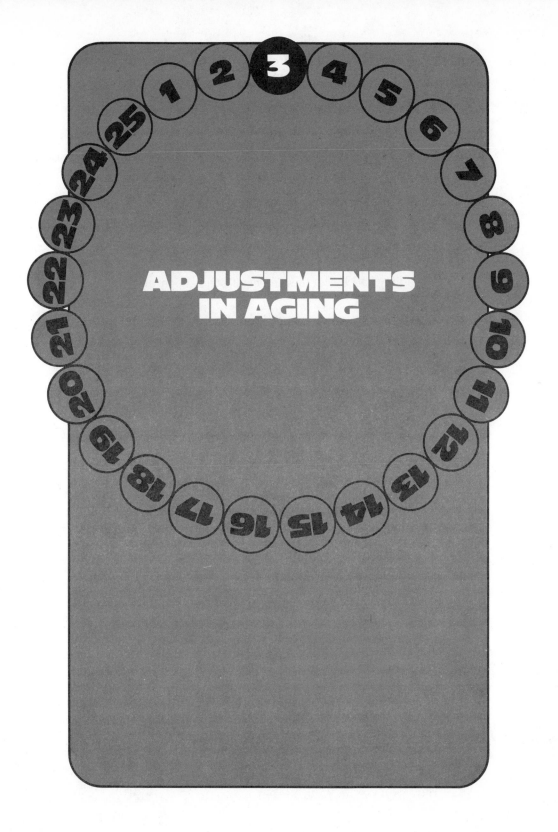

ADJUSTMENTS IN AGING

Growing old is not easy. Various changes and losses during the aging process demand multiple adjustments requiring much stamina, ability, and flexibility. Frequently, there are more simultaneous changes than experienced during any other period of life although in "coping" ability, it appears that the old surpass their younger counterparts by far. Many adults find it exhausting enough to keep pace with technological advancements, societal changes, cost-of-living fluctuations, and labor market trends. Imagine how complex and complicated life can be for older individuals, who must also face retirement, reduced income, possible housing changes, frequent losses through death of significant persons, and declining ability to function. To promote an awareness and appreciation of the complex and arduous adjustments involved, the sections below consider some of the factors which affect the successful management of the multiple changes associated with aging and the achievement of satisfaction and well-being during the later years.

RETIREMENT

One of the major adjustments to be made as an individual ages is the loss of a work role through retirement. For many, this is when the impact of aging is first experienced. Retirement is especially difficult in a society like ours, where an individual's worth is commonly judged by his or her productivity. Work is often viewed as the dues required for active membership in a productive society. The attitude that unemployment, for whatever reason, is an undesirable state is adhered to by many of today's aged persons, who were raised under the omnipresent cloud of the "puritan work ethic."

Occupational identity is largely responsible for an individual's social position and for the social role attached to that position. Although it is known that individuals function differently and individually in similar roles, some behaviors continue to be associated with certain roles, promoting stereotypes. How frequently do certain stereotypes assigned to various roles continue to be heard: the tough construction worker; the immoral go-go dancer; the fair judge; the righteous clergyman; the learned lawyer; and the doctor as healer. The realization that these associations are not consistently valid does not prevent their propagation. Too frequently, individuals are described in terms of their work role rather than their personal characteristics, for example, "the nurse who lives down the road" or "my son the doctor." Considering the extent to which social identity and behavioral expectations are derived from the work role, it is not surprising that an individual's identity is threatened when retirement occurs. During childhood and adolescence, we are guided toward an independent, responsible adult role, and in academic settings, we are prepared for our professional roles; but where and when are we prepared for the role of retiree?

Gerontological nursing is concerned with the welfare of both the current aged population and future aged populations. A lifetime of poor health care practices is a handicap that cannot be remedied in old age. Assisting aging individuals with their retirement preparations is preventive intervention, maximizing the potential for health and well-being in old age. As a part of such intervention, aging individuals should be encouraged to establish and practice good health habits, such as proper diet, the avoidance of alcohol, drug, and tobacco abuse, and regular physical examinations.

When one's work is one's primary interest, activity, and source of social contacts, separation from work leaves a significant void in one's life. Aging individuals should be urged to develop interests that are not related to work. Retirement is facilitated by learning how to use, appreciate, and gain satisfaction from leisure time throughout an employed lifetime. In addition, enjoying leisure time is a therapeutic outlet for life stresses throughout the aging process.

Gerontological nurses must understand the realities and reactions encountered when working with retired persons. Insight into this complicated process may be gained by considering the phases of retirement developed by Robert Atchley (1975). Not all retirees go through all phases.

Remote phase: Early in the occupational career, future retirement is anticipated, but rational preparation is seldom done.

Near phase: When the reality of retirement is evident, preparation for leaving one's job begins, as does fantasy regarding the retirement role.

Honeymoon phase: Following the retirement event, a somewhat euphoric period begins whereby fantasies from the preretirement phase are tested. Retirees attempt to do everything they never had time for simultaneously. A variety of factors (finances, health, etc.) limit this, leading to the development of a stable life-style.

Disenchantment phase: As life begins to stabilize, a letdown, sometimes a depression, is experienced. The more unrealistic the preretirement fantasy, the greater the degree of disenchantment.

Reorientation phase: As realistic choices and alternative sources of satisfaction are considered, the disenchantment with the new retirement routine can be replaced by developing a life-style that provides some satisfaction.

37

Stability phase: An understanding of the retirement role is achieved, and this provides a framework for concern, involvement, and action in one's life. Some enter this phase directly after the honeymoon phase, and some never reach it at all.

Termination phase: The retirement role is lost as a result of either the resumption of a work role or dependency due to illness or disability.

It is obvious that different nursing interventions may be required during each phase. Some of the preretirement planning recommendations discussed earlier can be employed during the remote phase. Counseling regarding the realities of retirement may be part of the near phase, whereas helping retirees place their new found freedom into proper perspective may be warranted during the honeymoon phase. Being supportive of retirees during the disenchantment phase without fostering self-pity and helping them identify new sources of satisfaction may facilitate the reorientation process. Appreciating and promoting the strengths of the stability phase may reinforce an adjustment to retirement. For general nursing there are many considerations related to the phases of retirement. For example, when the retirement phase is terminated due to disease or disability, the tactful management of dependency and the respectful appreciation of losses are most important.

Nurses' self-evaluation of their own attitudes toward retirement are an essential part of their role in the retirement process. Does the nurse see retirement as a period of freedom, opportunity, and growth? or of loneliness, dependency, and meaninglessness? Is the nurse intelligently planning for her own retirement? or denying it, by avoiding encounters with retirement realities? Nurses' views of retirement have an impact of the retiree-nurse relationship, and gerontological nurses can be especially good models of constructive retirement practices and attitudes.

FAMILY CHANGES

The family unit is the major source of satisfaction for many older people and contrary to the belief of many persons, most of the aged have regular, frequent contact with family members. The love and companionship of a spouse, the rewards and pride derived as offspring develop into independent adults, the deepened—and often renewed—relationships with siblings, and the joy of grandchildren and great-grandchildren can be essential ingredients for a satisfying old age. The family can be a key source of support, as well, cushioning the multiple losses and changes associated with aging while instilling hope and interest for a meaningful future.

The parental role is a dynamic one which frequently changes to meet the growth and development needs of both parent and child. During middle and late life, parents must adjust to the independence of their children as they become responsible adult citizens and leave home. Today, the first child usually leaves home and establishes an independent unit 22 to 25 years after the parents were married. For persons who have invested most of their adult lives nurturing and providing for their offspring, a child's independence may have significant impact. Although parents freed from the responsibilities and worries of rearing children have greater time to pursue their own interests, they are also freed from the meaningful, purposeful, and satisfying activities associated with child rearing, and this frequently results in a profound sense of loss.

A woman in late middle age or old age today was influenced by a historical period that emphasized the role of wife and mother. For instance, to provide job opportunities for men returning from World War II, women were encouraged to focus their interests on raising a family and to forfeit the scarce jobs to men. Unlike many of today's younger women, who combine (and in some situations equally value) employment and motherhood, these women centered their lives on their families, from which they derived their sense of fulfillment. Having developed few roles from which to achieve satisfaction other than that of wife and mother, many of today's older women feel a definite void when their children are grown and gone. To compound this problem, the highly mobile life-style of many young persons limits the degree of direct contact she has with her children, who are now adults, and with her grandchildren.

The older man shares many of the same feelings as his wife. Throughout the years, he feels he has performed useful functions, which made him a valuable member of society. He may have fought for his country in undisputably honorable wars. Most likely, he worked hard to support his wife and children, and his masculinity was reinforced with proof of his ability to beget and provide for offspring. With his children grown, he is no longer required to provide—a mixed blessing in which he may sense relief and purposelessness. In addition, he learns that the rules have changed; his pride at being a war hero may have been shattered by antiwar advocates; his ability to support a family without the need for this wife to work is now viewed as oppressive by feminists; his efforts to replenish the earth are scorned by today's zero population proponents; and his attempt to fill the masculine role for which he was socialized is considered "macho" or inane by today's standards.

Although the extended family was not as widespread or perfect as many thought, it was more prevalent in days gone by. It provided immediate support systems, shared responsibilities, economic benefits, and other advantages to both the young and old family member. Grand-

39

parenting was an active role which provided a sense of usefulness and satisfaction for the aged, who, in turn, could feel secure that the family unit would be responsible for their growing needs and increased requirements for assistance.

The emergence of today's nuclear family units changed the roles and functions of the individuals in a family. The aged are expected to have limited input into the lives of their adult children. Children are not required to meet the needs of their aging parents for financial support, health services, or housing. Moreover, parents increasingly do not depend on their children for their needs, and the belief that children are the best old-age insurance is a fading one. In addition, grandparenting, although very satisfying, is not usually an active role, especially since grandchildren may be scattered throughout the country. These changes in family structure and function are not necessarily negative. Most children do not abandon or neglect their aging parents, but maintain regular contact. Separate family units may help the parent-child relationship develop on a more adult-to-adult basis—to the mutual satisfaction of young and old. Although the advantages of nuclear family living are often seen primarily as a benefit to younger adults, older adults also enjoy the independence and freedom from responsibilities nuclear family life offers.

A common event that alters family life for the aged is the death of a spouse. The loss of that individual who has shared more love and life experiences, more joys and sorrows, may be intolerable. How, after many decades of living with another human being, does one adjust to the sudden absence of that person? How does one adjust to setting the table for one, to coming home to an empty house, or to not touching that warm, familiar body beside him or her in bed? Adjustment to this significant loss is coupled with the demand to learn the new task of living alone.

Death of a spouse affects more women than men since most older men are married and most older women are widowed—a situation which is projected to continue in the future. Unlike many of today's younger women, who have greater independence through careers and changed norms, most of today's older women have lived family-oriented lives and been dependent on their husbands. Their age, limited education, lack of skills, or long period of unemployment while raising their families are handicaps in a competitive job market. If these women can find employment, adjusting to the new demands of a work role may be difficult and stressful. On the other hand, the unemployed widow may learn that pensions or other sources of income may be reduced or discontinued when the husband dies, necessitating an adjustment to an extremely limited budget. In addition to financial dependence, the woman may have depended on her husband's achievements to provide her with gratification and identity. (Frequently, the achievements of

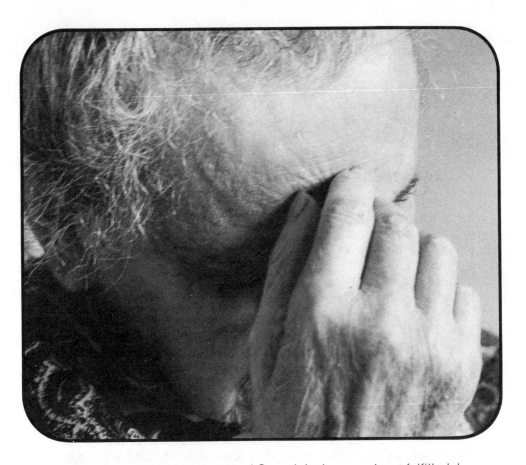

children serve this same purpose.) Sexual desires may be unfulfilled due to lack of opportunity, fear of repercussions from children and society, or residual attitudes from early learnings about sexual mores. If a woman's marriage promoted friendships with other married couples and only inactive relationships with single friends, the new widow may find that her pool of single female friends is scarce.

For the most part, when the initial grief of the husband's death passes, most widows adjust quite well. The high proportion of older women who are widowed provides the availability of friends who share similar problems and life-styles; this is especially true in urban areas. Old friendships may be revived to provide sources of activity and enjoyment. Some widows may discover that the loss of certain responsibilities associated with their partner's death, such as cooking, laundering, and cleaning for a husband, brings them a new and pleasant freedom. With alternative roles to develop, sufficient income, and choice over lifestyle, many women are able to make a successful adjustment to

41

widowhood. The nurse may facilitate this adjustment by identifying sources of friendships and activities—such as clubs, volunteer organizations, or other groups of widows in the community—and by helping the widow understand and obtain all the benefits to which she is entitled. This may require reassuring her that enjoying her new freedom and desiring relationships with other men is no reason to feel guilty, and supporting her as she learns to adjust to the loss of her husband and the new role of widow.

AWARENESS OF MORTALITY

Widowhood, death of friends, and the recognition of declining functions make older persons more aware of the reality of their own death. During their early years, individuals intellectually understand that they will not live forever, but their behaviors deny this reality. The lack of a will and absence of burial plans may be indications of this denial. As the reality of mortality becomes acute with advancing age, interest in fulfilling dreams, deepening religious convictions, strengthening family ties, providing for the ongoing welfare of one's family, and leaving a legacy are often apparent signs.

The significance of a life review in interpreting and refining our past experiences as they relate to our self-concept and help us understand and accept our life history has been well discussed by Robert Butler (1963; 1971). Rather than being a pathological behavior, discussing the past may be quite therapeutic and necessary for the aged. The thought of impending death may be more tolerable if people feel that their life had depth and meaning. Unresolved guilt, unachieved aspirations, perceived failures, and other multitudinous aspects of "unfinished business" may be better understood and perhaps resolved. Although the condition of old age may provide limited opportunities for excitement and achievement, there may be satisfaction in knowing that there *were* achievements, and many excitements as well, in other periods of life. The old woman may be frail and wrinkled, but she can still delight in remembering how she once drove the young men insane. The retired old man may feel that he is useless to society now, but he realizes his worth through the memory of wars he fought to protect his country and the pride he feels in knowing he supported his family through a depression.

The young can benefit from the reminiscences of the aged, growing in depth and gaining a new perspective on life as they learn about their ancestry. Imagine the impact of hearing about slavery or immigration or epidemics or industrialization or wars from an older relative who has been part of making that history. What history book's description of the Great Depression can compare with hearing one's grandparents describe events one's own family experienced—such as going to bed hungry at night? In addition to their place in the future, the young can fully realize their link with the past when the desire of the aged to reminisce is appreciated and fostered.

Older persons should be encouraged to discuss and analyze the dynamics of their lives, and listeners should be receptive and accepting. Poems and autobiographies, as unsophisticated as they may be, should be recognized as significant legacies from the old to the young. I am reminded of my own father-in-law, who at age 71 started a family scrapbook for each of his children. Any photograph, newspaper article, or announcement pertaining to any family member was reproduced and included in every album. The family patiently tolerated this activity—reluctantly sending him copies of graduation programs and photographs for every scrapbook. The family viewed the main value of this activity as providing something benign to keep this old man occupied. It was not until years after his death that the significance of this great task was appreciated as a priceless gift. Such tangible items may serve as an assurance to both young and old that the impact of an aged relative's life will not cease upon death.

DECLINING FUNCTION

The obvious changes in appearance and bodily function which occur during the aging process make it necessary for the aging individual to adjust to a new body image. Colorful soft hair turns gray and dry; flexible straight fingers become bent and painful; body contours are altered and height decreases. Stairs which were once climbed several times daily demand more time and energy to negotiate as the years accumulate. As subtle, gradual, and natural as these changes may be, they are recognized and, consequently, body image and self-concept is affected.

The manner in which individuals perceive themselves and function can determine the roles they play. A construction worker who has less strength and energy may forfeit his work role; a club member who cannot hear speech may forfeit his or her role; fashion models may forfeit that role when they perceive themselves as old. Interestingly, some persons well into their sixth and seventh decades refuse to join a senior citizen club and accept the role associated with being a member of such a club because they do not perceive themselves as being old. The nurse will gain insight into the self-concept of older persons by evaluating what roles they are willing to accept and what roles they reject.

It is sometimes difficult for the aging person to accept the declining efficiency of the body. Poor memory, slow response, easy fatigue, and altered appearance are among the many frustrating results of declining function, and they are dealt with in a variety of ways. Some older people deny them and often demonstrate poor judgment in an attempt to make the same demands on their bodies as they did when younger. Others try to resist these changes by investing in cosmetic surgery, beauty treatments, miracle drugs, and other expensive endeavors that diminish the budget but not the normal aging process. Still others exaggerate these effects and impose an unnecesarily restricted life-style on themselves. Societal expectations frequently determine the adjustment individuals make to declining function.

Common results of declining function are illness and disability. Most older people have one or more chronic diseases (Brody, 1974) and more than a third have some disability which is serious enough to limit major activities, such as work and housekeeping (Riley and Foner, 1968). A fear that the aged have is that their illness or disability may cause them to lose their independence. Becoming a burden to one's family, being unable to meet the demands of daily living and having to enter a nursing home are some of the fears associated with dependency. Children and parents may have difficulty exchanging dependent-independent roles. The physical pain which an illness produces may not be nearly as intolerable as the dependency it causes.

Nurses should help aging persons understand and accept the normal physical decline associated with advanced age. Factors which can promote optimum function should be encouraged, including proper diet, paced activity, regular physical examination, early correction of health problems, and avoidance of alcohol, tobacco, and drug abuse. Assistance should be offered with attention to preserving as much of the individual's independence and dignity as possible.

REDUCED INCOME

Financial resources are important at any age since they affect our diet, health, housing, safety, and independence and influence many of the choices we face in life. The economic profile of many aged persons is dim. Retirement income is less than half the income earned while fully employed. For a majority of the aged, social security income, originally intended as a *supplement*, is actually the *primary source* of retirement income—and it has not even kept pace with inflation. Less than one-fifth of the aged have income from a private pension plan, and those who do often discover that the fixed benefits established when the plan was subscribed to have almost no value because of inflation. (Of the workers who are currently active in the labor force, more than one-half will not have pension plans when they retire.) More than one-fourth of the aged live in poverty; only a minority are fully employed or financially comfortable. Few olderly persons have accumulated enough assets during their lifetime to provide financial security in old age.

44

TABLE 3-1: RETIREMENT BUDGET: INCOME SOURCES

Income Sources	Current Monthly Income	Income After Retirement
1. Salary	_____	_____
2. Pension	_____	_____
3. Other (savings, rents, investments, etc.)	_____	_____
4. Second job	_____	_____
5. Social security	_____	_____
6. Spouse's income	_____	_____
7.		
8.		
Total		

A reduction in income is a significant adjustment for many older persons, as it triggers off a whole series of other adjustments that must be made. An active social life and leisure pursuits may have to be markedly reduced or eliminated. Relocation to less expensive housing may be necessary, possibly forcing the aged to leave many family and community ties. Dietary practices may be severely altered and health care may be viewed as a luxury over which other basic expenses, such as food and rent, take priority. If the older parent has to depend on children for supplemental income, an additional adjustment in thinking may be needed.

The importance of making financial preparations for old age many years prior to retirement is clear. Nurses should encourage aging working people to determine whether their retirement income plans are keeping pace with inflation. Aged individuals need assistance in obtaining all the benefits they are entitled to and in learning how to manage their income wisely. Nurses should be aware of the impact economic welfare has on health status and should actively involve themselves in political issues that promote adequate income for all individuals.

LONELINESS

Loneliness and desolation emphasize all the misfortunes of people who are growing old. Children are grown and gone, friends and spouse may be deceased, and others who could allay the loneliness may avoid the aged individual because they find it difficult to accept the changes they see or to face the fact that they too will be old some day. Location in a sparsely populated rural area can geographically isolate older persons, and when they live in an urban area, they may be fearful of going

45

TABLE 3-2: RETIREMENT BUDGET: EXPENSES

Living Requirements	Current Monthly Expenses	Expenses After Retirement
Living accommodations		
Mortgage or rent	_____	_____
Utilities (gas, electricity, water)	_____	_____
Taxes	_____	_____
Maintenance	_____	_____
Telephone	_____	_____
Food and other necessities	_____	_____
Clothing	_____	_____
Medical (doctor, dentist, medicine)	_____	_____
Insurance		
Life	_____	_____
Health	_____	_____
Auto	_____	_____
Other	_____	_____
Loans and other credit	_____	_____
Automobile expenses (gas, oil, repairs)	_____	_____
Entertainment	_____	_____
Subtotal	_____	_____
Other expenses (10% of subtotal)	_____	_____
Total	_____	_____

outdoors. Hearing and speech deficits and language differences, which present communication barriers, can also foster loneliness. Insecurity resulting from multiple losses can cause suspiciousness of others and lead to a self-imposed isolation. At a time of many losses and adjustments, personal contact, love, extra support, and attention are needed—not isolation. These are essential human needs. Isn't it likely that a failure to thrive will occur in adults who feel unwanted and unloved just as it does in infants, who display anxiety, depression, anorexia, and behavioral and other difficulties when they perceive love and attention to be inadequate?

Nurses should attempt to intervene when isolation and loneliness are detected in an aged person. There are programs that provide telephone reassurance or home visits as a source of daily human contact, and the person's church may also provide assistance. Nurses can help the person identify and join social groups and sometimes even accompany him or her to the first meeting. A change in housing may be called for to provide a safe environment that is conducive to social interaction. If the aged person speaks a foreign language, relocation to an area in which members of the same ethnic group live can often remedy loneliness. Even pets are frequently very significant and effective companions to the aged.

It should be emphasized that being alone is not synonymous with being lonely. Periods of solitude are essential at all ages, providing us with the opportunity to reflect, analyze, and better understand the dynamics of our lives. Older individuals may want periods of solitude to reminisce and review their lives. Some individuals, young and old, prefer and choose to be alone and do not feel isolated or lonely in any way. Of course, attention should also be paid to the correction of hearing, vision, and other health problems which may be the cause of social isolation.

SOCIETAL PREJUDICE

It is not difficult to detect overt ageism in our society. Rather than showing appreciation for the vast contributions of the aged and their wealth of resources, society is beset with prejudices and lacks adequate provisions for them, thus derogating their dignity. The same members of society that oppose providing sufficient income and health care benefits for the aged enjoy an affluence and standard of living that was provided through the efforts of the aged.

Although the aged constitute the most diverse and individualized group, they continue to be stereotyped by misconceptions such as the following:

Old people are sick and disabled.

Most old people are in nursing homes.

Senility comes with old age.

Old people are unhappy.

People either get very tranquil or very cranky as they age.

Old people have lower intelligence and are resistant to change.

Old people aren't able to have sexual intercourse and aren't interested in sex anyhow.

There are few satisfactions in old age.

Since for a majority of older persons the above statements are not true, increased efforts are necessary to make the members of society aware of the realities of aging. Groups such as the Gray Panthers have done an outstanding job of informing the public about the facts regarding aging and the problems and rights of older adults. More advocates for the aged are needed.

Erik Erikson says that the last stage of the life cycle is concerned with integrity versus despair. Integrity results when the older individual

47

derives satisfaction from an evaluation of his or her life. Disappointment with one's life and the lack of opportunities to redo one's past bring despair. The experiences of our entire lifetime determine whether our old age will be an opportunity for freedom, growth, and contentment, or a miserable imprisonment of our human potential.

REFERENCES

Atchley, Robert C. *The Sociology of Retirement.* Schenkman, Cambridge, Mass., 1975.

Brody, S. J. "Evolving Health Delivery Systems and Older People." *American Journal of Public Health,* 64:245, 1974.

Butler, Robert. "The Life Review: An Interpretation of Reminiscence in the Aged." *Psychiatry,* 26:65–76, 1963.

———"The Life Review." *Psychology Today,* 5:49–51, December 1971.

Riley, Matilda W., and Foner, Ann. *Aging and Society, Vol. I: An Inventory of Research Findings.* Russell Sage Foundation, New York, 1968, p. 214.

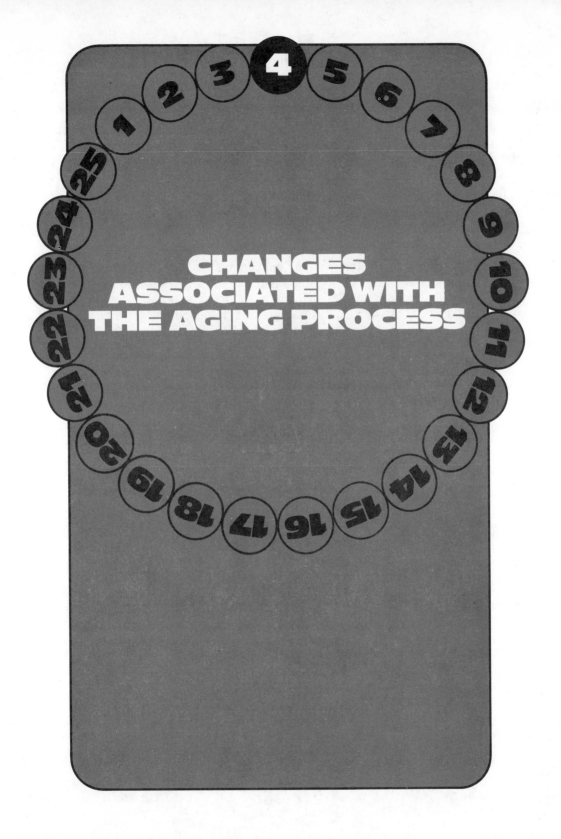

CHANGES
ASSOCIATED WITH
THE AGING PROCESS

Living is a process of continual changes. Infants become toddlers, pubescent children blossom into young men and women, and dependent adolescents develop into responsible adult members of society. The type, rate, and degree of physical, emotional, psychological, and social changes experienced during this life process are highly individualized, being influenced by genetic factors, environment, diet, health, stress, and a variety of other factors.

That the process of change continues into old age is natural and to be expected. The multitude of changes that have occurred, during the life span of those who achieve old age, make old people appear physically, psychologically, and socially different in certain ways. However, they continue to share characteristics with younger individuals, and thus remain linked with all human beings. Understanding the changes experienced during the aging process will assist the nurse in caring for older individuals. Such an understanding will provide a foundation for the nurse's assessment and guidance and for adjusting the care plan and implementing it. The following pages will highlight some of the common changes.

PHYSICAL CHANGES IN STRUCTURE AND FUNCTION

The aging process shows its effects on the basic cellular level, with a gradual loss in the number of cells (Freeman, 1965). An older individual may have 30 percent fewer cells than the younger adult. Although the cells are fewer in number, they are larger in size, and consequently there is less of a reduction in cellular mass. The proportionate increase in body fat as the cell mass decreases leaves a somewhat similar appearance of the total body mass (Goldman, 1971). As the body fat atrophies with advanced age, the body's contours gain a bony appearance along with a deepening of the hollows of the intercostal and supraclavicular spaces, orbits, and axillae. Intracellular fluid decreases, although there is no significant changes in the extracellular fluid, and there is a decrease in the total body fluid (Figure 4-1). The cells tend to combine in irregular patterns as one ages, giving altered structure to the body tissues. These cellular changes influence virtually every body system.

Cardiovascular System

The heart itself does not significantly change in structure, although marked inactivity is known to promote cardiac atrophy (McKeown, 1965). It is not uncommon for an aged heart to be smaller in size and pigmented with lipofuscin granules. The valves of the heart become thick and rigid as a result of sclerosis and fibrosis, compounding any cardiac disease present in the individual (McMillan and Lev, 1964). The vessels lose their

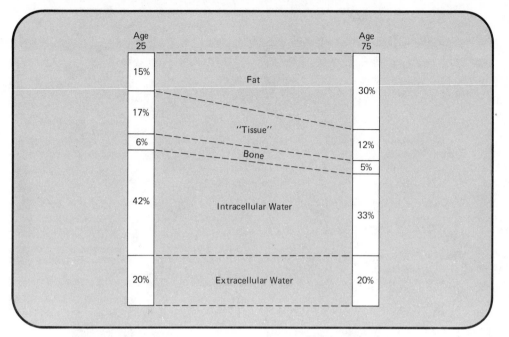

Figure 4·1. Distribution of major body components with age. (Source: R Goldman, *American Geriatric Society Journal*, 18 (765), 1970.

elasticity, and muscular arteries in the head, neck, and extremities become more prominent.

There are various physiologic changes in the cardiovascular system that occur. A slower heart rate and decreased stroke volume cause decreases in cardiac output as high as 40 percent between the ages of 25 and 65 years (Brandfonbrener, Landowne, and Shock, 1955). Sudden stress is not managed well by the aged heart, as demonstrated by a lesser increase in pulse rate and a prolonged time for return to the previous rate (Goldman, 1971). The stroke volume may increase to compensate for this situation, which results in an elevation in blood pressure—although it is possible for the blood pressure to remain stable as a tachycardia progress to heart failure in the elderly (Harris, 1974). Oxygen utilization is less efficient, which may contribute to prolonged tachycardia in older individuals (Harris, 1974). There is a wide range into which the pulse rate may fall—from 44 to 108 beats per minute (Harris, 1974). Increased peripheral resistance contributes to a rising blood pressure, affecting both the systolic and diastolic pressures (Master and Lasser, 1961). Although Harris has considered hypertensive levels in the aged as being persistent elevations over 170 mmHg systolic and 95

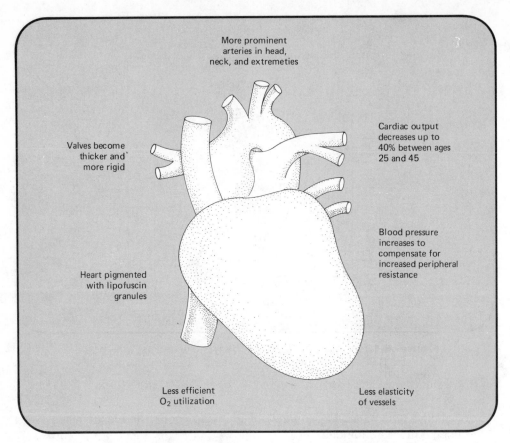

More prominent
arteries in head,
neck, and extremeties

Valves become
thicker and
more rigid

Cardiac output
decreases up to
40% between ages
25 and 45

Blood pressure
increases to
compensate for
increased peripheral
resistance

Heart pigmented
with lipofuscin
granules

Less efficient
O_2 utilization

Less elasticity
of vessels

Figure 4-2. Cardiovascular changes with aging.

mmHg diastolic, Harris, Caird and Judge (1974) offer slightly higher
upper limits of blood pressure (Table 4-1) and discourage treating blood
pressures lower than these levels as hypertensive.

Respiratory System

The aged lung tends to be larger on inspection due to a loss of
elasticity. This results in an increase in residual capacity of approximately 50 percent by age 90 (Mithoefer and Karetzky, 1968). The number
of alveoli are reduced and are of increased size, as are the bronchioles
and alveolar ducts. As the residual volume increases, the vital capacity
is lowered (Norris, et al., 1956). The maximum breathing capacity is
reduced. Total lung capacity is not significantly different in older
individuals, however.

Age does not influence the blood carbon dioxide level (pCO_2)

52

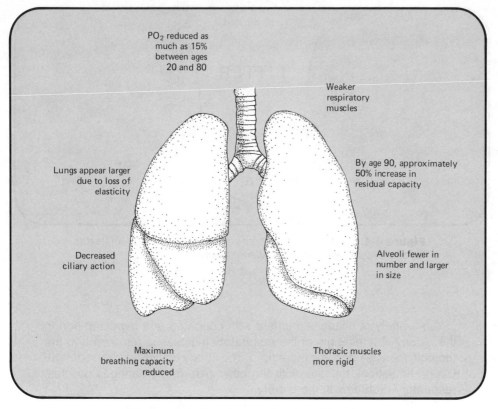

PO$_2$ reduced as
much as 15%
between ages
20 and 80

Weaker
respiratory
muscles

Lungs appear larger
due to loss of
elasticity

By age 90, approximately
50% increase in
residual capacity

Decreased
ciliary action

Alveoli fewer in
number and larger
in size

Maximum
breathing capacity
reduced

Thoracic muscles
more rigid

Figure 4-3. Respiratory changes with aging.

which remains at approximately 40 mmHg, but it does decrease the
arterial blood oxygen level (pO$_2$) by 10 to 15 percent between the ages
of 20 and 80 (Mithoefer and Karetzky, 1968). Thus an older individual
may have a blood oxygen level of 75 mmHg.

TABLE 4-1: SUGGESTED UPPER
LIMITS OF BLOOD PRESSURE IN OLD AGE

Age	mmHg for Men		mmHg for Women	
	Systolic	Diastolic	Systolic	Diastolic
60–69	195	100	200	110
70–79	195	105	210	110
80+	195	105	210	115

Source: F. I. Caird and T. G. Judge, *Assessment of the Elderly
Patient,* Pitman Medical Publishing Co., New York, 1974, p. 34.

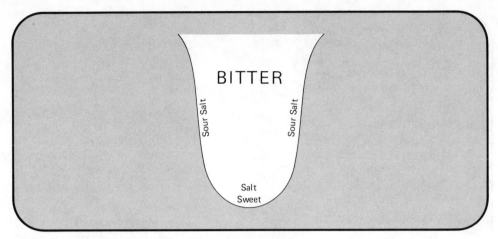

Figure 4-4. Taste sensations lost with age. Sweet and salt flavors tend to be lost before bitter and sour flavors.

A variety of changes interfere with coughing and expectoration in the elderly. The strength of the respiratory muscles is reduced and the thoracic muscles become more rigid. The ciliary activity is also reduced. Cough limitations together with the other respiratory changes promote respiratory problems in the elderly.

Gastrointestinal System

Although not as fatal as cardiovascular or respiratory problems, gastrointestinal problems are more discomforting and bothersome to older individuals. A contributing factor is the common loss of teeth due to poor dental care, environmental influences, or changes in gingival tissues. After age 30, peridontal disease is the major cause of tooth loss, and it is rare to find an individual who has not suffered severe tooth loss by age 70. The teeth in older adults may have a flatter surface and appear to be longer due to resorption of the gum tissue around the tooth's base. Taste sensation decreases with age, due to chronic irritation (as with pipe smoking) or to a wearing out or atrophy of taste buds. There is a tendency for the sweet sensations on the tip of the tongue to be lost earlier than the sour, salt, and bitter taste sensations (Figure 4–4).

Esophageal motility is decreased and the esophagus tends to become dilated. The lower esophageal sphincter relaxes and esophageal emptying is slower (Soergel et al., 1964). The stomach is

54

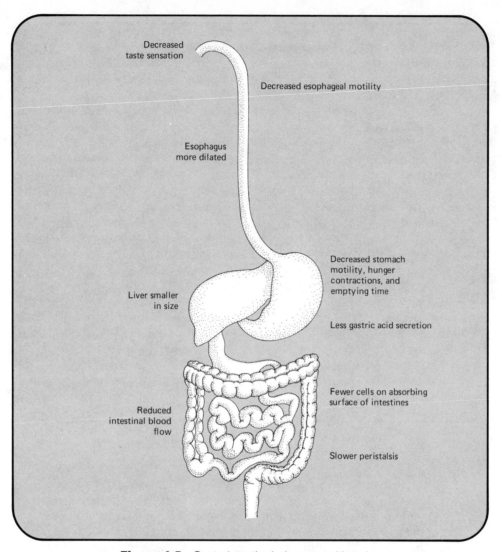

Decreased
taste sensation

Decreased esophageal motility

Esophagus
more dilated

Liver smaller
in size

Decreased stomach
motility, hunger
contractions, and
emptying time

Less gastric acid secretion

Reduced
intestinal blood
flow

Fewer cells on absorbing
surface of intestines

Slower peristalsis

Figure 4-5. Gastrointestinal changes with aging.

believed to have decreased motility, along with decreases in hunger contractions, gastric acid secretion, and emptying time (Sklar, 1974). Some atrophy occurs throughout the small and large intestine, although research regarding the changes in the intestine is limited; constipation, common in the older population, is thought to be a result of slower colonic peristalsis. Absorption may be decreased due to change in

55

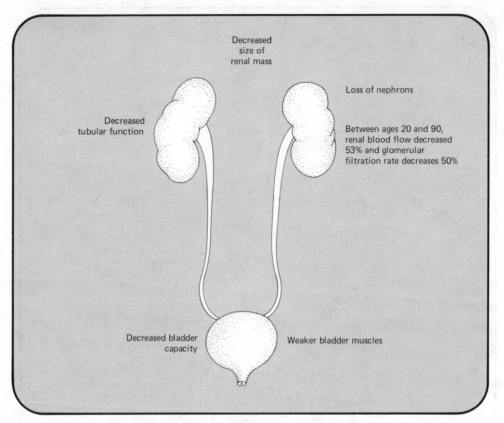

Figure 4-6. Urinary tract changes with aging.

gastric acid secretion, decreased motility, reduced intestinal blood flow, and fewer cells on the absorbing surface. Some researches have determined an absence of external anal sphincter reflexes as a major factor in fecal incontinence in the aged (Alva et al., 1967).

The liver is smaller in size with advancing age, and research has shown a reduction in splanchnic blood flow (Sherlock et al., 1971) and a decreased storage capacity (Calloway and Merrill, 1965). Total serum bilirubin, SGOT (serum glutamic oxalectic transaminase) SGPT (serum glutamic pyruvic transaminase), and alkaline phosphate values are not significantly altered with age.

Genitourinary System
The renal mass decreases in size with age, attributable to the loss of nephron units (Goldman, 1971). Renal tissue growth declines with age (Oliver, 1952), and atherosclerosis may promote atrophy of the kidney.

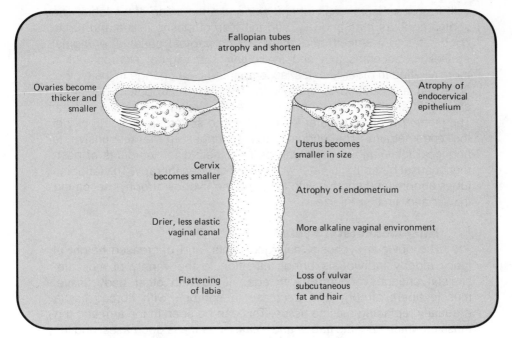

Ovaries become thicker and smaller

Fallopian tubes atrophy and shorten

Atrophy of endocervical epithelium

Cervix becomes smaller

Uterus becomes smaller in size

Atrophy of endometrium

Drier, less elastic vaginal canal

More alkaline vaginal environment

Flattening of labia

Loss of vulvar subcutaneous fat and hair

Figure 4-7. Changes in the female genitalia with aging.

These changes will alter renal function in a variety of ways. Renal blood flow decreases 53 percent and the glomerular filtration rate at age 90 is almost 50 percent less than it was at age 20 (Davies and Shock, 1950). Tubular function also decreases, demonstrated by increased problems in concentration of urine. The maximum specific gravity at age 80 has been shown to be 1.024, whereas at younger ages the maximum was 1.032 (Goldman, 1971). Decreased tubular function also affects reabsorption from the filtrate, making a 1+ proteinuria in the aged, which is of no diagnostic significance (Kahn and Snapper, 1974). Decreased renal functioning is further displayed by an average blood urea nitrogen (BUN) of 21.2 mg% at age 70, whereas from ages 30 to 40 the average is 12.9 mg% (Kahn and Snapper, 1974).

The bladder undergoes changes during the aging process, including weakening of the bladder muscles and a decreased bladder capacity. Emptying of the bladder is more difficult and retention of a large volume of urine may result.

Prostatic enlargement is present in most elderly men, although rate and type varies with individuals. Three-fourths of the men over age 65 have some degree of prostatism (Jaffee, 1974). The female genitalia demonstrate many changes with age (Agate, 1963; Jeffcoate, 1967). The vulva, affected by hormonal changes, gains an atrophic appearance, with loss of subcutaneous fat and hair and a flattening of the labia. The vagina appears pink and dry, and the loss of elastic tissue and rugae contributes to a smooth and shiny looking vaginal canal. The vaginal epithelium becomes thin and avascular. The vaginal environment is more alkaline in older females, accompanied by a change in the type of flora and a reduction in secretions. The cervix atrophies, becoming smaller in size, and an atrophy of the endocervical epithelium occurs. The uterus becomes smaller in size also and suffers from an atrophy of the endometrium. The endometrium continues to be responsive to hormonal stimulation, which can be responsible for incidents of post-menopausal bleeding in older women on estrogen therapy. The fallopian tubes atrophy and shorten with age, and the ovaries atrophy, becoming thicker and smaller in size.

Musculoskeletal System

The obvious kyphosis, enlarged joints, and decreased height of many elderly individuals brings attention to the variety of musculo-skeletal changes occurring with age. Along with other body tissue, muscle fibers atrophy and decrease in number, with fibrous tissue gradually replacing muscle tissue. This can be seen in the arm and leg muscles which become flabby and weak. Bone mass decreases, and the amount of bone mineral is reduced, contributing to the brittleness of older bones. While long bones do not significantly shorten with age, thinning disks and shortening vertebrae reduce the length of the spinal column. Height is reduced approximately two inches between ages 20 and 70 (Rossman, 1971). Varying degrees of kyphosis may occur, accompanied by a backward tilting of the head, and there are varying degrees of flexion at the wrists, hips, and knees.

In addition to structural change, slower movement is observed in older individuals. Muscle tremors may be present during resting states, believed to be associated with extrapyramidal system degeneration. The tendons undergo shrinkage and sclerosis, which causes a decrease in tendon jerks (Grob, 1974). Reflexes are lessened in the arms and nearly completely lost in the abdomen, but maintained in the knee. For a variety of reasons, muscle cramping may frequently occur.

Nervous System

It is difficult to describe with accuracy and exactness the nervous system's changes with age due to the dependence of this system's function on other body systems. For instance, cardiovascular difficulties may reduce cerebral circulation and be responsible for cerebral dys-function. Declining nervous system function may be unnoticed, as changes are often nonspecific and slowly progressing. There is a delay in response and reaction time—especially reaction associated with

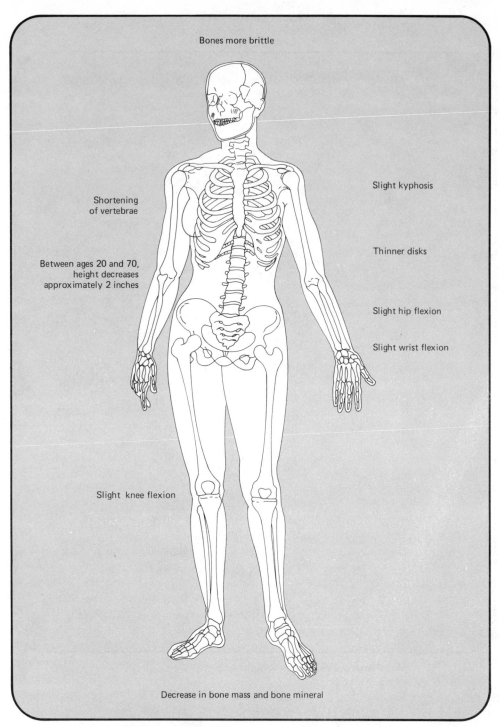

Bones more brittle

Slight kyphosis

Shortening
of vertebrae

Thinner disks

Between ages 20 and 70,
height decreases
approximately 2 inches

Slight hip flexion

Slight wrist flexion

Slight knee flexion

Decrease in bone mass and bone mineral

Figure 4-8. Skeletal changes with aging.

59

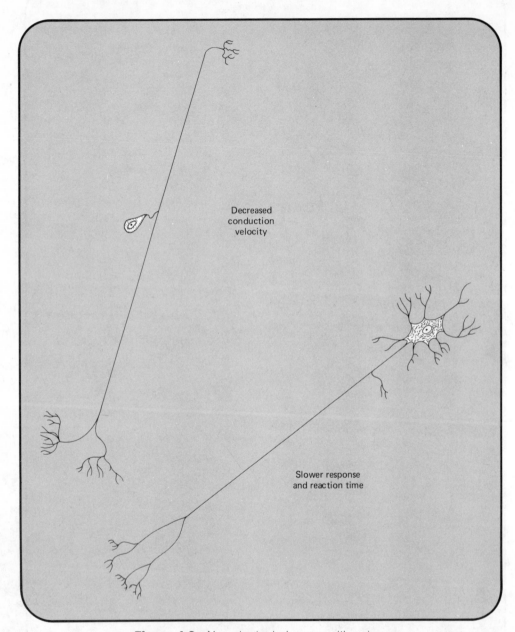

Decreased
conduction
velocity

Slower response
and reaction time

Figure 4-9. Neurological changes with aging.

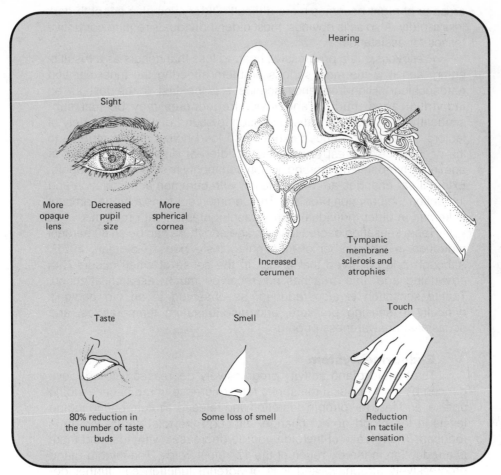

Figure 4-10. Sensory changes with aging.

stress. The conduction velocity has also been shown to decrease with age (Goldman, 1971).

Sensory Organs

The five senses becomes less efficient with increasing age, interfering in varying degrees with safety, normal daily functioning, and general well-being. Perhaps the greatest of such interferences results from changes in vision. Sclerosis of the pupil sphincter and a decrease in pupil size occur, making the pupil less responsive to light. The cornea becomes more spherical, and the lens opaque. Visual acuity decreases, as does the extent of the visual field, making peripheral vision more difficult. The light perception threshold increases and vision in dim

61

areas or at night becomes more difficult. Older eyes also adapt to dark less rapidly. Also as is obvious, most older individuals require corrective lenses for assistance.

Presbycusis is a progressive hearing loss that occurs as a result of aging, and it is the most serious problem affecting the inner ear and retrocochlear. High-frequency sounds are the first to be lost as an individual ages; middle and lower frequencies may be lost subsequently. This problem causes speech to sound distorted. A variety of factors, including continued exposure to loud noise, may contribute to the occurrence of presbycusis. The middle ear displays the effects of age in the tympanic membrane, which commonly is sclerotic or atrophic. External ear changes are insignificant, with cerumen accumulation and impaction the common problem. The cerumen contains a higher amount of keratin in older individuals which contributes to that problem.

Taste sensation decreases with age and there can be an 80 percent reduction in the number of functioning taste buds (Goldman, 1971). Although it is observed that a loss in the sense of smell occurs with advancing age, this area has not received much research attention. Tactile sensation is also reduced, as observed in an old person's difficulty in sensing pressure, and discriminating temperatures, and occasional unawareness of pain.

Endocrine System

The thyroid gland activity progressively decreases with age, evidenced by a lower basal metabolic rate, decrease in radioactive iodine uptake, and less thyrotropin secretion and release. Protein-bound iodine levels in the blood do not change, although the total serum iodide is reduced. The release of thyroidal iodide decreases with age, and there is a reduction in the excretion of the 17-ketosteroids. The thyroid gland progressively atrophies, and loss of adrenal function can further decrease thyroid activity (McGavack, 1974a).

Much of the secretory activity of the adrenal cortex is regulated by ACTH, (adrenocorticotropic) a pituitary hormone. As ACTH secretion decreases with age, secretory activity of the adrenal gland also decreases (McGavick, 1974a). Although the secretion of ACTH does not affect aldosterone secretion, it has been shown that less aldosterone is produced and excreted in the urine of older persons (Flood et al., 1967). The secretion of glucocorticoids 17-ketosteroids, progesterone, androgen, and estrogen, also influenced by the adrenal gland, are reduced as well.

Pituitary activity is altered by age in a variety of ways. The growth hormone (STH-somatotrophic or growth hormone) is present in older and younger individuals in similar amounts, although the blood level may be reduced. Decreases are seen in adrenocorticotropic (ACTH), thyroid-stimulating (TSH), follicle-stimulating (FSH), luteinizing (LH), and luteo-tropic (LTH) hormones to varying degrees (McGavick, 1974b). Gonadal secretion declines with age, including gradual decreases in testos-terone, estrogen, and progesterones (Pincus, 1956). With the exception of alterations associated with changes in plasma calcium level or dysfunction of other glands, the parathyroid glands maintain their function throughout life.

Integumentary System

In addition to the regular effects of the aging process, heredity, environment, diet, general health, activity, and exposure influence the condition of the skin. The changes in the integumentary system are easily recognized and include lines and wrinkles from the loss of subcutaneous fat; thinning, graying scalp hair; thicker hair in the nose and ears; skin pigmentation due to clustering of melanocytes; and less elastic and more delicate skin, due to decreased hydration and vascular-ity of the dermis (Burgeon and Burgeon, 1958). The fingernails become hard and brittle. The decrease in the number and function of the sweat glands results in a slight reduction in perspiration (Wells, 1954).

PSYCHOLOGICAL CHANGES

Psychological changes during the aging process cannot be iso-lated from concurrent physical and social changes. Sensory organ impairment can impede the interaction of older individuals both with their environment and with other persons, thus influencing their psycho-logical status. Likewise, feeling useless and socially isolated may obstruct optimum psychological function. General health status, genetic factors, educational achievement, and activity are among the factors which influence psychological changes during the aging process. In light of the involvement of other factors in the psychological functioning of older adults, and the awareness that psychological changes differ among aged individuals, some general findings can be discussed.

Drastic changes in basic personality do not commonly occur as one ages. The kind and gentle old person was most likely that way when younger. Likewise, the cantankerous old person was probably not mild and meek in earlier years. Excluding pathological processes, the personality will be consistent to that of earlier years, possibly with more open and honest expression. The alleged "rigidity" of older persons is more a result of physical and mental limitations, rather than a personality change. For example, an older person's insistence that furniture not be rearranged may be interpreted as rigidity, but to someone coping with poor memory and visual deficits, this may be a wise safety measure. Changes in personality traits may occur in response to events which alter

63

one's attitude toward oneself, such as retirement, death of a spouse, loss of independence, income reduction, and disability (Birren, 1964; Neugarten, 1968).

Memory may be altered with age, and usually memory for past events is superior to the retention and recall of more current information—even that presented seconds to minutes earlier. This explains why the older person who can't remember the name of the nurse who has cared for him all week can accurately recall the name of every member of his World War I outfit. Memory problems are more common in the presence of a poor health status. Evidence indicates changes in intelligence test scores with increasing age. Older individuals tend to generally do less well on intelligence tests involving spatial perception, decoding tasks, arrangement of geometric forms, and psychomotor performance in general. On the other hand, performance involving information, verbal comprehension, and arithmetic operations improves with age through the sixth decade (Botwinick, 1967). There is a correlation between the health status of the older individual and intelligence test scores.

In general, it is wise to interpret the findings related to intelligence and the aged with much caution, as results may indicate a problem with the measurement tool and method rather than with the person whose intelligence is being measured. Cross-sectional studies may be attempting to test similar information for different age groups; different environmental and educational advantages, as well as unique life experiences due to living in different periods of history, may cause the old and young to respond differently to similar questions and situations. Longitudinal studies are able to measure changes that occur in a specific generation as it ages; however, the costs and time involved with longitudinal studies have made this type of research scarce. In interpreting research associated with intelligence and the aged one must consider the aged population sampled. Were they representative of the aged population, or a sample from a nursing home? One must also consider the number sampled. Were the findings from 100 people generalized as representative of 20 million? The tool used for intelligence measurement is also a factor. Was it a written test with print too small for aged eyes to read? Did the test require the older person with a hearing deficit to listen for questions and directions? The relevancy of the test must also be determined. Was there a cultural or age bias in the items being tested?

Although learning ability is not seriously altered with age, other factors do interfere with learning in older individuals. These include motivation, attention span, problems in transfering information into the nervous system, perception deficits, and disease. Older individuals may display less readiness to learn and may depend on previous experience for solutions to problems rather than experiment with new problem-

64

solving techniques. Differences in the intensity and duration of the older person's physiological arousal may make it more difficult to extinguish previous responses and acquire new material. The early phases of the learning process tend to be more difficult for older individuals than younger ones; however after a longer early phase, they are then able to keep equal pace. While there is little difference between old and young in verbal or abstract ability, older persons show some difficulty with perceptual motor tasks. There is some evidence indicating a tendency toward simple association rather than analysis.

Since it is generally more difficult to learn new habits when old habits exist which must be unlearned, relearned, or modified, this is a particular problem for individuals with a lifetime accumulation of habits. Habit reversal, such as performing a task in reverse order, is more difficult (Botwinick, 1967). There is little decline in the psychomotor performance of simple tasks with age, although there is some problem with a series of tasks that is complicated, coordinated, and continuous in sequence. As motor performance is slower, due to decreased neuromuscular activity, poor judgment may be displayed by older persons. The alterations in an old person's psychological ability are an individual matter determined by the challenges he or she faces, the stresses imposed, and the education, activity, experiences, and health of the particular person.

REFERENCES

Agate, J. *The Practice of Geriatrics.* Thomas, Springfield, Ill., 1963.

Alva, J., Mendeloff, A. I., and Schuster, M. M. "Reflex and Electromyographic Abnormalities Associated with Fecal Incontinence." *Gastroenterology,* 53:101, 1967.

Birren, J. E. *The Psychology of Aging.* Prentice-Hall, Englewood Cliffs, N.J., 1964.

Botwinick, J. *Cognitive Processes in Maturity and Old Age.* Springer, New York, 1967.

Brandfonbrener, M., Landowne, M., and Shock, N. W. "Changes in Cardiac Output with Age." *Circulation,* 12:577, 1955.

Burgeon, C. F. Jr., and Burgeon, J. S. "Aging and the Cutaneous System." Geriatrics, 13:391, 1958.

Caird, F. I., and Judge, T. G. "Assessment of the Elderly Patient." Pitman Medical Publishing Co., New York, Eng., 1974, p. 34.

Calloway, N. O., and Merrill, R. S. "The Aging Adult Liver, I: Bromsulphalein and Bilirubin Clearances." *Journal of the American Geriatrics Society*, 13:594, 1965.

Davies, D. F., and Shock, N. W. "Age Changes in Glomerular Filtration Rate, Effective Renal Plasma Flow and Tubular Excretory Capacity in Adult Males." *Journal of Clinical Investigation,* 29:496, 1950.

Flood, C., Gherondache, C., Pincus, G., Tait, J. F., Tait, S. A. S., and Willoughby, S. "The Metabolism and Secretion of Aldosterone in Elderly Subjects." *Journal of Clinical Investigation,* 46:960, 1967.

Freeman, J. T. "Body Composition in Aging." In Freeman, J. T. (ed.), *Clinical Features of the Older Patient.* Thomas, Springfield, Ill., 1965.
Goldman, Ralph. "Decline in Organ Function with Aging." In Rossman, I. (ed), *Clinical Geriatrics.* Lippincott, Philadelphia, 1971, pp. 19–21, 24, 30, 41.
Grob, David. "Common Disorders of Muscles in the Aged." In Chinn, A. B. (ed.), *Working with Older People: A Guide to Practice, Vol. IV: Clinical Aspects of Aging,* USPHS Pub. No. 1459, Rockville, Md., U.S. Health Services and Mental Health Administration, 1974, pp. 156–162.
Harris, R. "Special Features of Heart Disease in the Elderly Patients." In Chinn, A.B. (ed.), *Working with Older People: A guide to Practice, Volume IV: Clinical Aspects of Aging,* USPHS Pub. No. 1459, Rockville, Md., U.S. Health Services and Mental Health Administration, 1974, pp. 83, 89.
Jaffe, J. W. "Common Lower Urinary Tract Problems in Older Adults." In Chinn, A. B. (ed.), *Working with Older People: A Guide to Practice, Vol. IV: Clinical Aspects of Aging,* USPHS Pub. No. 1459, Rockville, Md., U.S. Health Services and Mental Health Administration, 1974, p. 142.
Jeffocoate, T. N. A. *Principles of Gynecology,* 3rd ed. Prentice-Hall (Appleton), Englewood Cliffs, N.J., 1967.
Kahn, A. I., and Snapper, I. "Medical Renal Diseases in the Aged." In Chinn, A. B. (ed.), *Working with Older People: A Guide to Practice, Vol. IV: Clinical Aspects of Aging,* USPHS Pub. No. 1459, Rockville, Md. U.S. Health Services and Mental Health Administration, 1974, p. 132.
McGavick, T. H. "Endocrine Changes with Aging Significant to Clinical Practice." In Chinn, A. B. (ed.), *Working with Older People: A Guide to Practice, Vol. IV: Clinical Aspects of Aging.* USPHS Pub. No. 1459, Rockville, Md. U.S. Health Services and Mental Health Administration, 1974, (a) p. 198, (b) p. 195.
Master, A. M., and Lasser, R. P. "Blood Pressure Elevation in the Elderly." In Breast, A. M., and Moyer, J. H. (eds.), *Hypertension: Recent Advances.* Lea & Febiger, Philadelphia, 1961.
McKeown, F. *Pathology of the Aged.* Butterworth, London, 1965.
McMillan, J., and Lev, M. "The Cardiopulmonary System in the Aged." In Powers, J. D. (ed.), *Surgery of the Aged and Debilitated Patient.* Saunders, Philadelphia, 1968, chap. 5.
Mithoefer, G. C. and Karetzky, M. S. In Powers, J. D. (ed.): *Surgery of the Aged and Debilitated Patient.* Saunders, Philadelphia, 1968 Chap. 5.
Neugarten, B. L. (ed.). *Middle Age and Aging.* Univ. of Chicago Press, 1968.
Norris, A. H., Shock, N. W., Lansdowne, M., and Falzone, J. S. "Pulmonary Function Studies: Age Differences in Lung Volume and Bellows Function." *Journal of Gerontology,* 11:379, 1956.
Oliver, J. "The Growth and Decline of the Renal Tissues." In Lansing, A. I. (ed.), *Cowdry's Problems of Aging,* 3rd ed. Williams & Wilkens, Baltimore, 1952.
Pincus. G. "Aging and Urinary Steroid Excretion." In Engle, E. T., and Pincus, G. (eds.), *Hormones and the Aging Process.* Academic Press, New York, 1956, pp. 1–18.
Rossman, I. *Clinical Geriatrics.* Lippincott, Philadelphia, 1971, p. 6.
Schonfield, David, and Robertson, Elizabeth A. "Memory Storage and Aging." *Canadian Journal of Psychology,* 20:228–236, 1966.
Sherlock, S., Beorn, A. G., Billing, B. H., and Patterson, J. C. S. "Splanchnic Blood Flow in Man by the Bromsulphalein Method: The Relation of Peripheral Plasma Bromsulphalein Level to the Calculated Flow" (J. Lab. Clin. Med., 35:923, 1950). In Rossman, I. (ed.), *Clinical Geriatrics.* Lippincott, Philadelphia, 1971, p. 34.

Sklar, M. "Gastrointestinal Diseases in the Aged." In Chinn, A. B. (ed.), *Working with Older People: A Guide to Practice, Volume IV: Clinical Aspects of Aging,* USPHS Pub. No. 1459, Rockville, Md., U.S. Health Services and Mental Health Administration, 1974, p. 124.

Soergel, K. H., Zboralske, F. F., and Amberg, J. R. "Presbyesophagus: Esophageal Mobility in Nonagenarians." *Journal of Clinical Investigation,* 43:1472, 1964.

Wells, G. C. "Senile Changes of the Skin in Man." *Journal of the American Geriatrics Society,* 2:535, 1954.

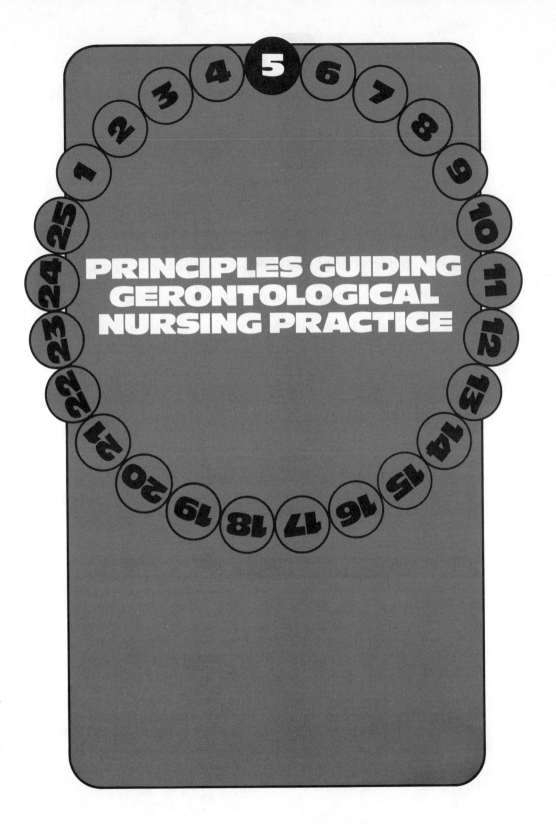

PRINCIPLES GUIDING GERONTOLOGICAL NURSING PRACTICE

Scientific data regarding theories, life adjustments, and general changes associated with the aging process combined with selected information from psychology, sociology, biology, and other physical and social sciences are utilized in accurately, intelligently, and effectively applying the nursing process to the older population. It is the responsibility of the professional nurse to use these scientific data as the foundation for nursing practice and to make sure through educational and supervisory means that others to whom responsibility for care is delegated also utilize them.

Data from the variety of disciplines is incorporated also in the development of nursing principles—proven facts or theories that are accepted by society and that direct nursing actions. In addition to the general principles utilized in the delivery of care to all individuals, there are specific principles for the care of individuals in certain age groups or with particular health problems. The principles guiding gerontological and geriatric nursing practice, discussed in this chapter, are the following:

1. Aging is a natural process common to all living organisms.
2. Heredity, nutrition, health status, life experiences, environment, activity, and stress are factors which influence the normal aging process and demonstrate unique effects in each individual.
3. Scientific data related to normal aging and unique psychobiosocial characteristics of aged individuals are combined with general nursing knowledge in the application of the nursing process to the aged population.
4. Aged individuals share similar universal self-care demands with all other human beings.
5. Each aged individual has unique capacities and limitations regarding his or her ability to fulfill universal self-care demands.
6. The focus of gerontological and geriatric nursing is to take action in a planned, organized, and therapeutic manner:
   a. To strengthen the individual's self-care capacities
   b. To eliminate or minimize self-care limitations
   c. To provide direct care services by acting for, doing for, or partially assisting the individual when universal self-care or therapeutic demands cannot be independently fulfilled

1. **Aging—a natural process common to all living organisms.**
Every living organism begins aging from the very time of conception. The process of growing old helps the individual achieve the mature cellular, organ, and system functioning that is necessary for the accomplishment of developmental tasks throughout life. Constantly and continuously, every cell of every organism ages. Many people discuss and approach aging as though it were a pathological experience. When

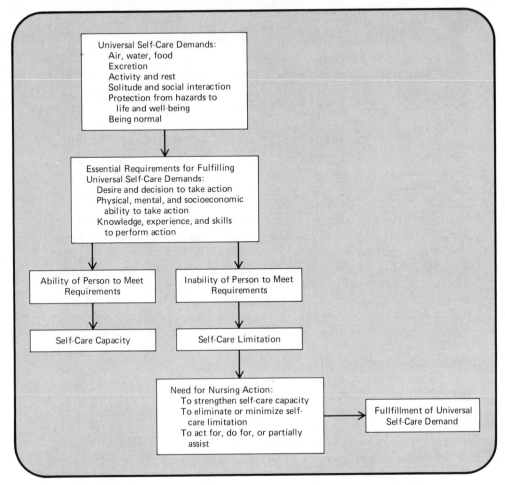

Figure 5-1. Relationship between nursing and the total self-care system.

asked what aging means to them, they usually respond with typical statements:

"Getting senile"
"Looking gray and wrinkled"
"Losing health and independence"
"Becoming inflexible, demanding, and disinterested"
"Having less satisfaction and happiness"
"Returning to childlike behavior"
"Suffering losses"

71

Although each of the above responses may be true for a given older individual, they cannot be generalized as descriptive of aging in most people. Aging is not a crippling disease and although some limitations may be imposed as the body systems lose efficiency in function, aging itself does not reduce the opportunity for happiness, fulfillment, and independent function. An increased understanding of the aging process may promote a more positive attitude toward old age.

2. Factors that influence the normal aging process. Heredity, nutrition, health status, life experiences, environment, activity, and stress demonstrate unique effects in each individual. Among the variety of factors either known or hypothesized to alter the usual pattern of aging, inherited factors are believed by some researchers to produce chromosomal alterations that cause cells to age at a particular rate. In addition, malnourishment hastens the ill effects of the aging process, and laboratory studies of eating patterns have demonstrated that fish and rats have a longer than usual life span when they are underfed. Illness may hasten the aging process, reduce the human life span, or exaggerate certain limitations of advancing age. Exposure to environmental toxins and certain viruses may cause a more rapid aging of the human organism, as may overexertion and stress. On the other hand, mental, physical, and social activity may reduce the rate and degree of declining function with age.

Every person ages in a very individualized manner, although some general characteristics may be evident among most people in a given age category. Just as we wouldn't assume all 30-year-olds to be identical and would evaluate, approach, and communicate with each in a different and individualized manner, we must recognize that no two 60-year-olds, 70-year-olds, or 80-year-olds are alike. It is a responsibility of the nurse caring for the aged person to recognize the effects of various factors on a particular individual's aging process and how these effects are consequently displayed in the individual. An awareness of the unique aging patterns among people and a more individualized approach will enhance nursing practice with the older person.

3. Data and knowledge used in applying the nursing process to the aged population. In nursing the aged, the scientific data related to normal aging and the unique psychobiosocial characteristics of aged individuals are combined with a general knowledge of nursing. The nursing process provides a systematic approach to the delivery of nursing service. It affirms that nursing actions are deliberate and purposeful, involving a combination of intellectual, interpersonal, and technical skills (Yura and Walsh, 1973). The scope of nursing includes more than following a medical order or performing an isolated task; the nursing process involves a wholistic approach to individuals and the care they require. Four activities are components of the nursing process: assessment, planning, implementation, and evaluation.

As discussed in previous chapters, the unique characteristics and changes associated with the aging process require that certain adjustments be made in the application of the nursing process to the aged. In addition to handling differences in laboratory values, data analysis, priorities, nursing techniques, etc., the nurse caring for the older individual must thoroughly understand the physiological and psychological differences and the unique socioeconomic problems and must utilize this knowledge when assessing, planning, implementing, and evaluating care. Chapter 6 provides a more thorough examination of the application of the nursing process to aged individuals.

4. Self-care demands. Aged individuals share similar universal self-care demands with all other human beings. Every human being has certain basic requirements for the optimum and integrated functioning of the total individual. These needs, or life's demands, categorized in a variety of ways, have been described by Dorothea Orem (*Nursing: Concepts of Practice*) as air, water, food; excretion; activity and rest; solitude and social interaction; avoidance of hazards to life and well-being; and being normal.

Through self-care practices, the individual performs activities independently and voluntarily to meet these universal life demands. Age, illness, and disability may interfere with an individual's ability to do so, and assistance may be required perhaps in the form of nursing services. Some explanation of the effects of aging on an individual's universal self-care demands, and related nursing considerations are discussed in Chapter 7.

5. Capacities and limitations regarding self-care. Each aged individual has unique capacities and limitations regarding his or her ability to fulfill universal self-care demands. Not all individuals can, do, or will meet their universal self-care demands similarly or equally. A variety of factors will determine the success with which these needs are met. Individuals are said to have *self-care* capacity when they are able to be independent and take responsibility for meeting these needs. When the individual's ability to fulfill a demand is partially or totally restricted, he or she is said to have a self-care limitation. Whether the aged person can handle the universal demands of daily living and the actions required to meet specific therapeutic demands, such as the self-administration of medications and complying with a low-sodium diet, depends on several factors, including (a) the desire and decision for action; (b) the required physical, mental, and socioeconomic means for

73

taking action; (c) the knowledge, experience, and skills needed to perform the action.

a. ***Desire and decision for action.*** The value a person sees in performing the action, as well as the person's knowledge, attitudes, and beliefs, and degree of motivation influence the desire and decision for action. Limitations result if a person lacks desire or decides against action. If an individual isn't interested in preparing and eating meals because of social isolation and loneliness, a dietary deficiency may develop. A hypertensive individual's lack of desire and decision to forfeit potato chips and pork products in his or her diet because he or she does not think it is worth the benefit may pose a real threat to his or her health. The person who is not informed of the importance of physical activity may not realize the need to arise from bed during an illness, and consequently may develop complications. A dying individual, viewing dying as a natural process, may decide against medical intervention to sustain his or her life and may not comply with prescribed therapies.

Values, attitudes, and beliefs are deeply established and not easily altered. While the nurse should respect the right of individuals to make decisions affecting their life, if limitations restrict their ability to meet self-care demands, the nurse can help by explaining the benefit of a particular action, providing information, and developing motivation. In some circumstances, as with an emotionally ill or mentally incompetent person, desires and decisions may have to be superceded by professional judgments.

b. ***Physical, mental, and socioeconomic means.*** Aged individuals may be able to remain active and involved in life if they have adequate financial resources. A person will be able to prevent contractures if he or she is physically able to have unrestricted motion. On the other hand, if individuals lack the finances to obtain necessary health care services or the energy to ambulate and feed themselves or the mental faculties to cross a street safely, self-care will be limited.

It is the responsibility of nursing to minimize or reduce limitations imposed by physical, mental, and socioeconomic restrictions. Nursing services that assist in the reduction of limitations will be more fully discussed in Chapter 7.

c. ***Knowledge, experience, and skills.*** Limitations exist when the knowledge, experience, or skills required for a given self-care action are inadequate or nonexistent. An individual with a wealth of social skills is capable of a normal, active life that

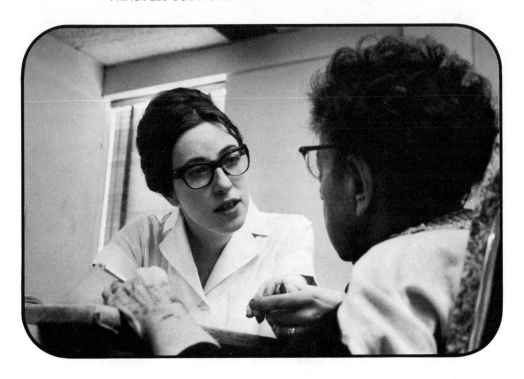

includes friendships and other social interaction. People who have knowledge of the hazards of cigarette smoking will be more capable of protecting themselves from health problems associated with this habit. On the other hand, an older man who is widowed may not be able to cook and provide an adequate diet for himself if he depended on his wife for meal preparation. The diabetic person who lacks skill in self-injection of insulin may not be able to meet his or her therapeutic demand for insulin administration. Specific nursing considerations for enhancing self-care capacities will be offered in other chapters.

6. Planned, organized, and therapeutic nursing action. The nurses actions are directed toward (a) strengthening the individual's self-care capacities; (b) eliminating or minimizing self-care limitations; and (c) providing direct care services by acting for, doing for, or assisting the individual when universal self-care or therapeutic demands cannot be independently fulfilled.

An individual unaffected by illness, disability, advanced age, or limited resources may be fully able to perform the necessary actions related to universal self-care demands. These individuals may have no need for nursing services. Even when self-care actions cannot be

75

performed and a limitation is present, nursing services can sometimes increase the individual's self-care capacity and reduce the limitation. At times, the self-care capacity cannot be temporarily or permanently improved and the self-care limitation cannot be eliminated. In these situations the nurse may have to perform the action, partially or totally, or assist other personnel or family members in performing the action. The following case will exemplify some types of needs an aged person has regarding universal self-care demands. It should be remembered that this sort of example is not all inclusive.

The Case of Mrs. D
Mrs. D, 78 years old, was admitted to a hospital service for acute conditions with the identified problems of a fractured neck of the femur, malnutrition, and a "disposition problem." Initial observation revealed a small-framed, frail-looking lady, with obvious signs of malnutrition and dehydration. She was well oriented to person, place, and time, and able to converse and answer questions quite coherently. Although her memory for recent events was poor, she selcom forgot to inform anyone who was interested that she neither liked nor wanted to be in the hospital. Her previous and only other hospitalization had been 55 years earlier!

Mrs. D had been living with her husband and an unmarried sister for more than 50 years when her husband died. For the five years following she had depended heavily on her sister for emotional support and guidance. Then, her sister died, which promoted feelings of anxiety, insecurity, loneliness, and depression. Living alone, she cared for her six-room home in the county with no assistance other than that from a neighbor who did the marketing for Mrs. D and occasionally provided her with transportation. A year later, on the day of her admission to the hospital, Mrs. D fell on her kitchen floor, weak from her malnourished state. Discovering her hours later, her neighbor called an ambulance which transported Mrs. D to the hospital. Once the diagnosis of fractured femur was established, plans were made to perform a nailing procedure and to correct her malnourishment and find a new living arrangement since her home seemed to demand more energy and attention then she was capable of providing.

Based on an assessment of Mrs. D's self-care capacities and limitations, a variety of nursing actions were planned to assist her in fulfilling the general universal self-care demands and specific therapeutic self-care demands imposed by her problems.

Nursing Actions Related to Universal Requirements

The chart that follows describes the nursing actions that are necessary in fulfilling the universal requirements for (1) air, food, and water; (2) excretion; (3) activity and rest; (4) solitude and social interaction; (5) avoiding hazards to life and well-being; and (6) being normal. These procedures can be related to caring for Mrs. D in the case described above.

UNIVER-SAL REQUIRE-MENT	RELATED NURSING ACTION	TYPE OF ACTION
AIR		
	1. Maintain normal respirations	
	Preventing blockage of airway, or any other interference with normal breathing	Partially assisting
	Observing for and detecting respiratory problems early	Partially assisting
	2. Promoting active and passive exercises	
	Teaching and encouraging turning, coughing, and deep-breathing exercises	Strengthening self-care capacity
	Encouraging active exercises, such as using blow bottles and deep-breathing	Strengthening self-care capacity
	Performing passive range of motion exercise	Doing for
	3. Avoiding external interferences with respiration	
	Providing good room ventilation	Doing for
	Avoiding restrictive clothing, linens, or equipment	Doing for
	Positioning in manner conducive to best respiration	Partially assisting
	Preventing anxiety-producing situations, such as delays in answering call bell	Doing for
FOOD AND WATER		
	1. Stimulating appetite	
	Planning diet according to person's preferences, consisting with therapeutic requirements	Partially assisting
	Providing quiet, pleasant environment that allows for socialization with others	Doing for
	Stimulating appetite through appearance and seasoning of foods	Minimizing self-care limitation
	2. Planning meals	
	Reading menu selection to patient	Partially assisting
	Guiding choice of high-protein, carbohydrate, and vitamin- and mineral-rich foods	Minimizing self-care limitation
	Assessing food preferences and including them in menu selections	Acting for

UNIVER-SAL REQUIRE-MENT RELATED NURSING ACTION	TYPE OF ACTION
3. Assisting with feeding	
Conserving energy and promoting adequate intake by preparing food tray, encouraging rest periods, and feeding when necessary	Strengthening self-care capacity, doing for, and partially assisting
4. Preventing complications	
Not leaving solutions, medications, or harmful agents in location where they may be mistakenly ingested (especially when assessment indicates visual limitations)	Acting for
Checking temperature of foods and drinks to prevent burns (especially when assessment indicates decreased cutaneous sensation)	Acting for
Assisting in the selection of foods conducive to bone healing and correction of malnutrition	Partially assisting
Observing fluid intake and output for early detection of imbalances	Minimizing self-care limitation
Assessing general health status frequently to detect new problems or improvements that have resulted from changes in nutritional status (weight changes, skin turgor, mental status, strength, etc.)	Acting for and minimizing self-care limitation

EXCRETION

1. Promoting regular elimination of bladder and bowels	
Guiding the selection of a diet high in roughage and fluids	Partially assisting
Observing and recording elimination pattern	Acting for and minimizing self-care limitation
Assisting with exercises to promote peristolsis and urination	Partially assisting
Arranging schedule to provide regular time periods for elimination	Acting for
Assisting with hygienic care of body surfaces	Partially assisting
Providing privacy when bedpan is used	Acting for
2. Developing good hygienic practices	
Teaching importance and method of cleansing perineal region after elimination	Strengthening self-care

UNIVER- SAL REQUIRE- MENT RELATED NURSING ACTION	TYPE OF ACTION
3. Preventing social isolation Preventing, detecting and cor- recting body odors resulting from poor hygienic practices	Acting for, minimizing self- care capacity
ACTIVITY AND REST	
1. Adjusting hospital routines to indi- vidual's pace	Strengthening self-care capacity
Spacing procedures and other activities	Acting for
Allowing longer periods of time for self-care activities	Minimizing self-care limitation
2. Providing for energy conservation Promoting security and relaxation through the avoidance of frequent changes of personnel	Acting for
Allowing for short rest periods sev- eral times a day	Strengthening self-care capacity
Controlling environmental noise, light, and temperature	Acting for
3. Preventing complications asso- ciated with immobility (such as decubiti, constipation, renal cal- culi, contractures, hypostatic pneumonia, thrombi, edema, and lethargy)	
Encouraging frequent change of position	Minimizing self-care limitation
Motivating and rewarding activity	Strengthening self-care capacity
Teaching simple exercises to pre- vent complications and improve motor dexterity	Strengthening self-care capacity
Planning activities to increase independence progressively	Acting for and strengthening self-care capacity
SOLITUDE AND SOCIAL INTERACTION	
1. Controlling environmental stimuli Scheduling the same personnel to care for person	Acting for
Maintaining a regular daily schedule	Strengthening self-care capacity
Arranging for a roommate with similar interests and background	Acting for and strengthening self-care capacity
Regulating the amount of visitors	Acting for
Spacing activities and procedures	Acting for and minimizing self-care limitation

UNIVERSAL REQUIREMENT / RELATED NURSING ACTION	TYPE OF ACTION
2. Promoting meaningful social interactions	
Instructing others to speak clearly and sufficiently loud while facing the person	Strengthening self-care capacity
Planning activities in which person can be involved	Strengthening self-care capacity
Promoting and maintaining an oriented state	Strengthening self-care capacity and minimizing self-care limitation
Displaying interest in person's social interactions and encouraging their continuation	Strengthening self-care capacity
Initiating contacts with community agencies to develop relationships that can continue after discharge	Acting for and minimizing self-care limitation
Assisting with grooming and dressing	Partially assisting and minimizing self-care limitation
3. Providing opportunities for solitude	
Providing several preplanned time periods during the day in which person can be alone	Acting for
Providing privacy by pulling curtains around bed and making use of facilities such as chapel	Minimizing self-care limitation and partially assisting
AVOIDING HAZARDS TO LIFE AND WELL-BEING	
1. Compensating for poor vision	
Reading to person	Doing for and minimizing self-care limitation
Writing information and labeling with large letters and color coding when possible	Minimizing self-care limitation
Removing obstacles that could cause accidents, such as foreign objects in bed, clutter on floor, and solutions which could be mistaken as water	Minimizing self-care limitation and acting for
Communicating this problem to other personnel	Acting for
Initiating an ophthalmology referral	Acting for
2. Compensating for decreased ability to smell:	
Preventing and correcting odors resulting from poor hygienic practices	Partially assisting and minimizing self-care limitations

80

UNIVERSAL REQUIREMENT	RELATED NURSING ACTION	TYPE OF ACTION
	Detecting unusual odors early (may be symptomatic of infection)	Acting for
	3. Compensating for hearing loss	
	Speaking clearly and loudly while facing person	Minimizing self-care limitation
	Utilizing feedback techniques to make sure person has heard and understood	Minimizing self-care limitation
	Initiating referral to ear, nose, and throat clinic	Acting for
	4. Maintaining good skin condition	
	Inspecting for rashes, reddened areas, and sores	Doing for
	Assisting with hygienic practices	Partially assisting
	Giving back rubs, changing person's position frequently, and keeping person's skin soft and dry	Doing for / Partially assisting and minimizing self-care limitation
	5. Preventing falls	
	Supporting person who is ambulating or being transported	Partially assisting
	Maintaining muscle tone	Strengthening self-care capacity
	Keeping bed rails up and supporting person in wheelchair	Doing for
	Providing rest periods between activities	Strengthening self-care capacity and minimizing self-care limitation
	Placing frequently used objects within easy reach	Partially assisting
	6. Maintaining proper body alignment	
	Utilizing sandbags, trochanter rolls and pillows	Minimizing self-care limitation and partially assisting
	Supportive person's affected limb when it is lifted or moved	Partially assisting and minimizing self-care limitation
	7. Seeking safe living arrangements in preparation for person's discharge	
	Evaluating patient's preferences, capacities, and limitations, in order to suggest appropriate arrangements	Acting for and partially assisting
	Initiating referral to social worker	Acting for

BEING NORMAL

    1. Improving physical limitations where possible

UNIVER-SAL REQUIRE-MENT	RELATED NURSING ACTION	TYPE OF ACTION
	Assisting with reeducation for ambulation	Partially assisting and strengthening self-care capacity
	Exercising body parts to maintain function	Partially assisting and minimizing self-care limitation
	Encouraging patient to consume an adequate diet	Strengthening self-care capacity
	Initiating referral for audiometric examination to explore utility of hearing aid	Acting for Minimizing self-care limitation
	Initiating ophthalmology referral to explore utility of corrective lenses	Acting for and minimizing self-care limitation
2. Maintaining familiar components of life-style		
	Adjusting hospital routine to person's home routine as much as possible	Acting for and minimizing self-care limitation
	Encouraging person to wear own clothing	Minimizing self-care limitation
	Providing person with personal items from home, pillow, blanket, photographs, and tea cup	Minimizing self-care limitation
	Providing leisure activities person is accustomed to	Minimizing self-care limitation and strengthening self-care capacity
3. Promoting active participation		
	Providing person with opportunities to make own decisions whenever possible	Strengthening self-care capacity
	Involving person in care	Strengthening self-care capacity
	Stimulating and encouraging communication	Strengthening self-care capacity

The above principles of gerontological nursing practice are basic to the nursing care of older persons. These principles lay a solid foundation upon which specialized nursing actions for the aged can be developed. A truly professional gerontological nurse demonstrates a distinct and effective blend of cognitive and technical skills to achieve excellence in gerontological care. Only by utilizing sound valid data can nurses surpass the technical level of caring for the aged, and attain the realm of intelligent care of the aged.

REFERENCES

Orem, Dorothea E. *Nursing: Concepts of Practice.* McGraw-Hill, New York, 1971.

Yura, Helen, and Walsh, Mary B. *The Nursing Process: Assessing, Planning, Implementing and Evaluating,* 2nd ed. Prentice-Hall (Appleton), Englewood Cliffs, N.J., 1973.

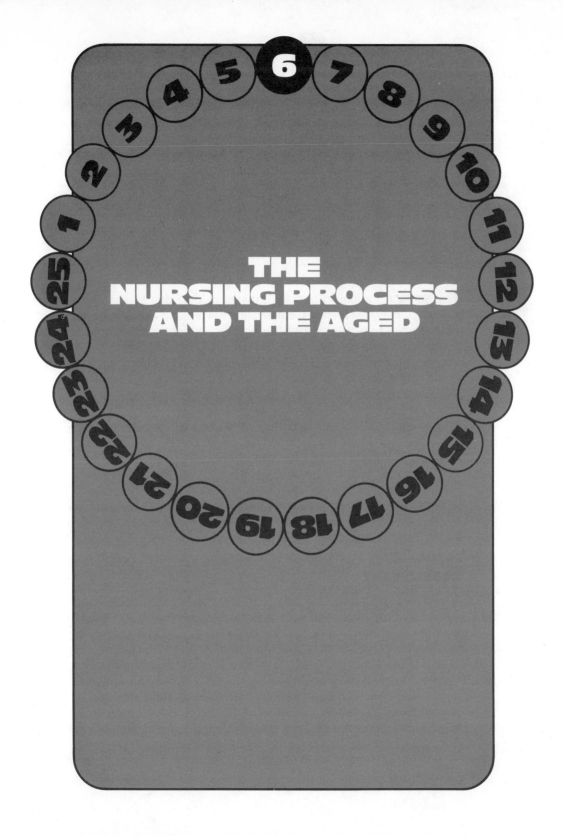

THE NURSING PROCESS AND THE AGED

As mentioned in the previous chapter, the nursing process requires an orderly, organized, and intentional approach to the delivery of nursing services. When knowledge regarding both normal aging and the specific differences of aged persons is added, the result is a complete system of nursing care for aged individuals. There are four phases of the nursing process: (1) an initial assessment, (2) specific planning to compensate for limitations and to maintain and strengthen the capacities of the individual, (3) implementation of these plans through a variety of selected nursing actions, and (4) evaluation of the effectiveness of these actions in achieving the desired outcomes. This evaluation, in turn, provides feedback that may stimulate a reassessment and establishment of new plans, and so on. This sequence would apply to one isolated problem as follows:

Assessment: Patient frequently urinates in bed due to short time interval between feeling the sensation to void and actual voiding.

Plan: Prevent voiding in bed by walking patient to bathroom at regular intervals.

Implementation: Patient is walked to bathroom q 2h during daytime with assistance of nurse.

Evaluation: Patient did not void in bed entire day but was too fatigued to participate in other activities.

Assessment: Q 2h walks to bathroom expend the energy required for other activities, although it does prevent patient from voiding in bed.

Plan: Prevent voiding in bed by assisting patient to bedside commode q 2h during daytime and walking to bathroom with assistance of nurse once per shift.

Each phase is described in the sections that follow.

ASSESSMENT

Assessment pertains to the collection and review of data pertaining to the physical, emotional, and socioeconomic status of the individual. Not only are capacities and limitations determined during this activity, but required nursing actions are also identified. Although assessment is the first step of the nursing process, it is not an activity that is done once and forgotten. Instead, it is an ongoing process, whereby all observations and interactions are utilized to collect new data, recognize changes, and analyze needs.

Many nurses view assessment as an isolated nurse-client activity solely for data gathering. This is frequently observed during a clinic visit when a patient is initially interviewed or completes a questionnaire pertaining to health status. In institutional settings, the nurse may plan the first encounter with the patient and his or her family to include an interview and examination for baseline data collection. It is perfectly appropriate for this activity to be a separate one in some situations. However, it is also possible to integrate data collection into other activities, such as during an informal conversation at mealtime or during a back rub. Nurses who have an understanding of the type of essential information necessary for comprehensive and individualized care planning and delivery may know how to integrate the physical, emotional, and socioeconomic assessment with other contacts with individuals and their families, documenting their assessment later. Some nurses, due to individual preference or inexperience, may be inclined to use a nursing-history tool to guide them in their information gathering. Regardless of the approach, it is essential that standard, comprehensive, baseline data be collected and documented for all aged individuals, and that assessment be viewed as a dynamic process, rather than limited to an initial activity of the nurse-client relationship.

Of the various skills required in assessment, good communication is especially important if honest and thorough information is to result. The nurse must communicate the reason the information is being sought, how it will be used, and an assurance it will be managed discreetly and respectfully. Many persons have had limited experience in being interviewed by service agencies, and many may be reluctant to share their personal problems of financial status with "strangers." Time must be provided for the establishment of trust in the nurse in order for the individual to be willing to share information. In addition, language may have to be adjusted to meet the needs of the particular individual. For instance, a person may respond negatively when asked Do you ever expectorate in the morning? But when asked Do you ever bring up phlegm in the morning? or Do you ever have to cough or spit up in the morning? the person may better understand the question and respond accurately. Using common jargon can help the nurse obtain more accurate information. Many patients who do not understand the term *diuretics* know what is meant by *fluid pills.*

Patients may think of medications as being only those drugs prescribed by a physician and not contribute the information that they regularly take aspirin, antacids, or laxatives when asked if they're taking any medications. Identifying such lack of understanding or misconceptions during the assessment has important implications for care planning and delivery, especially in terms of the educational needs of the patient. The manner in which a question is presented can influence the accuracy of the response. Asking Do you ever have to use a laxative? may elicit a negative response because the person may believe it is wrong to do so and be unwilling to make the admission. Rephrasing the question to How

85

often do you have to use a laxative? may convey understanding that the person may have to occasionally use a laxative and make him or her more willing to give an honest response.

When asked for their age, elderly persons may forget whether they are 77 or 79 years old; but if asked for their birthdate, they may rapidly recall the exact day, month, and year. Instead of inaccurately labeling the person as confused, the nurse might make an assessment that memory for recent events is poor, and seek more information related to that characteristic. Emotional and neurological status, attention span, language barriers, and hearing, vision, and speech deficits can also be detected through the keen use of communication skills during the assessment process. The interview with the aged individual is complemented by, or sometimes, by necessity, substituted for, an interview with the individual's family. This not only creates a potential for further collection of information, but also actively involves the family in the person's care.

Physical examination of the aged person is part of the assessment process and, like the interview, is either separately defined or integrated into other care activities. The physical assessment by a nurse serves a different purpose from the physical examination by a physician. The physician may diagnose a specific degree of hearing loss. The nurse *recognizes* this loss and attempts to *assess* how this loss is managed by the patient and the way the care may have to be altered to compensate for this limitation. Likewise, the physician may be concerned with identifying the extent of disability caused by arthritic fingers. The nurse would be more concerned with identifying relief and supportive measures. The focus of the nurse's physical examination is to recognize capacities, limitations, and pathology, and also to establish how these factors will be managed, to analyze the effects of these factors on the individual's ability to fulfill universal self-care demands, and to identify nursing actions which may be required.

A nursing-history tool may be used as a guide to standardized and comprehensive data collection, and as a source for documenting the assessment in a consistent, organized, and easy manner. The tool utilized will vary to meet the needs of the individual agency and should be flexible enough to meet the unique needs of the client and the nurse in a particular situation. Some baseline data, beneficial to incorporate in the assessment may include the items discussed below.

1. Profile of patient. Identifying information includes full name, sex, race, religion (including name and location of church, synagogue, etc.), date of birth, address, telephone number, languages spoken, and name of spouse or nearest contact person.

2. Profile of family. If the spouse is living, information should be obtained pertaining to his or her full name, date of birth, address, telephone number, occupation, and length of marriage. An assessment of the spouse's health status is also beneficial, not only in order to identify problems, but to evaluate the ability of this person to assist the patient should the need arise. If the spouse is deceased, it is useful to know the date and cause of death. Sometimes through exploring this information with the patient, unresolved grief, guilt, or other feelings are surfaced.

Names and addresses of children add helpful information to the record as do their ages and health status, which provide a realistic estimate of their ability to assist the patient. It is becoming increasingly common to find such situations as an ill 85-year-old whose only source of assistance with daily home care is an ill 68-year-old. (One in five aged individuals has a child over the age of 65!) Deceased children and the date and cause of death should also be explored, and profiles of any other members of the household should be obtained. Just because the aged person may have no living family does not mean that friends or boarders in the household aren't providing a strong support system.

The relationship with family members is useful to know. There are situations in which an elderly person would prefer living in a shabby room alone rather than in the new home of a daughter with whom he or she never got along. Likewise, if an elderly couple have had a satisfying marriage and have never been apart, the health team could make sure that when they are admitted to a nursing home, it is one in which they can share the same room and have their relationship respected.

3. Occupational profile. If the individual is employed, information pertaining to the type of work, length of time at the present job, and working hours should be collected. The type of work can give clues to occupationally caused illnesses and indicate the type of diversionary activities the patient may prefer. It may be useful to explore the individual's reason for working if he or she is of retirement age. Continuing employment due to the satisfactions obtained from the job and a sincere desire in wanting to remain employed will have different implications from disliking one's job but having to work due to financial necessity. If the person is unemployed or retired, it is useful to evaluate the reason. Being unemployed because one desires to retire and travel has different implications from unwanted mandatory retirement or being unemployed due to poor health. The length of unemployed time and the means of income are valuable to know and may help the nurse assess factors such as interests and financial concerns. Here again, the nurse should question the patient as to his or her occupational history.

87

4. Home profile. The patient's home environment is essential to know, although this information is often overlooked by those who provide care for the aged in institutional settings. The home profile should include the type of dwelling, number of levels, location of bathroom and patient's bedroom, stairs climbed in an average day, location of nearest neighbor, availability of a telephone, type of community, safety hazards, and whether the person owns or rents the home. The capacity of the individual to fulfill responsibilities in the home should also be explored.

The nursing history should reflect the presence of pets in the household. This may appear to be an insignificant consideration, but to the aged individual a pet may provide an important source of satisfaction and companionship. Some aged individuals may resist an emergency hospitalization or new housing due to their concern about the welfare of their pet. Knowledge pertaining to the cause of certain health problems, allergies for instance, may also be revealed by collecting information regarding pets.

5. Economic profile. Various sources and amounts of income and whether the person is receiving all the benefits to which he or she is entitled should be ascertained. Sometimes the elderly aren't aware that they may qualify for certain benefits, or they may have been unable to understand the application process for these benefits. The monthly income should be balanced with the monthly expenses to evaluate the capacity of the individual to meet financial obligations. While obtaining this data, the nurse may learn that the aged person is eating a poor quality diet due to budget constraints or that he or she is fearful of losing a home through inability to pay the annual property tax. Clues to specific financial concerns should be sought while questioning the person about his or her financial status.

6. Health insurance. The type of health insurance and policy number is basic information. If there is no insurance, measures can be taken to enroll the person in a program suited for his or her needs. The lack of health insurance sometimes discourages people from seeking health care; it can be a source of stress should hospitalization be required.

7. Currently used health and social resources. The names and locations of other physicians, social workers, visiting nurses, public health nurses, clinics, and hospitals involved with the individual should be recorded. They can provide additional insight into the patient and should be kept informed to promote continuity of care. It is important to obtain information and avoid duplication regarding community resources utilized by the patient, such as home health aides or delivered meals.

8. Social and leisure activities. Knowing what organizations the person belongs to and his or her hobbies and interests helps guide the nurse in planning the care and also indicates the person's health status, energy level, and opportunities for socialization. Sometimes organizations to which the individual has belonged will provide visits and continued communication, should the individual be hospitalized or enter a nursing home.

9. Health history. The health history of an aged person need not explore every childhood disease or minor health problem that has ever existed, unless this information is significant to the current health status. Information pertaining to a family tendency toward stroke, diabetes, heart disease, cancer, or hypertension may be more relevant. Health problems of current concern, or for which treatment is being obtained, should be recorded. A history of diabetes, hypertension, tuberculosis, and cancer should be indicated, even if the patient states that he or she is free of the disease at present. Major hospitalizations, surgeries, and fractures in the past may give insight into current problems and should be explored. Women should be questioned as to the number and course of pregnancies. Allergies to foods and other items and drug sensitivities should be recorded.

10. Current health status. Current health problems should be recorded, and the patient's and family's knowledge and understanding of these problems should be ascertained. Perceptions regarding these problems should be indicated if significant—for example, the belief by an individual that his cancer was "caught" from his wife who recently died of the disease. Any limitations in functions or inability to perform the activities of daily living should be assessed, as well as the methods in which these problems are managed and coped with. Any particular appliance or prosthesis used in the management of health problems should be listed. The main concerns and goals of the patient and family in relation to the health status should be discussed and reflected in the assessment.

11. Medications. The name and dosage of all medications which the older person is taking is vital information. The nurse should explore how and why the medication was obtained. The aged are as guilty as the young of self-prescription of medication! The time and method in which the medication is taken and the patient's understanding

89

of the medication, its action, and its adverse effects should be indicated. Exploring this information with the individual will often give clues to errors in drug administration and drug related symptoms which he or she may be displaying. The nurse may also detect discrepancies. For example, a physician at one clinic may have prescribed a medication that combats the effect of a drug another physician has concurrently prescribed. The patient should be instructed to take all medications along when visiting a health facility or physician.

12. Physical status. Assessment of physical status requires an examination of the person as well as an interview. Baseline values for vital signs should be established when the person is well in order to have comparative data available should the person's health status change. Although one of the vital signs may be severely altered in the aged, it may still fall within normal limits for the general adult population. For instance, normal body temperature in the aged may be as low as 95° F and a temperature of 98° F would be a severe elevation for that person, but it could be missed because it is a low normal for younger adults. Such a missed diagnosis can delay correction of the problem. The normal body temperature should be established, and the individual should be informed of his or her norm. Sometimes ancillary personnel who obtain a thermometer reading of 96° F in aged persons, believe there was an error in the way they performed the procedure, and record the temperature as 98.6° F to avoid "criticism" of their procedure. All nursing staff should understand that a lower body temperature in aged individuals can be the normal value for that person.

Unless the patient is unable to satisfactorily hold a thermometer in place sublingually, this should be the means of obtaining body temperature. Recent research indicates that for general assessment purposes, the most accurate recording of the body temperature is obtained by using the sublingual site. This site reflects temperature changes faster than the rectal site. Reduced blood flow to the lower bowel and the possible presence of feces may cause inaccurate rectal temperature readings. If the sublingual site cannot be used, the nurse can then use the axilla, if there is a stable and controlled environmental temperature. When no other site is possible or practical, a rectal temperature should then be obtained. Research indicates that an accurate oral reading is obtained by leaving the thermometer in place at least seven minutes. Rectal thermometers need only two minutes for an accurate reading in rooms of at least 72° F or greater, and three minutes in rooms under 72° F (Nichols and Kucha, 1972).

The rate, rhythm, and volume of the pulse should be noted during assessment of the older adult. The acceptable range for pulse rate is 50 to 100 beats per minute, although the elderly may occasionally have rates which fall beyond those boundaries. Irregularity of pulse rhythm is not uncommon in the aged, but it should be evaluated if the irregularity is due to digitalis toxicity, an electrolyte imbalance, or a disease process. A full, bounding pulse may occur in the presence of volume excess while a volume deficiency or electrolyte imbalance is demonstrated by a weak, thready pulse. The arteries of the aged may feel tortuous due to the loss of elasticity and smoothness with advancing age.

The rate, rhythm, and depth of the aged's respirations should be noted. The number of respirations may range within 14 to 18 per minute, although slower rates are not unusual in the aged. Irregularities of rhythm are not unusual either, and respirations similar to Cheyne-Stokes respirations may be evidenced during sleep. Depth of respirations is lessened as a result of reduced strength of the respiratory muscles and rigidity of the thoracic cage. An increase in respiratory rate and depth may indicate metabolic acidosis, while the opposite, accompanied by an irregular rhythm, occurs with metabolic alkalosis.

Increased peripheral resistance results in higher systolic and diastolic blood pressures in older individuals. Hypertensive levels in the aged are considered persistent elevations of 170 mmHg systolic and 95 mmHg diastolic, or greater. A shortening of the vertebral column also occurs with age and accompanies slight hip and knee flexion to produce a decreasing height. There is a tendency for weight gain in the fifth and sixth decades, which plateaus in the late sixth and seventh decades, and is followed by a gradual loss thereafter. Although the total body weight decreases in old age, there is an increase in the amount of body fat with age.

A urine sample should be evaluated as part of the individual's assessment. The color and clarity of the specimen should be noted, as well as the presence of any unusual characteristics. Due to the declining efficiency of the kidneys, several differences may be noted in the urine of the aged. A proteinuria of 1+ may result from decreased reabsorption from the filtrate and is usually of no diagnostic significance in the aged. An increased renal threshold for glucose may result in high blood glucose levels without evidence of glycosuria, decreasing the accuracy of urine testing for glucose. Older adults also have a lower specific gravity due to decreased ability to concentrate urine.

The entire surface of the body should be examined to assess the condition of the skin. Any skin breakage or wound should be described as to location and size. Specific measurements should be used; instead of describing a decubitus ulcer on the heel as being "small," give the exact measurement whenever possible in inches or centimeters. Rashes should also be distinctly described, and the location and characteristics of any discolored areas noted.

Hair should be described as to condition and amount. Whether the

TABLE 6-1: NORMAL RANGE OF JOINT MOTION FOR THE AGED

Joint	Range of Motion
Neck	Flexion, 45° Extension, 45° Rotation, 60° Laterat bend, 45°
Shoulder	Flexion, 150° Hyperextension, 30° Abduction (hand supine), 160° Abduction (hand prone), 110°
Elbow	Flexion, 160°
Wrist	Palmar flexion, 80° Dorsal flexion, 70° Ulnar flexion, 60° Radial flexion, 10° Rotation (internal and external), 90°
Thumb	Proximal phalange flexion, 70° Distal phalange flexion, 90°
Finger	Proximal phalange flexion, 90° Proximal phalange hyperextension 30° Middle phalange flexion, 120° Distal phalange flexion, 80°
Hip	Extension (lying prone), 5° Extension (standing), 30° Flexion (knee bent), 120° Flexion (knee straight), 90° Abduction, 35° Adduction, 30°
Knee	Flexion, 100° Hyperextension, 5°
Ankle	Dorsiflexion, 10° Plantar flexion, 40° Eversion, 25° Inversion, 35°
Great toe	Proximal phalange flexion, 35° Proximal phalange hyperextension, 75° Distal phalange flexion, 50°
Other toes	Proximal phalange flexion, 30° Proximal phalange hyperextension, 75° Middle phalange flexion, 80° Distal phalange flexion, 45°

hair is matted or well groomed may give clues to other problems, such as the inability to comb hair due to an immobile joint or a negative self-concept. Nails should be examined for breakage, discoloration, curving, and the presence of a fungal infection.

Assessment of mobility should consider not only individuals' ability to ambulate, but also the characteristics of their gait, the type of assistance required for ambulation, the length of time a person is able to ambulate without discomfort and fatigue, the ability to rise from a chair and toilet, and the ability to climb stairs. The capacity and limitation in regard to each factor should be described. The function of all limbs should be evaluated, with attention to the location and degree of any contracture, arthritis, paralysis, painful movement, and spasm. The nurse should attempt to identify the measures the older person employs to assist with or relieve any limitations in extremity function. It is also helpful to note which is the dominant hand of the individual. Table 6-1 shows the degrees of joint motion that are normal in aged individuals.

In regard to respiratory function, the older person should be questioned as to a history of orthopnea, dyspnea, shortness of breath, wheezing, asthma, coughing, and any other respiratory disturbance. The frequency of occurrence, precipitating factors, and the extent to which they limit the individual should be ascertained, as well as the measures used to assist with or relieve the problem. The present and past smoking history of the individual should be reviewed. A sputum specimen should be obtained and its characteristics noted. Circulatory function should be reviewed, and a history recorded of chest pain, tachycardia, edema, extremity cramps, palpitations, or any other symptom of poor cardiac function. The extent to which any problem limits the individual should be explored, as well as measures used to assist with or relieve the problem. The extremities should be examined for color, temperature, and equality of pulse. The presence of a pacemaker should be noted.

The nutritional status of the older person should be assessed by reviewing the quality and quantity of food and fluid intake. Food preferences, restrictions, and intolerances should be indicated, in addition to the usual meal pattern for the individual. Factors which cause and relieve indigestion, constipation, and diarrhea should be explored. Since poor dental status can restrict food intake and threaten nutritional status, part of the nutritional assessment should include an examination of teeth and/or dentures. Any adjustments that must be made for eating, such as nasogastric feedings or pureeing foods, should be made known.

Bladder function should be assessed with attention to the presence of nocturia, frequency, burning, urgency, incontinence, stress incontinence, and retention. The voiding pattern should be reviewed in regard to frequency and amount. The length of time any indwelling catheter or ostomy has been present should be recorded, and the technique of care should be described.

The frequency and characteristics of bowel movements should be ascertained, with consideration to any recent change in either. The frequency of occurrence and management of diarrhea and constipation should be explored. The presence of hemorrhoids, fecal incontinence, or an ostomy should be described in terms of length of time present and management.

Assessment of the older person's sensory status is vital and extremely beneficial to care delivery. The ability of the individual to hear regular sounds should be evaluated first. Can he or she hear a telephone ring or a door close? Does he or she understand all conversation? The ability to hear high-frequency sounds should then be evaluated; these sounds, which are most problematic for the aged, include the consonant sounds *f,z,s* and *sh.* To make sure lipreading isn't taking place, questions should be asked from the side of the person or from behind. The use of a hearing aid should be noted. Ears should be examined for cerumen impactions, not uncommon in the aged.

Visual capacities and limitations should be carefully reviewed, and the type, age, and source of corrective lenses should be noted as well as an assessment of night vision, peripheral vision, color discrimination, depth perception, and reading ability. The status of other senses is also important. Taste sensation can be evaluated by testing the individual's ability to differentiate among sweet, sour, salty, and bitter substances. Likewise, a variety of substances can be used in determining the individual's ability to detect different odors and temperatures. With the individual's eyes closed, the nurse can determine if the person can sense differences between hot and cold temperatures, sharp and dull sensations. Assessment of speech includes whether a speech is laryngeal or esophageal, or if aphasia exists. The location, degree, and type of any pain should be described with explanations of effective relief measures.

It is helpful to know rest and sleep patterns and the factors that interfere with or promote each. A thorough review of medications and other measures used to induce sleep may reveal other problems of which the nurse should be aware, such as alcohol or drug abuse or misuse. It should be remembered that more rest and less sleep is required by older people.

In assessing the reproductive systems of a woman, the date of her last gynecological examination should be obtained and she should be examined for the presence of any vaginal discharge, itching, lesions, breast masses, nipple discharge, and breast pain. (Older females have a more alkaline vaginal environment, predisposing them to more vaginal infections.) History of a mastectomy should be indicated, including the

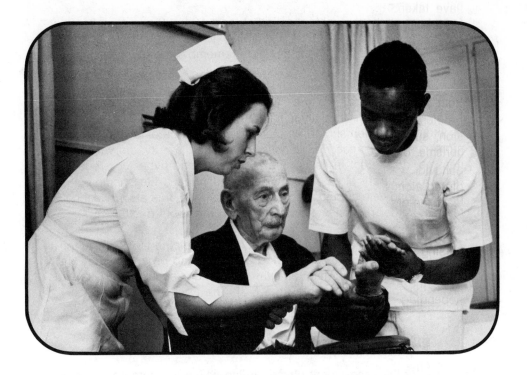

use of a prosthesis. Men should be evaluated for scrotal swelling, lesions, discharge, and impotency. A sexual history is useful to include. Attempts should be made to determine sexual interest, frequency of sexual activity, factors limiting sexual expression (psychosocial as well as physiological), attitude, and presence of dyspareunia.

13. Mental status. Mental status can be evaluated throughout the assessment process by observing how alert the individual is, how well and how rapidly he or she responds to stimuli, and how lucidly he or she behaves. Orientation to person, place, and time can be determined indirectly throughout the interview or by questions such as Where do you live? What is the day and date? Why did you visit the hospital today? Who is your primary nurse? and Who is now president of the United States? Memory should also be assessed. *Old memory,* recall of events that have taken place in the past, can be assessed by asking questions such as What year did World War II end? This type of memory is usually good in the aged. *Short-term memory,* recall of events occurring up to 10 minutes after the information is introduced, can be assessed by techniques such as introducing yourself or giving a simple direction and immediately asking the individual to repeat what you said. The aged have more of a problem than the young have with this type of memory.

95

Long-term memory, events recalled at least 10 to 20 minutes after they have taken place, would be the ability to describe the medication schedule taught the previous day or to remember the day one visited a friend last week. This type of memory declines with age as well.

14. Emotional status. Nursing observations and information from older persons and their family may indicate specific emotional problems. Attention should be paid to the presence of anxiety, depression, suspiciousness, fearfulness, emotional lability, nervous mannerisms, disinterest in self or life in general, and hyper or hypoactive behavior. Current stress factors in the individual's life should be explored along with coping mechanisms employed. It is also revealing to learn the older person's attitude and concerns about death.

Compilation of data. If the information obtained is compiled on a nursing history form, it will provide guidance and organization in data collection and ease in data retrieval. A sample of such a form is provided in the following pages (Table 6-2). The type of format will vary, depending on the type of information and the use to which it is put.

PLANNING

After the assessment phase, during which the nurse collects and analyzes quantitative and qualitative data pertaining to the individual, plans can be made for using nursing measures to alleviate the specific problems and needs that have become apparent. Since aged individuals may be experiencing a variety of physiological, psychological, and socioeconomic losses, some of their problems may require more immediate attention or be of greater concern than others. It is therefore necessary to establish *priorities* when planning for care, and if possible, to enlist the active participation of the individual for whom care is being planned. This approach respects the right of the individual to make decisions affecting his or her life. It also avoids conflicts that can arise from the differing opinions of individuals and nurses regarding priorities and avoids wasting human and material resources. The following case illustrates

A visiting nurse was concerned about the housing situation of the 72-year-old woman she was caring for. The house this woman lived in was too large for the woman to clean adequately and consequently was unclean and cluttered. Leaking faucets, peeling wallpaper, and roaches added to the nurse's impression that it was necessary to seek new housing for the woman.

The nurse worked diligently with the local housing authorities and social services department to locate an affordable apartment in a

TABLE 6-2: NURSING HISTORY FOR OLDER ADULTS

1. PROFILE OF PATIENT
Name _____ Sex _____ Race _____ Religion _____ Date of birth _____
Address _____ Telephone _____
Language spoken _____ Nearest contact person _____

2. PROFILE OF FAMILY

Spouse
_____ Living
    Health status:
    Age:
    Occupation:
_____ Deceased
    Year deceased:
    Cause of death:
Others in household:

Children
_____ Living
    Names and addresses:
_____ Deceased
    Year deceased:
    Cause of death:

3. OCCUPATIONAL PROFILE

_____ Employed
    Type of Work:
    Length of employment
    Working hours:
    Sources of income:

_____ Unemployed
    Reason:
    Length of unemployment:
    Feelings about unemployment:
    Previous occupations:

4. HOME PROFILE

_____ Single dwelling
_____ Multiple dwelling
_____ Own
_____ Rent
_____ Telephone
_____ Pets

Number of levels:
Location of bathroom:
Location of bedroom
Nearest neighbor:
Household responsibilities

5. ECONOMIC PROFILE
Sources of income:
Monthly income:
Monthly expenses:
Financial concerns:

6. HEALTH INSURANCE
_____ Medicaid
_____ Medicare
_____ Blue Cross/Blue Shield
_____ Other:
Policy number:

7. HEALTH AND SOCIAL RESOURCES CURRENTLY UTILIZED
_____ Private M.D.   _____ H.M.O.   _____ Social worker
_____ Hospital   _____ Visiting Nurse   _____ Meals on wheels
_____ Clinic   _____ Public health nurse Other:

8. SOCIAL/LEISURE ACTIVITIES
Organization Membership:
Hobbies/Interests:

9. HEALTH HISTORY
_____ Allergies   _____ Hospitalizations:
    Food: _____ Surgery:
    Drug: _____ Fractures:
    Other: _____ Major health problems:
_____ Diabetes
_____ Hypertension
_____ Cancer

97

TABLE 6-2: NURSING HISTORY FOR OLDER ADULTS (Cont'd)

10. CURRENT HEALTH STATUS
Knowledge and Understanding of Health Problems:

Limitations of function or   Management of Limitations:
performance of ADL:

Health goals:

11. MEDICATIONS

Name	Dosage	How and When Taken	How Obtained	Knowledge and Understanding of Medication

12. PHYSICAL STATUS

T ____ (A,O,R)   Height ____   Urine:
P ____   Weight ____ (recent changes:)   S/A: ____
R ____   BP _____ (sitting, standing, lying)   Specific gravity:
                                                          How obtained:
                                                          Characteristics:

Skin condition
____ Intact   ____ Rash (describe)   ____ Wounds (describe)
____ Dry   ____ Discoloration (describe)

Hair condition: | Nail condition:

Mobility
____ Ambulatory   ____ Able to rise from chair or toilet
____ Nonambulatory   ____ Able to climb stairs
____ Ambulatory with assistance: (specify)

TABLE 6-2: NURSING HISTORY FOR OLDER ADULTS (Cont'd)

Extremity function

	Location	Degree of Limitation	Assistive/Relief Measures
Contracture			
Arthritis			
Painful movement			
Paralysis			
Spasm			
Amputation			
Dominant hand			

Respiration

	Precipitating Factors	Degree of Limitation	Assistive/Relief Measures
Orthopnea			
Dyspnea			
Shortness of breath			
Wheezing			
Asthma			
Coughing			

Sputum characteristics:
Smoking history: _____ Tracheostomy

Circulation

	Precipitating Factors	Degree of Limitation	Assistive/Relief Measures
Chest Pain			
Tachycardia			
Edema			
Cramping in extremities			

Equality of pulse, temperature, and color in extremities:

TABLE 6-2: NURSING HISTORY FOR OLDER ADULTS (Cont'd)

Nutrition

Teeth:	Dentures:	Chewing problems:
Number:	____ Partial—Complete	Swallowing problems:
Status:	Fit:	Feeding tube:
Date last dental exam:		

	Precipitating Factors	Assistive/Relief Measures
Indigestion		
Constiptation		
Diarrhea		

Usual meal pattern:	Fluid intake:
	Alcohol use:
Food preferences:	Food restrictions:

Bladder

____ Nocturia	____ Burning	____ Incontinence	____ Catheter
____ Frequency	____ Urgency	____ Stress incontinence	____ Ostomy

Voiding pattern:
Urine characteristics:

Bowel

____ Hemorrhoids	____ Pain during movement	____ Chronic constipation	____ Incontinence
____ Straining	____ Recent change in pattern	____ Chronic diarrhea	____ Ostomy

Stool

Bowel movement pattern:
Characteristics:

	Frequency of Use and Results Obtained	
Laxatives		
Suppositories		
Enemas		

Sensory status		
	Degree of Limitation	Assistive/Relief Measures

TABLE 6-2: NURSING HISTORY FOR OLDER ADULTS (Cont'd)

Hearing
    All sounds
    High frequency

Vision
    Full vision
    Night vision
    Peripheral vision
    Reading
    Color discrimination
    Depth perception

Taste

Smell

Touch
    Feels pressure and pain
    Differentiates temperature
    Speech
    Pain

| _____ Hearing aid | _____ Eyeglasses | Date last vision exam: |
| Other sensory data: | _____ Contact lenses | Date last hearing exam: |

Rest and sleep
    _____ Insomnia (describe)   Medicines and alcohol used to induce sleep:
    _____ Night restlessness   Factors interfering with rest:
    _____ Night confusion   Usual sleep and rest pattern:

Female reproductive factors:		Male reproductive factors
_____ Vaginal discharge	_____ Nipple discharge	_____ Scrotal swelling
_____ Itching	_____ Breast pain	_____ Lesions
_____ Lesions	_____ Mastectomy	_____ Discharge
_____ Breast mass	(indicate right or left)	_____Impotency
_____	_____ Prosthesis	
Date last exam:		

Sexual profile

| _____ Interest | _____ Dyspareunia | Attitude: |
| _____ Sexually active | _____ Limitations: | Frequency: |

13. **MENTAL STATUS**

    _____ Alert   Orientation
    _____ Rapid response to verbal stimuli   _____ Person
    _____ Slow response to verbal stimuli   _____ Place
    _____ Confused   _____ Time
    _____ Stuporous   Attention span:
    _____ Comatose
Memory of recent events: Memory of past events:

TABLE 6-2: NURSING HISTORY FOR OLDER ADULTS (Cont'd)

14. EMOTIONAL STATUS

___ Anxious	___ Hyperactive	___ Disinterest in life
___ Fearful	___ Hypoactive	___ Emotionally labile
___ Depressed	___ Suspicious	___ Suicidal

Self concept: | Current stress factors:

Attitude and concerns about death:

Other data:

Informant

___ Patient
___ Other (specify)

Signature of Nurse   Date

modern facility. She felt positive about her efforts to arrange for a housing improvement that would maintain the independence of the elderly woman in a community setting.

With excitement, the nurse shared her accomplishment with the old woman, anticipating that the woman would express delight at the improvement the new housing would bring to her life. Needless to say, the nurse was shocked to hear the woman refuse the new apartment. Didn't this woman understand? Was she confused? How could she deny an opportunity to leave her shabby house and move to a modern apartment?

If the participation of the elderly woman had been elicited initially in establishing plans for her housing problem, the nurse may have saved herself and others much time and energy and delivered more efficient and effective care. To this 72-year-old, maintaining the same house in which she had spent most of her lifetime was of utmost importance. The familiar furnishings, the memories, the yard in which her dog could romp, her friendly neighbor of long standing were all part of that old house. Of course, she didn't like the dirt and roaches either; but even though her limited efforts couldn't control the situation, maintaining her own home was worth the price. If the nurse had explored these factors with the elderly lady, and if they had jointly established priorities, perhaps the nurse's efforts could have focused on arranging a homemaker's service or exploring church groups or other local resources to obtain a handyman to make the necessary repairs at a nominal cost.

When developing plans, nurses should also enlist the cooperation of other professionals who will be involved in the care of the individual, such as the physician, social worker, physical therapist, nutritionist and paraprofessionals. Since older persons often have several interwoven problems, a multidisciplinary approach is essential. It is confusing to the older individual if each discipline exerts efforts toward different and sometimes conflicting goals. This reduces the therapeutic value of the care and is an ineffective and inefficient use of the time, energy, and human and financial resources of the various disciplines. Multidisciplinary interdependence, cooperation and respect are requirements for intelligent care of the aged.

The nurse should not only focus the care on management of existing problems, but also on the prevention of problems. Consideration is given to each of the universal self-care demands with this preventive planning, utilizing the data obtained from the nursing history. For example, from the assessment the nurse may have learned that the individual has occasional periods of depression which can lead to eating problems. Although there may be no current nutritional problem, planning can include arranging for the person to attend a senior citizen lunch program to provide an opportunity for socialization and enjoyment, in order to prevent poor eating habits from developing. Likewise, an older person's skin may be in fine intact condition when he or she is admitted to a hospital and placed on complete bedrest. To maintain this skin condition, the nurse would plan to turn the individual frequently, offering massages and using a bath oil when bathing the person.

In some agencies, plans are translated into nursing orders, which give specific direction to nursing actions by specifying exactly what is to be done, by whom, when, how, and where. Nursing orders provide for consistency and continuity in care through the selective identification and explicit description of particular nursing actions required for a given individual. In some agencies, nursing orders are sanctioned the way physician's orders have traditionally been sanctioned. Examples of nursing orders are:

Ambulate the patient from bedroom to dayroom q4h during daytime, with a staff member providing support on each side.

Reduce fluid intake to 300 ml between 6 P.M. and 6 A.M.

Instruct patient's daughter on wound-dressing technique and have her change dressings with nurse's assistance when she visits on Wednesdays.

Provide warm basin of water at bedside qAM in which patient can soak hands.

Wheel patient to room of Patient X at mealtime for a two-hour visit.

Arrange for staff member to assist patient's wife in taking patient outside in wheelchair this Sunday for two to three hours.

103

Call Social Service Department to arrange round-trip transportation and an escort for patient's clinic visit Friday at 10 A.M.

Obviously, the above nursing orders provide a greater understanding of what actions are required for the individual than vague directions, such as instruct family in care, encourage activity, provide socialization, prevent unnecessary incontinence.

Any staff member reading the nursing order knows exactly what the care planner had intended and also has a means of evaluating the effectiveness of the action. For example, if the nursing care plan stated "reduce fluid intake at bedtime," one care giver could interpret this as meaning only 100 ml after 9 PM, another could interpret it as 500 ml after dinner, while to another it could mean no fluids after midnight. It would be difficult to evaluate the effectiveness of reducing fluid intake at bedtime to prevent nocturnal incontinence as there is no daily consistency or continuity of approaches. On the other hand, from the nursing order to "reduce fluid intake to 300 ml between 6 PM and 6 AM," the nurse can judge the effectiveness of the particular plan and identify exactly any change needed to result in the desired outcome.

Whether nursing orders or a nursing care plan form is used in a given agency, it is important to have plans in a written form and in a manner that is clearly understood and provides specific directions to anyone caring for the individual.

IMPLEMENTATION

Implementation involves action; it is the phase in which care planning is made operational. Whereas the assessment and planning phases of the nursing process require the use of more intellectual and interpersonal skills than technical ones, the implementation phase necessitates a proficient blend of all these skills. During the discussion of the focus of gerontological and geriatric nursing in the previous chapter, it was indicated that nursing actions are taken to (1) strengthen the individual's self-care capacities; (2) eliminate or minimize self-care limitations; and (3) provide direct care services by acting for, doing for, or partially assisting the individual when universal self-care or therapeutic demands cannot be independently fulfilled. When nurses are not directly responsible for all these actions, they can encourage and supervise any other individuals who perform them. The family or a neighbor or other personnel may be performing certain actions on behalf of the individual, and the nurse can provide guidance and coordinate actions. In such situations it is essential for the nurse to communicate to those responsible, providing significant data and relating the care plan with thoroughness.

Part of the nurse's responsibility will be to recognize when changes in the individual's capacities and limitations require a different provider of care for a given activity. Perhaps the patient has recovered from an illness and has restored energy and no longer requires an aide to assist with bathing; in this situation, the patient is the new care provider. On the other hand, if an aged individual becomes more limited in the ability for self-injection of insulin due to arthritic fingers, a visiting nurse may have to administer the insulin as the new care provider for this requirement. The nurse must be aware not only of the changing requirements for actions, but also of the changing requirements for persons to perform the actions.

EVALUATION

The fourth step in the nursing process is that of evaluation, whereby the degree to which plans and actions were effective in achieving desired outcomes is judged. If plans and actions continue to be effective and result in the desired outcomes, no change is necessitated. Some actions may have proven ineffective in achieving desired results, and specific alterations may be required in the care plan. Oversights or omissions may be detected, and additions may have to be made to the care plan. Thus, the evaluation process can result in no change, an alteration of the original plan, or an addition of new plans.

The individual for whom care is being provided, his family, and other care providers should be included in the evaluation process. It may be learned that although the action is bringing about the desired outcome, the action itself is not satisfactory to the individual or his care providers; perhaps a different action achieving the same result is necessary. For example, let us say the goal was to provide increased opportunities for socialization to an elderly widow living alone, and the actions planned included daily attendance at a senior citizen center. If the women has attended daily and developed friendships, the nurse can evaluate this action as effective in reaching the desired outcome. However, if the widow feels that visitng the center daily fatigues her to the extent that she is unable to perform her household responsibilities and is too expensive in terms of transportation costs, different plans to achieve a similar goal may be warranted. The nurse can alter the plan to provide a different means of transportation, to arrange for visits to the center on alternate days and for visitors to her home in between, and to obtain assistance for household chores. The nurse must not assume that a desired outcome has been necessarily achieved in the most preferable and beneficial manner to the individual.

Through evaluation, it is learned whether accurate, effective, and efficient planning and actions have taken place. Nursing audits are becoming an increasingly common means to evaluate nursing care. Several audit tools, such as the Slater Nursing Competencies Rating Scale and Phaneuf Audit are available to assist in this process. Increased research in the area of effective geriatric nursing practice is necessary to develop specific standards by which the application of the nursing process to aged individuals can be evaluated. Time, energy, and money can be saved by the aged person and the provider when useless plans and actions are recognized and replaced by those which will achieve the desired results.

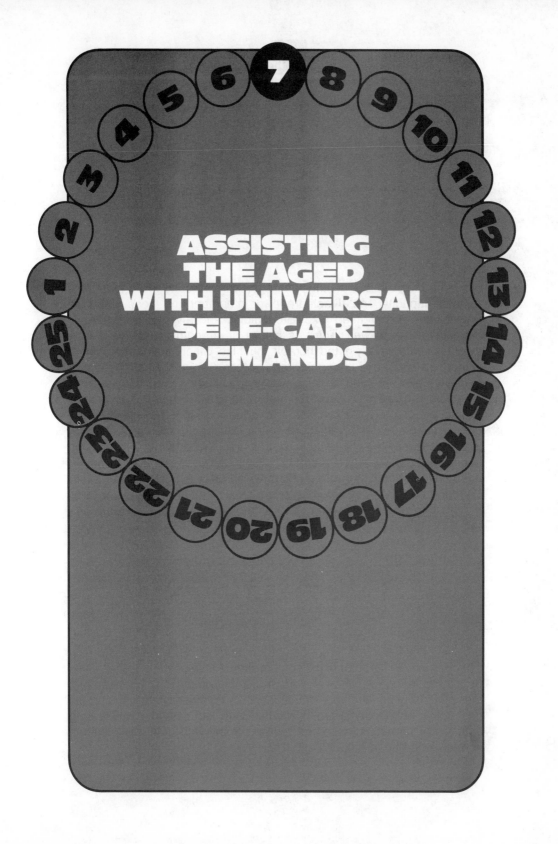

ASSISTING THE AGED WITH UNIVERSAL SELF-CARE DEMANDS

The nurse providing quality care for the older individual thinks and acts in a manner which demonstrates knowledge of (1) the unique psychobiosocial characteristics of aging; (2) the principles guiding gerontological and geriatric nursing practice; (3) the nursing process; and (4) expert clinical skills.

In this chapter, these areas of knowledge are combined to provide guidance in caring for aged persons. Each universal self-care demand is reviewed. The norms for fulfilling each demand and the limitations and potential capacities of aged individuals to do so are discussed. Measures which can assist the aged individual or the person providing care are presented.

AIR

The lungs lose elasticity with age, which results in an increased residual capacity. The alveoli are fewer in number and those which are present are of increased size. Bronchioles and alveolar ducts are of increased size as well. There is a loss of strength in the respiratory muscles and a rigidity of the thoracic muscles. Ciliary action is lessened with age also. These changes produce less respiratory activity, which gives an older person greater risk of developing upper respiratory infections. To prevent upper respiratory infections, respiratory activity should be promoted. Exercises, individually planned in view of the unique capacities and limitations of the individual, should be encouraged; these may benefit the total well-being of the individual, in addition to his respiratory function. Deep breathing exercises should be encouraged several times throughout the day with emphasis to forced expiration (Figure 7-1). The older person should attempt to cough and expectorate sputum following deep breathing exercises. Providing balloons or an inflatable toy to blow will assist in these exercises.

The aged should be advised to seek medical attention promptly, should any sign of a respiratory infection develop. Frequently, older people do not experience the chest pain associated with pneumonia to the same degree as younger adults, and they can be afebrile while possessing an infection. Thus, by the time symptoms become obvious, pneumonia can be in an advanced stage. The susceptibility of older people to drafts necessitates that indirect ventilation be utilized. Fibrositis, common in the aged, can be aggravated by chilling and drafts. Changes in the character of the sputum should also be reported, as it will be altered in the presence of certain disease processes. For example, the sputum will be tenacious, translucent, and grayish white with chronic obstructive pulmonary disease; purulent and foul smelling with a lung abscess or bronchiectasis; and red and frothy with pulmonary edema and left-sided heart failure.

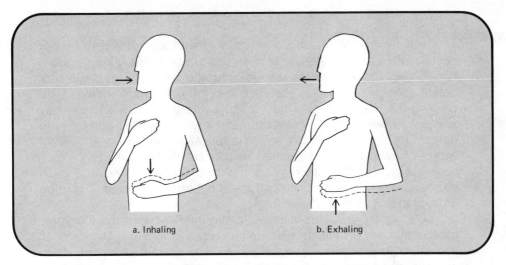

a. Inhaling   b. Exhaling

Figure 7-1. Breathing exercises for the aged should emphasize forced expiration: (a) With one hand below the ribs on the stomach and the other over the middle anterior chest, the individual should inhale to the count of one. The hand over the stomach should fall as the stomach moves downward; the hand over the chest should not move. (b) Exhale to the count of three. The hand over the stomach should rise as the stomach moves upward; the hand over the chest should not move.

The aged should be cautioned against periods of inactivity and bed rest due to the higher risk of upper respiratory infections. Some aged persons have been raised with the belief that when one is sick, one should go to bed. Family members with good intentions may encourage bed rest and inactivity for the aged person who is sick. Education by the nurse is required to teach the public the multitude of problems associated with immobility.

Approximately 80 percent of the aged have some degree of chronic obstructive pulmonary disease; thus, a higher amount of carbon dioxide retention can occur. The nurse should teach deep breathing exercises with forced expiration and encourage the person to do these exercises regularly. Carbon dioxide retention can cause adverse reactions to oxygen therapy, and the nurse should understand this and keenly observe for symptoms of carbon dioxide narcosis. These include confusion, muscle twitching, visual defects, profuse perspiration, hypotension, progressive degrees of circulatory failure, and cerebral depression, which may be displayed by increased sleeping to a deep comatose state. The nurse should be sure that oxygen is used prudently with the aged, that symptoms of carbon dioxide narcosis are recognized

109

early, and that blood gases are frequently evaluated when oxygen therapy is indicated.

Hair in the nostrils becomes thicker with age and may readily accumulate a greater amount of dust and dirt particles during inspiration. Unless these particles are removed and the nasal passage kept patent, there may be an interference with the normal inspiration of air. Blowing the nose and mild manipulation with the use of a tissue may adequately rid the nostrils of these particles. When these particles are difficult to remove, a cotton tipped applicator, moistened with warm water or normal saline solution may help loosen them. Caution should be taken not to insert the cotton tipped applicator too far into the nose since trauma can result. Any nasal obstruction not easily removed should be brought to a physician's attention.

Circulatory problems in the aged may interfere with the full oxygenation of all body tissues. It is known that less efficient oxygen utilization is a factor in prolonged tachycardia in many aged persons. Efforts to promote good circulation should be encouraged. Activity, range of motion exercises, frequent change of position, warmth, skin massage, gentle friction during bathing, and the avoidance of circulation interferences (such as garters or tight fitting shoes), will assist in improving circulation. Hypotension should be prevented, as this reduces cerebral circulation and subsequently decreases the amount of oxygenation to that tissue; this is an important consideration for the older person on antihypertensive therapy. Aged persons and those who care for them should be aware that blood pressure normally rises with age, and what may be a hypertensive level for a 40-year-old may fall within a normal boundary for the older adult.

FOOD AND WATER

Painless, intact gums and teeth will promote the ingestion of a wider variety of food. The ability to meet nutritional requirements in old age is influenced by basic dental care throughout one's lifetime. Poor dental care, environmental influences, poor nutrition, and changes in the gingival tissue commonly contribute to severe tooth loss in older persons. After the third decade of life, periodontal disease becomes the first cause of tooth loss, and by age seventy, a majority of people have lost all their teeth. Obviously, a lifetime of poor dental care cannot be reversed. Geriatric dental problems should be prevented early in the individual's life. Geriatric dentistry is a young specialty, but unfortunately those who have access to this service do not always have the financial means to avail themselves of it.

Through education, the nurse should make the public aware of the importance of good, regular dental care and oral hygiene at all ages and that aging alone doesn't necessitate the loss of teeth. The use of a tooth-brush is more effective in improving gingival tissues and removing soft debris from the teeth than are swabs or other soft devices. However, care should be taken not to traumatize the tissues, as they are more sensitive in the aged and easily prone to irritation. Dental problems should be readily corrected as they can affect virtually every system of the body. Loose teeth should be extracted as they can possibly be aspirated and cause a lung abscess.

Many aged persons believe that having dentures eliminates the necessity for dental care. The nurse should correct this misconception and encourage continued dental care for the individual with dentures. Lesions, infections and other diseases can be detected by the dentist and can lead to the prevention of serious complications. Also, changes in tissue structure may have affected the fit of the dentures and necessitate a readjustment. Poor fitting dentures need not always be replaced; sometimes they can be lined to ensure a proper fit. This should be made known to the older person who may resist correction out of concern for the expense involved. Most importantly, dentures should be used and not kept in a pocket or dresser drawer! Wearing dentures will allow proper chewing and may encourage including a wider variety of foods in the diet.

A poor appetite resulting from decreased taste sensation can also have adverse effects on the aged's nutritional status. Taste receptors are lost with age due to atrophy of the taste buds, chronic irritation, or general wearing out. The receptors on the tip of the tongue lose the most sensation, and these include the taste receptors for sweet and salt. The taste buds for bitter and sour tastes remain which make old people think most foods taste bitter. Those involved with the aged should recognize this factor and understand the reason why an older person may add seemingly excessive amounts of salt and sugar to their food. These taste deficiencies compound the difficulties in adjusting to a limited sodium or sugar diet, which is so frequently prescribed for the aged. The use of salt and sugar substitutes and other flavoring, such as lemon, should be considered to compensate for this taste limitation. Special efforts should be made to serve food attractively, and the use of wine to stimulate the appetite may prove beneficial.

Indigestion and food intolerance are common in the aged due to decreased stomach motility, less gastric secretion, and a slower emptying time. The older person frequently attempts to manage these problems by using antacids or limiting food intake—both potentially predisposing the person to other risks. Other means to manage these problems should first be explored. Several smaller meals may help reduce indigestion and promote a regular blood glucose level through-out the day, from which various benefits may also be realized. Fried

111

foods may be replaced by broiled, boiled, or baked ones. If an intolerance to a particular food exists, substitution with a tolerable food of equal nutritional value should be made. Sitting in a high Fowler's position will increase the size of the abdominal and thoracic cavities, provide more room for the stomach, and facilitate swallowing and digestion. Adequate fluid intake and activity will also promote digestion.

Constipation is a common problem among the aged due to slower peristalsis, inactivity, and less bulk and fluid in the diet. If food intake is reduced to relieve discomfort, this can threaten nutritional status. Laxatives, another relief measure, can result in diarrhea, which is also threatening to the aged's nutritional status. Constipation should be recognized as a frequent problem of the aged and preventive measures should be emphasized. Plenty of fluids, fruits, vegetables, and activity should be encouraged, as should providing regular and adequate time allowances for a bowel movement. Laxatives should be considered after other measures have proven ineffective, and then should be used with discretion. Mineral oil should not be used by the aged, as the fat soluble vitamins A, D, and E can dissolve in and be excreted with this substance, producing deficiencies of these vitamins.

Since malnourishment is a potential threat to the aged, it should be carefully observed for. The variety of factors contributing to this problem include decreased taste and smell sensations for food; reduced mastication capability; slower peristalsis; decreased hunger contractions; reduced gastric acid secretion, causing poor absorption of nutrients and minerals; and less absorption of nutrients due to reduced intestinal blood flow and fewer cells on the absorbing surface of the intestines. Socioeconomic factors are commonly responsible for malnourishment in the aged as well. The appearance of the aged may be misleading and cause a malnourished state to be undetected. An aged person who appears obese due to the presence of increased amounts of adipose tissue can actually be malnourished.

Malnourishment in the aged may be first demonstrated through symptoms of mental confusion, easily judged as senility and mistakenly treated as a separate problem. The nurse should carefully explore the quality as well as the quantity of food intake and engage in diet instruction as needed. The ability of the person to market and to purchase and prepare foods should be examined to assess the need for food stamps, delivered meals, or the service of a home health aide. Participation in a senior citizen lunch program or the arrangement of a mealtime visitor can eliminate poor eating habits resulting from social isolation. A review of the individual's budget may reflect the need for financial assistance to provide adequate money for food expenses.

The diet of the aged should reflect a *lower quantity* and *higher quality* of food (Figure 7-2). Less carbohydrates and fats are required in

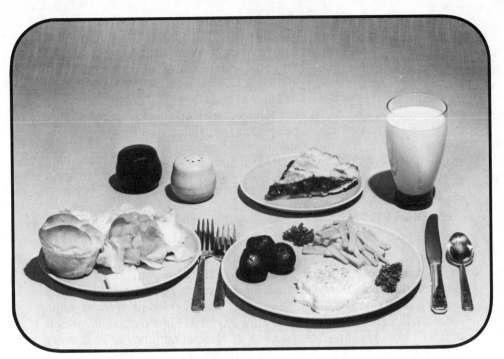

Figure 7-2. The diet of the aged should reflect a lower quantity and higher quality of food. (U.S. Dept. of Agriculture)

the diets of older adults. The decreased ability of the older person to maintain a regular blood glucose level emphasizes the need for a reduced carbohydrate intake. Sometimes, a high carbohydrate diet stimulates an abnormally high release of insulin which in turn causes hypoglycemia. (Here again, mental confusion may be the symptom presented.) At least a gram of protein per kilogram of body weight is necessary for the renewal of body protein and protoplasm, and for the maintenance of enzyme systems. Several protein supplements are available commercially and may be useful additives to the elderly's diet. Although the ability to absorb calcium decreases with age, calcium is still required in the diet to maintain a healthy musculoskeletal system as well as to promote the proper functioning of the body's blood clotting mechanisms. Unless other problems dictate differently, older women should have approximately 1600 calories, and older men, 2200 calories in a well-balanced daily diet.

The fluid consumption of older adults should range between 2500 and 3000 ml daily. The aged's daily fluid intake should be carefully evaluated to ascertain if this requirement is being met. Lack of motivation, avoidance of nocturia and frequency of urination, fear of incontinence, and inability to independently obtain or drink fluids are among the factors which could restrict fluid consumption. This fluid restriction

113

can not only predispose the older person to infection, constipation, and decreased bladder distensibility, but can lead to a serious fluid and electrolyte imbalance. Dehydration, a serious threat to the older person due to the already reduced amount of body water, is demonstrated by dry, inelastic skin, dry brown tongue, sunken cheeks, concentrated urine, elevated blood urea (above 60 mg per 100 ml), and in some cases, mental confusion. The aged are also affected more by overhydration due to decreased cardiovascular and renal function—a consideration if there is ever a therapeutic need for intravenous fluids.

EXCRETION

Changes in the urinary tract with age may give rise to a variety of elimination problems. One of the great annoyances results from a decreased bladder capacity. Some aged bladders may only have the capacity to hold 200 ml or less, and frequency is common in older persons as a consequence. This factor should be kept in mind when individuals, unable to independently ambulate, are placed in wheel-chairs. If possible, they should be offered an opportunity to void every two hours to prevent incontinence. Trips and activities should also be planned to allow for bathroom breaks at frequent intervals. Not only do older people find more frequent voiding necessary throughout the day, but night frequency may pose a bothersome problem as well. Often, kidney circulation may be decreased when the aged individual is in an upright position. When the recumbent position is assumed, circulation improves, promoting kidney function. Thus, voiding may be required a few hours after the individual lies down, promoting nocturia.

With the increased light-perception threshold making night vision difficult, nocturia could predispose the aged individual to accidents and threaten safety. Night-lights should be present to improve visibility during trips to the bathroom, and any clutter or environmental hazards which could promote a fall should be removed. Reduced fluids several hours prior to bedtime may lessen episodes of nocturia; if several episodes of nocturia continue to occur nightly, the person may need medical evaluation to ensure that no urinary tract problem exists. The aged and those caring for them should be aware that the longer-acting diuretics, such as the thiazides, even when administered in the morning, can cause nocturia.

Bladder muscles weaken with age which may promote retention of large volumes of urine. Women may experience retention from a fecal impaction, and men from prostatic hypertrophy, which is present to some degree in most older males. Symptoms of retention include urinary frequency, straining, dribbling, a palpable bladder, and a feeling by the individual that the bladder has not been emptied. This retention may

114

predispose the older person to the risk of developing a urinary tract infection. Good fluid intake and efforts to enhance voiding should be emphasized. Attempts to tighten the muscles through contraction exercises, and mild massage over the bladder area may assist in preventing urinary retention. Sphincter control may be improved by exercises such as tightening the perineum muscles and stopping the urine flow midstream when voiding.

The efficiency of the kidneys in filtration functions decreases with age, an important factor in the elimination of drugs. The nurse should look for signs of adverse drug reactions resulting from an accumulation of toxic levels of the medication. Higher blood urea nitrogen levels may result from reduced renal function, causing lethargy, mental confusion, headache, drowsiness, and several other symptoms. Decreased tubular function may cause problems in the concentration of urine; the maximum specific gravity at 80 years of age has been shown to be 1.024 while the maximum for younger ages is 1.032. Decreased reabsorption from the filtrate makes a proteinuria of 1.0 usually of no diagnostic significance. The renal threshold for glucose is increased, a serious concern since an older person may then be hyperglycemic without evidence of glycosuria. False negatives in diabetic urine testing can occur for this reason. Urine screening for the presence of a urinary tract infection may also produce false negatives, as it may exist without evidence of proteinuria.

Bowel function is often a major concern of the aged, many of whom were raised with the belief that anything but a daily bowel movement is abnormal. Slower peristalsis, inactivity, reduced food and fluid intake, and the ingestion of less bulk foods are frequently responsible for constipation in the aged. Decreased sensory perception may cause the signal for bowel elimination to go unnoticed and promote constipation.

Laxative abuse as a reaction to constipation is common in the aged, and the habitual use of laxatives should be discouraged. Magnesia based preparations can reduce the already reduced amount of gastric acids, and the problem of vitamin depletion from the use of mineral oil has already been mentioned. There is the serious risk that the use of laxatives and enemas can predispose the older person to dehydration. Education is necessary to help the aged, and those providing care for them, understand that daily bowel elimination is not necessary.

A good fluid intake, a diet rich in fruits and vegetables, activity, and the establishment of a regular time for bowel elimination can be beneficial in maintaining a regular elimination pattern. As there is a tendency in the aged for incomplete emptying of the bowel at one time, time should be provided for full emptying, and for repeated attempts at subsequent times. Those caring for the older person should understand that there may be a need for the aged to have a bowel movement one-half to one hour after the initial movement. Sometimes, an older person's request to be taken to the bathroom or to have a bedpan for a bowel movement just after he has had one is viewed as an unnecessary demand and ignored; it is then wondered why fecal incontinence has occurred. It is useful for the aged to attempt to have a bowel movement following breakfast, as the morning activity following a period of rest and the ingestion of food and fluid stimulate peristalsis. Suppositories may occasionally be necessary to stimulate elimination, and they should be administered one-half hour before bowel elimination is desired. Fecal softeners are commonly prescribed to promote elimination in the aged.

Fecal impaction may occur as a result of constipation. Preventive measures to avoid constipation are the best approach to this problem. Observation of the frequency and character of bowel movements may indicate the development of fecal impaction; a defecation record is a must for the older person in a hospital or nursing home. Symptoms to note include distended rectum, abdominal and rectal discomfort, oozing of fecal material around the impaction (often mistaken as diarrhea), and palpation of a hard fecal mass during digital examination of the rectum. This problem should receive the attention of a health professional and be immediately corrected. Removal of fecal impactions should be attempted with care. Sometimes an oil retention enema will soften the impaction and facilitate its passage through the rectum. If this initial procedure is not effective, it may be essential to break up the impaction with a lubricated gloved finger. Inserting 60 ml of hydrogen peroxide prior to the digital attempt at removal will sometimes assist in breaking the impaction.

Itching and discomfort around the rectum may occur as a result of poor hygienic practices or dryness resulting from reduced secretions of the mucus membrane. Scratching and dryness can irritate the tissue and possibly lead to skin breaks and infection. Regular thorough cleansing with soap and water, followed by the application of a lubricant in small quantities, may prevent this problem. Coarse toilet tissue should always be avoided.

Flatulence, not uncommon in the aged, is caused by constipation, irregular bowel movements, certain foods, and poor neuromuscular control of the anal sphincter. Achieving a regular bowel pattern and avoiding flatus-producing foods may relieve this problem, as may the administration of certain medications intended for this purpose. Discomfort associated with the inability to expel flatus may occasionally occur in the aged. Increased activity may provide relief, as may a knee-chest position, if possible. A flatus bag consisting of a rectal tube with an attached plastic bag that prevents the entrance of air into the rectum can also be used (Figure 7-3).

Elimination of wastes through the skin must also be considered.

116

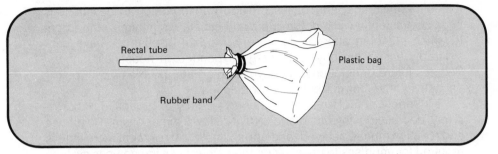

Rectal tube

Plastic bag

Rubber band

Figure 7-3. A flatus bag can be made by attaching a plastic bag to a rectal tube.

Perspiration and oil production is decreased with age, making less frequent bathing necessary for older adults. Reduced hydration and vascularity of the dermis make the skin less elastic and more delicate. Consequently, dryness, itching, and breakage of the skin can result from bathing too frequently. Unless another problem warrants a different pattern, complete bathing is not required more than every third or fourth day. Partial sponge baths to the face, axillae, and perineum on a daily basis should prevent odor and irritation. Neutral or superfatted soaps and bath oils should be used for bathing, followed by the application of skin softeners and moisterizers. Tub baths are not only effective for good cleansing, but enhance circulation and provide an opportunity to exercise stiff joints. (Safety considerations during tub baths will be discussed later in this chapter.) Showers may also be enjoyed by the aged and the use of shower chairs and other appliances may assist with this activity. The individual's unique bathing habits, schedule, and preferences should be appreciated and respected, as should the right to privacy and protection from exposure during bathing activities.

ACTIVITY

Through activity, many physical, psychological, and social benefits are gained. Physical activity aids respiratory, circulatory, digestive, excretory, and musculoskeletal functions. Mental activity maintains mental functioning and promotes a sense of normality. Multiple health problems, such as atherosclerosis, joint immobility, pneumonia, constipation, decubiti, and insomnia, can be avoided when an active state is maintained.

Maintaining a physically active state is a challenge not only for the aged, but for most of the adult population. Fewer and fewer occupations require hard physical labor, and those which still do usually utilize technological inventions to perform the more strenuous tasks. Television viewing and spectator sports are popular forms of recreation. Au-

117

tomobiles, taxicabs, and buses provide transportation to destinations once conveniently walked. Elevators and escalators minimize the extent to which climbing stairs is necessary. Modern appliances have considerably eased the physical energy expended in household chores. Perhaps future generations will have even greater problems with physical activity than our current aged population.

A variety of factors affect the aged's ability to be active. Progressively decreasing thyroid gland activity slows metabolism. Response and reaction time is delayed, and approximately 10 percent more time is required for impulses to travel along the pathways of the nervous system. Muscle fibers atrophy and decrease in number; fibrous tissue gradually replaces muscle tissue, evidenced in flabby and weak arm and leg muscles. Immobility, weakness, and pain of the joints often results from arthritis problems in aged persons. Hormonal changes contribute to thinning and weakening of the bones, and muscle cramping occurs more easily. Less blood is pumped by the heart due to decreases in cardiac function, causing the physical stress associated with activity to be poorly managed. Rising from a lying or sitting position may cause a 60 mm drop in blood pressure and lead to uncomfortable dizziness or fainting. Activity may be further reduced by urinary frequency or incontinence, sensory losses, social isolation, limited financial resources to participate in recreational activities, and inability to maintain pace with a hurried society.

Considering such interferences with activity, special efforts are demanded by the aged and those caring for them to maintain and promote an active state. Education should be provided to teach the public and care providers the importance of physical activity for the aged. Sometimes, families believe they are assisting their older family members by allowing them to be sedentary. Often, assisting with household responsibilities not only enhances good functioning of the body's systems, but promotes a sense of worth by providing an opportunity for productivity. Older people should be taught that although physical activity may be more uncomfortable or demanding than inactivity, additional health problems and disability may be spared in the future. Motivation is necessary at times to stimulate interest in physical activity. For instance, encouraging membership in a senior citizen's club can often motivate many other types of activity, such as providing the incentive to get out of bed, prepare a good breakfast, eat, bathe, dress, and travel to the club destination. Those involved with the aged can provide motivation by demonstrating a sincere interest in the individual's activities. Recognizing the person's housekeeping efforts, using his or her handmade gifts, commenting on a well-groomed appearance, and asking about the latest club activity are small but meaningful ways to reinforce the aged's positive efforts toward maintaining an active state.

Exercises are valuable at any age and are of much benefit to the elderly. Capitalizing on the regular activities of daily living is one means to provide exercise. During a shower or bath the older person can perform flexion and extention exercises under the guise of cleansing and drying various body parts. Dishwashing can be a means of exercising stiff finger joints with the assistance of warm water. Deep breathing and limb exercises can be incorporated into the period between awakening and rising from bed. Foot, leg, shoulder, and arm circling can be done while watching a regular television program. Often, a regular exercise schedule can be established and maintained with greater success when it is integrated into other routine activities since there is more tendency to forget or omit exercises when they are an isolated activity. Figure 7-4 depicts several exercises which may be beneficial to the aged.

Exercises should be paced throughout the day, and fatigue from exercising should be avoided because of chance of muscle pain and cramping. Morning exercises loosen stiff joints and muscles and encourage activity, while bedtime exercises promote relaxation and encourage sleep. If an older person is not accustomed to a great deal of physical activity, exercises should be introduced gradually and increased according to readiness. Some tachycardia may normally occur during the exercises and continue for several hours thereafter. Longer periods of time must be allowed for the older person to perform exercises, and rest periods should follow. Warm water and warm washcloths or towels wrapped around the joints may ease joint motion and facilitate exercising.

As the weaker, thinner, and more brittle bones of the elderly are more easily fractured, these persons should avoid forceful exercise of an immobilized joint, jumping and running exercises, and strenuous sports. Elderly persons with cardiac or respiratory problems should seek advice from their physician as to the amount and type of exercise best suited for their unique capacities and limitations. At times, the older person may need partial or complete assistance with exercises. The nurse or other care providers may find it helpful to remember these points:

1. All body joints should be exercised through their normal range of motion at least three times daily (see Table 6-1 in the previous chapter).
2. The joint and the distal limb should be supported during the exercise.
3. A joint should not be forced past the point of resistance or pain.

Figure 7-5 shows some equipment that can assist the nurse in moving and exercising the elderly.

Psychological activity is as vital to the total well-being of the elderly

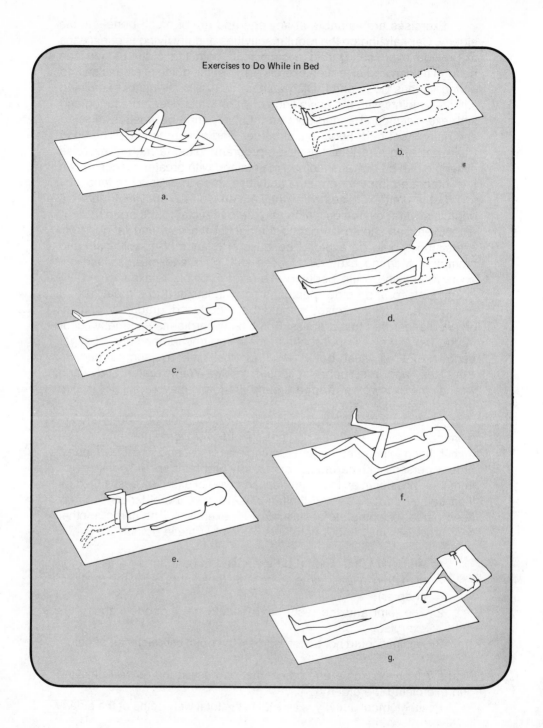

Exercises to Do While in Bed

a.

b.

c.

d.

e.

f.

g.

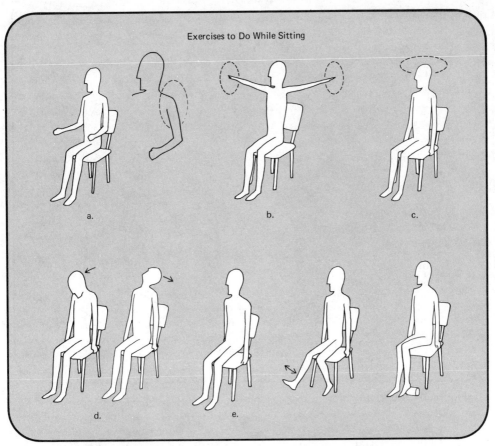

Figure 7-4. Exercises to do while in bed: (a) Flexing knee with opposite hand holding foot for assistance. (b) Rolling from side to side. (c) Scissorlike crossing of legs. (d) Raising chest. (e) Flexing knees while lying on abdomen. (f) Bicycling. (g) Lifting pillow over head with arms straight. Exercises to do while sitting: (a) Circling motion of shoulder joint with arm at side. (b) Circling arms. (c) Rotating head. (d) Flexing and extending neck. (e) Pushing up in chair with use of arms. (f) Kicking legs while sitting. (g) Rolling foot on tin can. All exercises can be built into regular activities. Exercises to do anytime: (a) Rolling pencil on hard surface. (b) Flexing fingers around pencil. (c) Exaggerating chewing motions. (d) Rubbing back with towel. (e) Tightening rectoperitoneal muscles. (f) Holding stomach in to tighten abdominal muscles.

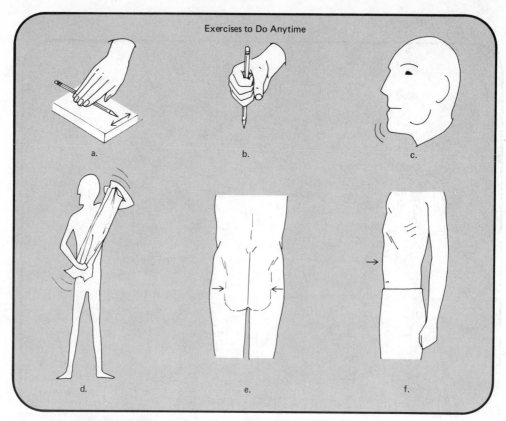

Exercises to Do Anytime

a.   b.   c.

d.   e.   f.

Figure 7-4 (continued)

as physical activity. Stimulation and challenges help the older mind maintain lucid functioning. Barring the existence of health problems, the personality and interests will remain consistent throughout an individual's lifetime. The assertive, independent young woman will most likely resent not having a role in decisions involving her and being addressed in a patronizing manner when she grows old. The couple who enjoyed nightclub entertainment throughout the years will not suddenly cease this activity when they begin to be considered old. Likewise, the individual who preferred privacy and solitude when young will most likely not live gregariously when aged. Activities for the aged should be planned according to the unique interests of the given individual. Old age may also be a time for the development of new hobbies and interests; *old people can learn and enjoy new activities.* As mentioned earlier, pets are frequently a source of interest, activity, and companionship for the elderly.

If it is expected that an aged person will be forgetful and confused, and if the person is treated as though this were true, he or she will most likely become forgetful and confused. On the other hand, if the person is expected to keep oriented to current events and relate on an equal basis with others, he or she will most likely remain alert, aware, and mentally active. Thus a self-fulfilling prophecy often dictates the activities in which old people will engage.

Two basic rules should guide those involved with psychological activity of the aged. First, the individual's psychological status should be assessed and psychological stimulation should be provided based on the person's unique capacities and limitations. In other words, *avoid stereotyping the aged*. Some aged individuals may derive psychological satisfaction from discussing a football game with friends at the local tavern, while others may seek satisfaction from completing a foreign language course at the local college. Individual differences, preferences, and abilities must be considered and appreciated. Second, adequate time and patience must be afforded the aged. Slower passage of impulses through the nervous system, sensory deficits, and the vast storehouse of information that is triggered off and has to be sorted through in response to psychological stimuli are just a few of the factors that interfere with rapid reactions in older people.

REST

Satisfying, regular activity promotes rest and relaxation. Greater amounts of rest are required by older people and should be interspersed with periods of activity throughout the day. Upon awakening, the older persons should spend several minutes resting in bed and stretching their muscles, followed by several more minutes of sitting on the side of the bed before rising to a standing position. This will reduce the morning stiffness of the muscles and prevent dizziness and falls resulting from postural hypotension. Some aged individuals may focus all of their activity in the early part of the day so that they will then have their evening free. For instance, the early morning hours may be invested in household cleaning, marketing, club meetings, gardening, cooking, and laundering so that these activities will be completed before evening. The evening hours may then be spent watching television, reading, or sewing. This pattern may be an outgrowth of many years of employment, whereby the individual worked eight hours during the early day and relaxed in the evening. Older people need insight into the advantages of pacing activities throughout the entire day and providing ample periods for rest and naps between activities. The nurse may need to review the daily activities and assist the person in developing a schedule that more equally distributes activity and rest throughout the day.

123

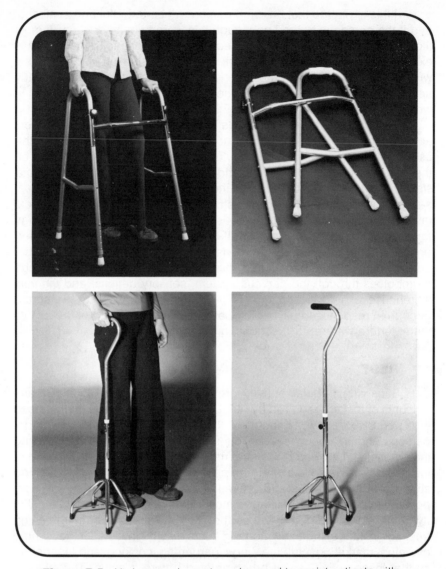

Figure 7-5. Various equipment can be used to assist patients with ambulation and transfer activities. (Courtesy of Maddak, Inc. Subsidiary of Bel-Art Products, Pequannock, N.J.)

Although more rest is required by the aged individual, the length of time required for sleep is reduced. Five to seven hours of night sleep is sufficient for the aged and longer periods may be harmful to their physical and mental functioning. The aged sleep less soundly and may frequently have their sleep interrupted by muscle cramps and tremors, environmental interferences, and nocturia. Older persons may be initially disoriented and confused when wakening in a dark room, and this possibility, combined with visual deficiencies and postural hypotension, may predispose them to accidents. A night-light should be provided in the person's bedroom, and if possible, bathroom lighting should remain on throughout the night. Clutter and furniture should not obstruct the pathway from the bedroom to the bathroom. It may be beneficial to provide a urinal, bedpan, or bedside commode in the older person's room if the bathroom is on a different floor of the house.

The attachment of side rails to the bed may be a beneficial protective measure for the older person at home. This not only prevents falls from bed, but it assists the individual with movement and provides a means of orientation to place. It is important for individuals to feel confident that they can remove these rails to get out of bed or that someone will be readily available to help them do so when necessary. Occasionally, hospital or nursing home patients will resist having side rails due to fear of staff delays in helping them out of bed. These patients need verbal and also behavioral reassurance that they are not trapped and unable to get up. Falls resulting from attempts to climb over the side rails may be prevented by prompt staff response to calls for assistance.

Vision and hearing limitations produce difficulties for care providers who need to communicate necessary questions, warnings, or directions during the night. Whispering to avoid awakening other sleeping individuals will not wake an aged person who has a reduced ability to hear or whose hearing aid is removed, and lipreading is difficult in dimly lit bedrooms. Focusing a flashlight on the lips of the speaker can help the individual read lips, and cupping the hands over the ear and speaking directly into it can aid hearing. A stethoscope can also be used to amplify conversation by placing the earpieces into the individual's ear and speaking into the bell portion.

It is not uncommon for the aged to have difficulty falling asleep. Much too often, the first means employed to encourage sleep is the administration of a sedative. Although the use of medications for the aged population is discussed in detail in Chapter 22, it is worthwhile to mention here that sedatives must be used with utmost care. Barbiturates should be used with extreme caution. They are general depressants, especially to the central nervous system, and they can significantly depress some vital body functions, lowering basal metabolic rate even more than it already is and decreasing blood pressure, mental activity, and peristalis to the extent that other problems may develop. The aged may be more susceptible to many of the adverse reactions to barbiturates. Nonbarbiturate sedatives are not without their problems either, and they should be used only when absolutely necessary. Due to the prolonged half-life of medications in the elderly, the effects of sedatives may exist into the daytime and result in confusion and sluggishness. (To compound the problem, these symptoms are sometimes treated with other medications!) Occasionally, sleeping medications will also reverse the individual's normal sleep rhythm. Sedatives may decrease body movements during sleep and predispose the older person to the many complications of reduced mobility.

Alternatives to sedatives should be used to induce sleep whenever possible. The activity schedule of the individual should first be evaluated. If he has been inactive in a bed or wheelchair all day, most likely he will not be sleepy at bedtime. Including more stimulation and activity during the day may be a solution. The amount of time alotted for sleep should also be evaluated. With a reduced demand for sleep, it should not be expected that the older person who goes to bed at 8 P.M. should be able to sleep until 8 A.M. the following day. A warm bath at bedtime can promote muscle relaxation and encourage sleep, as can a back rub, alleviating pain or discomfort, and finding a comfortable position. A quiet environment, at a temperature preferred by the individual, should be provided. Electric blankets can also promote comfort and relaxation.

Changes in sleep patterns may indicate signs of other problems in the elderly. Although early morning rising is not unusual for the aged, a sudden change to earlier awakening or insomnia may be symptomatic of emotional disturbance. Sleep disturbances may also arise from cardiac or respiratory problems which produce such difficulties as orthopnea and pain from poor peripheral circulation. Restlessness and confusion during the night may be a display of an adverse reaction to a sedative. Nocturnal frequency may be a clue to the presence of diabetes. It is important to assess the quality and quantity of sleep in the aged.

SOLITUDE AND SOCIAL INTERACTION

The axiom that people are social beings holds true for the aged as well. Through social interaction, we share our joys and burdens, derive feelings of normality, validate our perceptions, and maintain a link with reality. The aged, however, may face unique obstacles in their attempts to interact with others due to a variety of intrinsic and extrinsic factors.

The ability to communicate is an essential ingredient for social interaction, and sensory deficits in the aged may interfere with this process. Presbycusis may cause speech to be inaudible or distorted, as can impacted cerumen, a common problem in the aged. Older people may be quite self-conscious of this limitation and avoid situations in which they must interact. In turn, others may avoid them due to this difficulty. Telephone conversation can be affected by this problem, limiting social contact even further for the individual who may be socially isolated for other reasons. (Approximately one-tenth of the aged have some difficulty hearing on the telephone.) Corrective measures for hearing problems should be explored. An audiometric examination can determine whether the particular hearing problem can be improved by the use of a hearing aid, which should not be purchased without such an examination. It is not uncommon to find an older person attempting to correct a hearing problem independently by purchasing a hearing aid from a private party. Not only can this produce disappointing results, but it can waste hundreds of dollars from an already limited budget.

Inability to adjust to the presence of the aid and the distortion of sound caused by the amplification of environmental noise in addition to speech may cause rejection of its use. The nurse should encourage its use, offering support to the individual during this adjustment phase, suggesting that the aid be worn for progressively longer periods each day until the person feels comfortable with it and that it not be used in noisy environments such as airports, train stations, stadiums, etc. The aid should be checked to make sure that the earpiece is not blocked with cerumen and that the battery is working. This appliance may easily correct a hearing problem and reintroduce the older person to a socially active world. If a hearing aid will not solve the problem, efforts should be made to speak clearly and distinctly, in a low frequency but at an audible level while facing the individual. Shouting should be avoided, as it raises the high-frequency sounds, which the older person already has difficulty hearing, causing even greater hearing difficulties. Cupping the hands over the less deficient ear and talking directly into the ear may be helpful. Using gestures and pictures and pointing to items while talking about them can assist.

The nurse should examine the elderly's ears frequently for cerumen accumulation and gently irrigate the ear with a warm saline or hydrogen peroxide and water solution. The aged should understand that irrigation is superior to the use of cotton tipped applicators, which may push the cerumen back into the ear canal and cause an impaction. It is beneficial for the nurse to educate the public as to the effects of environmental noise on their health and their risk of developing presbycusis. Nurses should be actively involved themselves and encourage the involvement of others in legislation controlling noise pollution, as well as the enforcement of such legislation.

The ability to see is equally important to communication. Most elderly persons require some form of corrective lens and approximately half of the individuals identified as legally blind each year are 65 years

127

of age or older. Visual limitations can make communication quite problematic since facial expressions and gestures, which are just as important as the words, may be missed or misinterpreted. Lipreading to compensate for hearing deficits may be difficult and written correspondence may be limited because independent reading and writing become almost impossible tasks. Remaining aware of current events through newspapers and socialization through card playing and other games may thus be hampered. For visual deficit, one of the first assistive measures is a thorough eye examination, including tonometry, by an ophthalmologist. The importance of an annual eye examination, not only to detect vision changes and needs for alterations in corrective lenses, but also for early discovery of problems such as cataracts and glaucoma and other disease processes, must be stressed to the older person. Limited financial means and satisfaction with one's old pair of eyeglasses may cause the aged to neglect regular vision examinations.

To compensate for visual limitations, one should face the individual when speaking and exaggerate gestures and facial expressions. To compensate for the poor peripheral vision old people commonly have, one should approach the individual from the front and seat the person facing those with whom he is interacting. Ample lighting should be provided; several soft indirect lights are superior to a single bright glaring light. Interaction can be promoted by using games and playing cards with enlarged figures (see Figure 7-6), telephone dials with enlarged numbers that glow in the dark, and cassette recorders. Books and magazines with large print and recordings of current events and popular literature can provide a source of recreation and a means of keeping informed.

Because of declining physical function, the older person may have less energy to invest in social interaction. Urinary frequency and incontinence make the individual reluctant to engage in social activities, as do stiff, painful joints and other discomforts. Changes in appearance may alter the individual's self-concept and interfere with the motivation for and quality of social interaction. Although many of these problems cannot be eliminated, nursing intervention can help reduce the limitations they cause. Education of younger adults regarding the normal aging process can enhance their sensitivity and patience, and help them understand the socialization problems an aged person faces, perhaps thereby helping them learn how to minimize and manage these limitations when they grow old. Assuring the aged that their problems are shared by many others and that some of their limitations are a natural part of aging may help them feel "normal," and thus promote social interaction. The nurse can help review and perhaps readjust the person's activity schedule to conserve energy and maximize opportunities for social interactions. Medication schedules should be planned so that during periods of social activity analgesics will provide relief, tranquilizers won't sedate, diuretics won't reach their peak, and laxatives won't become most effective. This is common sense, but often overlooked. Likewise, fluid intake and bathroom visits prior to engagement in activities should be planned to reduce the fear or actual occurrence of "accidents," and activities planned for the aged should provide for frequent break periods for visits to the bathroom. Very often, the control of these minor obstacles can facilitate social interaction.

Given the capacity to interact socially and manage their own problems, the aged must then deal with social factors over which they have no control. Their circle of friends and relatives may become smaller through deaths, and a limited budget may necessitate giving food and shelter priority over social activities. A youth-oriented, fast-paced society may not provide an atmosphere conducive to active social involvement. If the disengagement theory is valid (see Chapter 2), how can the human need for social interaction be satisfactorily fulfilled by the aged? Nurses may discover the importance of influencing society in order to gain acceptance for the aged and obtain opportunities for them to remain socially active. Fortunately, most older people have close relationships with siblings, and most have at least one child less than an hour away whom they see at least weekly.

Solitude is also important for most human beings. It offers a rest from the many stimuli and interactions to which we are regularly exposed and provides for introspection, whereby insights into ourselves, others, and our environment are gained. Reflecting on and analyzing life's events help us to develop and to understand life. Periods of solitude are therapeutic to the aged. Unresolved feelings from earlier years may be worked through and resolved, resulting in personal satisfaction. In reminiscing, evaluating, and understanding the dynamics of life's earlier events and achievements, older people can find a satisfaction with the quality of their life that helps compensate for their multiple losses. They can also gain a new perspective on themselves and others. The death of friends, spouse, and others and the realization of one's own mortality necessitate thought regarding the reality of death and dying.

Time should be provided daily in which no interruptions interfere with solitude. How often are meaningful thoughts and resolutions to unfinished business interrupted by a care provider who wants to distribute a medication or take the individual to the dayroom or change bed linens? Often, busy care providers with a multitude of tasks to complete are not sensitive to the fact that elderly persons who appear to be doing nothing are performing a psychological task as important as any other task that might be performed for them at that time. Designated areas, such as a corner of the dayroom, or a bedroom, should be provided for privacy and respected as such. It must be remembered that solitude and loneliness

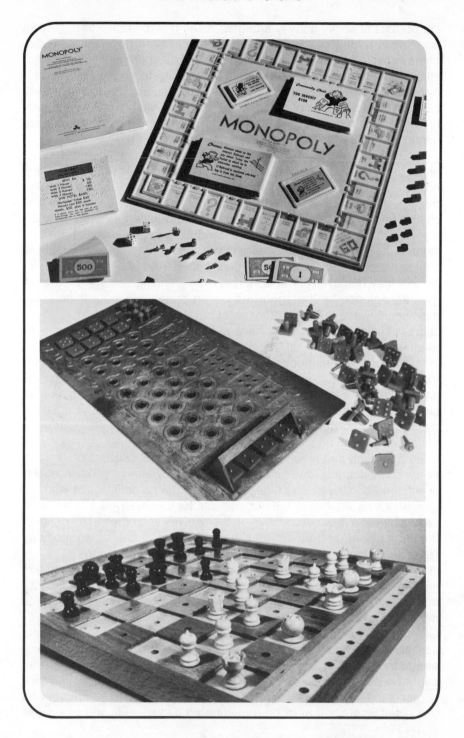

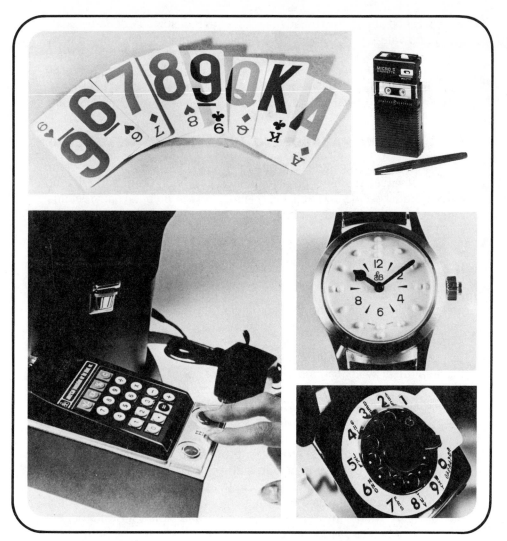

Figure 7-6. Special equipment can help the visually impaired engage in recreational activities: (a) Backgammon, Monopoly, dominoes, checkers, and dice sets with raised and depressed markings. (DiMartini, American Foundation for the Blind.) (MONOPOLY is Parker Brothers' registered trademark for its real estate trading game equipment (c) 1935, 1946, 1961. Photograph courtesy of Parker Brothers.) (b) Jumbo cards with oversized symbols and numbers, and portable radios and cassette recorders. (General Electric) (More information on aids and appliances for the visually impaired can be obtained from the American Foundation for the Blind, 16 West 16th St., New York, N.Y. 10011.)

131

are not synonymous. The nurse may discover that some aged individuals enjoy and value sitting alone in the park for hours and may forfeit a party invitation for a quiet evening at home. To *choose* solitude differs from being socially isolated and not have opportunities for social activity. The nurse must carefully assess the degree of solitude and social interaction and assist in achieving and maintaining a healthy balance of both.

AVOIDING HAZARDS TO HEALTH AND WELL-BEING

Protective measures to maintain health and well-being include regular physical examination; avoidance of alcohol, drug, and tobacco abuse; proper eating and activity; control of environmental hazards; and early correction of health problems. Due to lack of knowledge, ability, or good judgment, people occasionally expose themselves to, or neglect to protect themselves from, hazards to health and well-being. It is clear that neglecting regular Pap smears for the early detection and treatment of cervical cancer is a threat to a woman's life; that being unaware of the pollutants released from a local industry prevents the community from correcting the hazard; and that not having the benefit of regular dental care risks a child's health. While encountering similar problems to those of other age groups the aged face additional challenges that may pose unique threats and require special nursing considerations. Changes in the respiratory system create a greater risk of upper respiratory infection; changes in the urinary tract create a predisposition for a variety of urinary problems and infections; a more alkaline vaginal environment predisposes older females to some infections.

The lower body temperature of the aged can cause infectious processes to go unnoticed. The healing process is generally slower, and wounds that take 31 days to heal in a 20-year-old, take 55 days in a 40-year-old and 100 days in a 60-year-old (Manney). Normal absorption of food and excretion of waste products are altered, and there is a higher risk of malnourishment. Reduced pressure and ability to differentiate temperature create the danger of injury and breakage to the aged's more delicate and fragile skin. Brittle bones, resulting from reduced bone minerals, can fracture under the amount of stress that would not affect younger bones. Unrestricted activity is harder to achieve, and yet a multitude of problems associated with immobilization are quick to occur. Adverse reactions to drugs often occur and these problems remain untreated because mental confusion, the early sign of disease or drug problems, is often misjudged as senility. Those caring for the aged can help protect them from hazards to health and well-being by recognizing the potential threats discussed above and by understanding the following facts regarding normal values for this age group.

Body temperature is lower in the aged and may normally be as low as 95° F (35°C). The individual whose normal temperature is 96° F may be febrile at 99° F, but he or she may not be identified as such because this temperature is within a normal range for the general adult population. For every 1° F (0.6°C) temperature increase, the pulse increases from 7 to 10 beats per minute. If there is a delay in detecting the increase in metabolic, respiratory, and pulse rates which occur with an elevation in body temperature, serious complications can develop. Pulse rates can fall within a wide range, from 50 to 100 beats per minute, and frequently, the rhythm is irregular. Although an irregular rhythm may be of no diagnostic significance, there is a possibility that it is indicative of a problem, for example, digitalis toxicity.

Although the elderly may have a slow and irregular respiratory rate, the average number of respirations per minute ranges between 14 and 18. Systolic and diastolic blood pressures are higher in the aged as a result of increased peripheral resistance. Persistent elevations above 170 mmHg systolic and 95 mmHg diastolic are considered hypertensive levels in the elderly. (Caird and Judge suggest that normal upper limits can be 195/105 for a male over 80 years of age and 210/115 for a female, and that if these individuals are asytomatic, they need not receive antihypertensive therapy.). Attempting to reduce blood pressure to a level that is normal for younger adults can cause a reduction in cerebral blood flow and, consequently, a reduction in cerebral function. Health professionals should understand this phenomenon and not refer every older person with a blood pressure of 160/90 for treatment; this is costly to the older person and an inefficient use of a health professional's time. The nurse should inform the public of the higher blood pressure levels with advanced age during hypertension screening programs.

As can be seen, regular assessment is important in order to establish baseline norms for the aged individual and recognize changes in these norms. The aged person should be informed of the normal values of his or her vital signs, and these values should be documented on a permanent record. If an older person suddenly begins to display symptoms of senility, the cause may be hidden unless the previous norm for blood pressure has been established and is known by the health care provider. If examination reveals a blood pressure of 140/70, this could be interpreted as normal. However, if the previous blood pressure had consistently been 190/90, the person may now be hypotensive.

The older person's safety may also be threatened by certain visual changes with aging. Older eyes adapt less quickly to light and dark, see less well in dim areas, have greater difficulty with depth perception and peripheral vision, discriminate low-tone colors (such as blues and greens) less well, and may have more opaque lenses. These factors predispose the aged to many accidents. A small light should be left on throughout the night, and night driving should be discouraged. Bright lights and glare should be avoided by using several small lights instead of one large one, by filtering bright sunlight through sheer drapes or stained-glass windows, and by placing the older person's bed or chair so that it does not face a bright window.

To compensate for reduced peripheral vision, the individual should be approached from the front rather than from the back or side, and furniture and frequently used items should be arranged in full view. Altered depth perception may hamper the ability to detect changes in levels, and this may be helped by providing good lighting, eliminating clutter on stairways, painting the stairs a contrasting color, and using signals to indicate when a change in level is being approached. The filtering of low-tone colors should be considered when decorating areas for the aged; bright oranges and yellows and contrasting colors on doors and windows may be appealing and assistive. The problem with seeing low-tone colors should be considered when teaching urine testing to older diabetics since they must differentiate these colors to detect glycosuria. Cleansing solutions, medications, and other materials should be labeled in large letters to prevent accidents or errors.

Directions and warnings may also be missed due to poor hearing. Explanations and directions for diagnostic tests, medication administration, or other therapeutic measures should be explained in written as well as verbal form. The individual should live close to someone with adequate hearing who can tell him or her of fire alarms or other warnings. Decreased sense of smell may also cause the older person to miss life-saving warnings, such as the different scents of mouthwash and juice. Electric stoves may be helpful in preventing gas intoxication from the inability to detect a gas odor. The loss of taste receptors may cause the aged to use excessive amounts of sugar and salt in the diet, a possible health hazard. Reduced tactile sensation to pressure from shoes, dentures, or an unchanged position can cause skin breakdown, and inability to discriminate temperatures can cause burns.

Slower response and reaction times may prove to be safety hazards. Older pedestrians may misjudge their ability to cross streets as traffic lights change, and older drivers may not be able to react quickly enough to avoid accidents. Stove burns while cooking are also a danger, one compounded by visual problems. Slower movement and poor coordination subject the older person to falls and other accidents. Loose rugs, slippery floors, clutter, and poor-fitting shoes and slippers should be eliminated. Railings should be present on stairways and bathtubs. Rubber mats or nonslip strips are a must in the bathtub, where fainting and falls often occur as a result of reduced blood pressure—first from the warm bath water which dilates the peripheral vessels and then again from rising to a standing position. Using a stool in the tub and resting before rising are useful measures. Since poor judgment, denial, or lack of awareness of their limitations may prevent them from protecting their health and well-being, older people should be advised not to take risks such as window washing or climbing on a ladder.

With the vast number of medications used by older population, it is important to avoid inappropriate or unwise use of them. Feedback should be obtained to evaluate the understanding the individual has of his or her medications and their administration. All adverse reactions and special precautions should be written down and explained to the individual and the family. The necessity of the medication should be periodically reevaluated and it should be discontinued if there is no real therapeutic need for the drug any longer. Side effects may be demonstrated differently in the aged, and they should be anticipated and detected early. As many drugs are required in lower dosages for older persons, the lowest possible effective dose should be used. Additional problems and precautions with drug use in the elderly are discussed in Chapter 22. Since the aged are more susceptible to hazards, require a longer recovery period, and are prone to more complications when an illness develops, the most effective means of managing threats to health and well-being is to prevent them from occurring. The environmental checklist below suggests some preventive devices.

Environmental Checklist

Smoke detector
Telephone
Fire extinguisher
Vented heating system
Minimal clutter
Proper food storage
Adequately lighted hallways and stairways
Handrails on stairways
Even floor surface, easy to clean and requiring no waxing and free of loose scatter rugs and deep pile carpets
Unobstructed doorways, painted a different color from wall for easy visibility
Bathtub or shower with nonslip surface, safety rails, and no electrical outlets nearby
Windows easy to reach and open

Ample number of safe electrical outlets, preferably 3 feet higher than level of floor for easy reach
Safe stove with burner control on front
Shelves within easy reach to avoid need for climbing
Faucet handles that are easy to operate
For wheelchair use, doorways and hallways that are clear and wide enough for passage; ramps and/or elevators; bathroom layout to provide for wheelchair maneuvering; and sinks, stoves, tables, and cabinets low enough for reach from wheelchair

135

BEING NORMAL

The desire to be normal is important at any age. The aged, however, may find many unique challenges in achieving feelings of normality for two general reasons. First, our society's definition of normal is based upon a young model. Just observing advertisements and walking through a department store reflects our country's bias for the young. Those who can't keep pace or conform to the styles and activities of the young are in a sense viewed as abnormal. Second, knowledge of what is normal for the aged is rather recent and still developing. Not only lay people, but many health professionals don't know or understand norms for the aged. Consequently, wasted time, energy, and money is invested in achieving norms for the aged that are inappropriate or hazardous. Daily baths, shouting to compensate for hearing loss, inappropriate reduction of blood pressure, and determining fever by values used for the young are just several of the practices which may indicate poor utilization of existing knowledge. The nurse can be a more effective practitioner and a significant consumer advocate by educating others regarding normality in the aged.

Certain physiological changes may cause the aged to feel abnormal in reference to their appearance. A reduction in height occurs as thinning disks shorten the vertebral column. This is compounded by postural changes, such as slight hip and knee flexion, and in many individuals, kyphosis with a backward tilting of the head. Height reductions may even be more obvious because span and length of the upper extremities remain the same. With the exception of the face, body hair is lost and scalp hair commonly becomes thin and gray. The clustering of melanocytes causes some skin pigmentation to accompany the lines and wrinkles resulting from a loss of subcutaneous fat. Women may be disturbed at the facial hair and breast tissue atrophy what occurs with age, and men may find prostatic hypertrophy and baldness common problems. Tooth loss, dry skin, swollen joints, hard and brittle fingernails, and many other factors cannot be altered; but measures can be employed to promote a good appearance in the elderly.

Attractive clothing and jewelry may offset bodily changes. Cream-based cosmetics offer protection from sun and wind exposure and are also of psychological value. Shampooing the hair once or twice monthly can improve hair condition, and with regular brushing and scalp massage in between, this is all that is really necessary for the aged. Wigs can be worn and hair dyes may be used. (Rinses and vegetable dyes are less harmful than heavy metal and aniline-based dyes.) Facial hair can be removed by the use of tweezers, pumice stones, chemical agents or electric needles; mole hair should not be pulled but carefully cut with scissors to avoid trauma. Soaking will ease the task of cutting nails, and podiatry services may prove beneficial. Gauze or cotton placed gently under a curved nail may facilitate its straight growth. (These should be changed daily and removed for baths.) Creams and lotions may be used to soften skin. The aged should be motivated to practice good grooming habits and maintain an attractive appearance.

The effects of declines and alterations in body function on one's ability to feel and act normal should be considered by the nurse, and attempts should be made to provide the most normal life-style attainable in light of these limitations. Certain factors may make it difficult for the aged to adjust to the rapid rate of societal change and technological advancement. Performing a series of complicated, coordinated tasks may be problematic for the aged and reliance on previous experience may supersede creative problem-solving techniques. In addition, memory for past events may be far superior to memory of recent facts. Imagine how difficult it must be for an older person who has cooked with a gas stove for over 50 years to comprehend and learn the use of a microwave oven! Some of the normal daily demands of today's world may be difficult for the aged to fulfill.

Although a fuller discussion of sexuality and the aged is provided in Chapter 20, it may be useful to mention a few points here. It is normal for the aged to desire sexual satisfaction and be able to engage in sexual activity. Masters and Johnson have found through their research that sexual expression is more inhibited by social and psychological forces than by physical ability. The nurse should encourage older people to express their sexuality and should convey the importance of understanding and appreciating this to family members and others providing care for the aged. Ridicule, lack of privacy, and demeaning reactions to sexual behavior can prevent the aged from experiencing the psychological and physiological benefits of sexuality. Older males, whose responsiveness and intensity of pleasure may be reduced, should be encouraged to worry less about the actual performance of the sex act and to focus more on the importance of sharing love, warmth, and intimacy. This advice is applicable to older females as well. Hormonal imbalances may cause dyspareunia for the aged female, but hormonal replacement can often improve this problem. Health professionals and the public in general may have to change old attitudes and encourage sexual activity—if only for its therapeutic value alone.

In our society one's worth is often determined by one's productivity. Changing requirements for skills, the abundance of young workers, and rigid retirement policies often force the older worker out of the labor force, and the retired person may have feelings of worthlessness having no productive role to fill. Nuclear families and day-care centers often eliminate the traditional roles for grandparents. As a nonproductive member of society the aged individual often cannot help feeling abnormal. Some solutions to this problem are to discontinue discriminatory hiring practices and provide a capable older person with equal opportunity for employment; to abandon mandatory retirement practices; and to utilize the rich pool of wisdom and skills accumulated throughout the older person's lifetime by establishing employment or volunteer programs. Obviously, one can remain a valuable member of society when retired, and if society's attitude reflected this, the negative feelings associated with unemployment might be reduced. The financial security to live a full and satisfying life should also be something everyone can expect when retirement occurs.

Long-term goals should include programs to educate the public for aging. Youth should be helped to gain insight into the assets and problems of old age, and an appreciation and respect for the older members of society. Gaining an understanding of aging as a normal and natural process may encourage the development of a healthy attitude toward growing old. Learning how to prepare for old age through preventive health practices, the development of leisure activities, the accumulation of financial assets, periods of trial retirement prior to actual retirement, intelligent life planning, and increased legislation to promote health, security, and safety for the aged should be promoted.

REFERENCES

Caird, F. I. and Judge, T. G. *Assessment of The Elderly Patient.* Pitman, New York, 1974, p. 34.

Manney, James R. *Aging in American Society.* University of Michigan, Wayne State University, Ann Arbor, Mich., 1975, p. 27.

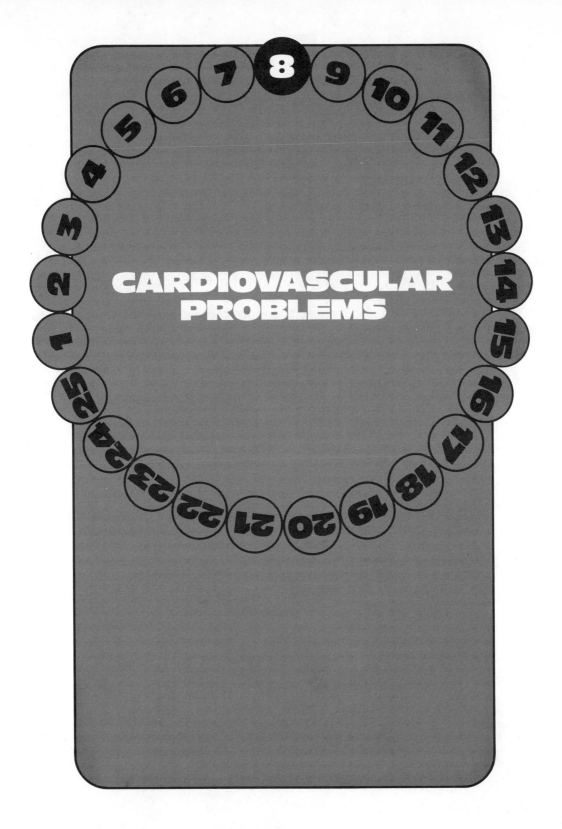

CARDIOVASCULAR PROBLEMS

The geriatric nurse frequently encounters persons with some form of cardiovascular disease. Heart disease increases with age and most deaths due to cardiovascular disease are in the aged population. The number one cause of death in individuals 65 years of age or older is cardiovascular disease. A review of some of the heart changes associated with the aging process promotes understanding of the reasons for cardiac problems in old age. The heart either remains the same or becomes smaller in old age than it was during middle adulthood, and the older heart has a deeper brown color. Subpericardial fat is present in greater amounts, and there is evidence of endocardial thickening and sclerosis. The aorta and arteries are less elastic, and the carotid artery may become kinked to the extent that it is mistaken for an aneurysm. The heart valves thicken and become more rigid.

The reduced efficiency of the heart is manifested in a variety of ways. Heart contractions may be weaker and cardiac output reduced. The lessened elasticity of the aorta and the presence of atrial atrophy produce problems in filling and emptying the heart. The utilization of oxygen is decreased, as are the cardiac reserve and the capacity for cardiac work. Despite these changes and reduced efficiency, the aged heart is able to meet the demands of daily life adequately. Under unusual circumstances, when stress places increased demands on the heart, the declining function of the heart is most apparent.

SYMPTOMS OF CARDIAC DISEASE

The gerontological nurse must be particularly alert to clues indicatint possible cardiac disease, either visible or as described by the patient.

Shortness of breath. The most common complaint associated with cardiac disease is shortness of breath. This symptom can be observed by the nurse when patients have to interrupt normal activities in order to "catch their breath" and when they become noticeably fatigued with minimal exertion. When patients refuse to participate in activities because they tire easily or indicate that a specific activity which never bothered them in the past, now causes them difficulty, the nurse should be suspicious of cardiac disease. An unjustified complaint that "there isn't enough air in the room to breathe" should also be viewed with suspicion. Sleep problems should be explored by the nurse since the inability to breathe fully, and the fear that death may occur while sleeping due to inadequate respirations may interfere with the individual's ability to relax and enjoy an entire night's sleep. Acute dyspnea should be brought to the physician's attention quickly as it can be a symptom of myocardial infarction in aged patients.

Chest pain. Acute or recurrent chest pain, a common complaint associated with cardiac disease, is difficult to assess. The pain described by the aged person may be atypical for cardiac disease as a result of altered pain sensation in old age. With the high prevalence of respiratory, gastric, and musculoskeletal problems in aged individuals, this symptom can also be attributed to some other existing disorder. The nurse should note the time of onset and the characteristics, location, duration, and other factors associated with incidents of chest pain.

Cheyne-Stokes respiration. This symptom is common in the aged and may be an indication of cardiac disease. The nurse should be alert in making observations and in noting patient's comments about having insomnia, which is frequently caused by Cheyne-Stokes respiration.

Changes in cerebral function. Occasionally, such changes are thought to be a result of the aging process, but this may actually be a symptom of cardiac disease and consequent poor cerebral circulation. The nurse should detect early the development of vertigo, mental confusion, change in mental status, or behavioral changes.

Edema. Edema is frequently a symptom of cardiac disease, especially with right-sided heart failure. Subtle clues which may be indicative of edema should be recognized, such as the inability to remove a previously removable wedding band, the complaint that shoes suddenly feel tight and an increase in weight.

Other Symptoms. Coughing and wheezing are symptoms which may reflect left-sided heart failure, and hemoptysis is frequently associated with congestive heart failure and pulmonary edema. As mentioned with chest pain, this group of symptoms may be attributed to respiratory disorders that are present in the aged individual. Some symptoms that occur with cardiac disease in younger adults, such as pain, anorexia, vomiting, frequency, and nocturia, occur less commonly in an old person with cardiac disease.

Since the early detection and diagnosis of cardiac disease can be difficult because of (1) a slow, gradual rate in the progress of symptoms,(2) an easy confusion of cardiac symptoms with those of other systems, and (3) an atypical manifestation of symptoms, keen, accurate nursing observations are especially important.

Electrocardiogram

A basic diagnostic aid in cardiovascular disease in the aged is the electrocardiogram. Even in the absence of disease, there are some

141

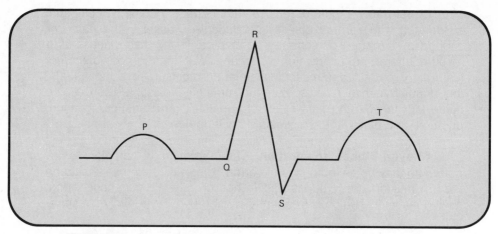

Figure 8-1. Normal adult EKG.

changes in the electrocardiogram of older persons with which the nurse should be familiar. For a basis of comparison, a normal adult EKG reading is shown in Figure 8-1, with parts labeled. In the aged, there is a reduced voltage of the waves and a slight prolongation of all intervals due to the slower conduction of impulses through the pacemaker, conduction system, and myocardium. Figure 8-2 shows a hypothetical EKG of an aged person superimposed on the normal adult EKG from Figure 8-1. The P wave may normally be smaller in the aged. The P-R interval shows no significant change while the QRS interval is slightly longer. The QT interval may show an increase, but it remains within the normal limit, and the T wave will appear lower. As can be seen, these changes do not produce a significant difference in the appearance of the EKG.

COMMON CARDIOVASCULAR DISEASES OF THE AGED

Although other cardiovascular diseases may occur in older persons, those most encountered by the gerontological nurse have been selected for this chapter. Only factors particularly relevant to the aged patient are discussed, and the nurse is encouraged to refer to medical-surgical textbooks for a complete review of the diseases presented.

Congestive Heart Failure

The incidence of congestive heart failure increases with age and is an especially potential complication in older patients with arteriosclerotic heart disease. The variety of conditions that can precipitate congestive heart failure in the aged include coronary artery disease, hyperten-

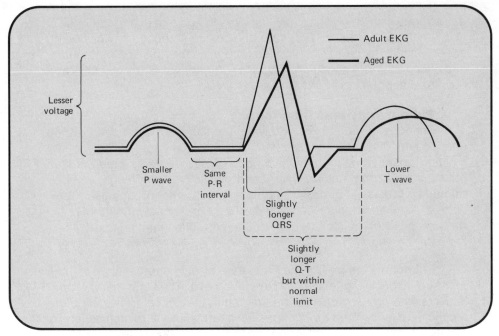

Figure 8-2. Age-related EKG changes superimposed on normal adult EKG.

sive heart disease, cor pulmonale, mitral stenosis, subacute bacterial endocarditis, bronchitis, pneumonia, congenital heart disease, and myxedema. Nurses should closely monitor patients with any of these conditions and detect indications of congestive heart failure. Symptoms of this problem which may develop in aged patients include mental confusion, insomnia, wandering during the night, agitation, depression, anorexia, nausea, weakness, shortness of breath, orthopnea, and bilateral ankle edema. The detection of any of these symptoms should be promptly communicated to the physician.

The management of congestive heart failure in the aged is basically the same as in middle-aged adults, commonly consisting of bedrest, digitalis, diuretics, and a reduction in sodium intake. The patient may be allowed to sit in a chair next to the bed; complete bedrest is usually discouraged to avoid the potential development of thrombosis and pulmonary congestion. The patient should be assisted into the chair and adequately supported. While sitting, the patient should be observed for signs of fatigue, dyspnea, changes in skin color, and changes in the pulse.

The nurse should be aware that the presence of edema and the

143

poor nutrition of the tissues associated with this disease, along with the more fragile skin of the aged, predisposes the patient to a greater risk of skin breakdown. Regular skin care and frequent change of positioning are essential. The nurse should also recognize that this is a frightening, and often recurring, condition requiring a great deal of reassurance and emotional support.

Pulmonary Heart Disease

Changes in the respiratory system associated with normal aging and certain disease processes in the aged can reduce pulmonary function, contributing to pulmonary heart disease. Factors which reduce pulmonary function include decreased elasticity of the lungs, alveolar dilation, fibrosis, kyphosis, emphysema, chronic bronchitis, tuberculosis, and mitral disease. The forms of pulmonary heart disease discussed below, pulmonary emboli and cor pulmonale, primarily affect the older person.

Pulmonary emboli. The incidence of pulmonary emboli is high in the aged, but the detection and diagnosis of it in this age group is rare. Patients who are in particular danger when they develop this problem are those with fractured hip, congestive heart failure, arrhythmias, and a history of thrombosis. Immobilization and malnourishment, frequent problems in the aged population, can contribute to pulmonary emboli. Symptoms which should be observed include mental confusion, apprehension, increasing dyspnea, slight temperature elevation, pneumonitis, and an elevated sedimentation rate. Older patients may not experience chest pain due to altered pain sensations, or their pain may be attributed to other existing problems. A lung scan or angiography may be done to confirm the diagnosis and establish the location, size, and extent of the problem. Treatment of pulmonary emboli in the aged does not significantly differ from that employed for the young.

Cor pulmonale. *Acute* cor pulmonale is usually a result of a massive pulmonary embolus, respiratory infection, atrial fibrillation, or chronic failure. This is often a problem experienced by older hemiplegics. With the exception of the use of morphine or barbiturates, treatment is the same as for younger adults. *Chronic* cor pulmonale is primarily a result of emphysema. This disease can develop into acute cor pulmonale, and nursing measures should focus on preventing this from happening. Treatment does not differ from that for the young, including antismoking education.

Coronary Artery Disease

Coronary artery disease is the popularly used phrase for ischemic heart disease. There is an increased prevalence of coronary artery disease with advanced age, so that some form of this disease exists in most persons 70 years of age or older.

Anginal syndrome. A symptom of myocardial ischemia, the angina syndrome presents itself in an atypical pattern, creating difficulty in detection. Pain may be diffuse and of a less severe nature than described by younger adults. The first indication of this problem may be a vague discomfort under the sternum, frequently following a large meal. The type of pain described and the relationship of the onset of pain to a meal may cause the patient, and the health professional, to attribute this discomfort to indigestion. As this condition progresses, the patient may experience precardial pain radiating down the left arm. The recurrence of anginal syndromes over many years can result in the formation of small areas of myocardial necrosis and fibrosis. Eventually diffuse myocardial fibrosis occurs leading to myocardial weakness and the potential risk of congestive heart failure.

Nitroglycerine has proved beneficial in the prevention and treatment of anginal attacks. As this drug may cause a drop in blood pressure, the patient should be cautioned to sit or lie down after taking this tablet to prevent fainting episodes and falls. To prevent swallowing the tablet and thus blocking its absorption, patients should be reminded not to swallow their saliva for several minutes following sublingual administration. Specific information on nitroglycerine is offered in Chapter 22. Long-acting nitrates are usually not prescribed for the aged. To prevent anginal syndromes, the patient should be taught and helped to avoid these factors which may aggravate this problem, such as cold wind, emotional stress, strenuous activity, anemia, tachycardia, arrhythmias, and hyperthyroidism.

Myocardial infarction. A cardiac problem frequently seen in older persons, especially in men with a history of hypertension and arteriosclerosis, myocardial infarction can have a delayed or missed diagnosis in the aged due to an atypical set of symptoms and the frequent absence of pain. Symptoms include pain radiating to the left arm, the entire chest, the neck, and abdomen; moist, pale skin; decreased blood pressure; low-grade fever; and an elevated sedimentation rate. Output should be observed since partial or complete anuria may develop as this problem continues. Arrhythmias may occur, progressing to fibrillation and death if untreated. Cardiac rupture may also occur, especially in older women.

The trend in treating myocardial infarction has been to reduce the amount of time in which the patient is on bedrest and to replace complete bedrest with allowing the patient to sit in an armchair next to the bed. The patient should be assisted into the chair with minimal exertion on his part. Arms should be supported to avoid strain on the heart. Not only does this armchair treatment help to prevent many of the complications associated with immobility, but it also prevents pooling of the blood in the pulmonary vessels, thereby decreasing the work of the heart.

Since aged persons are more susceptible to cerebral and intestinal bleeding, close nursing observation for signs of bleeding is essential if anticoagulants are used in the patient's treatment. Nurses should be alert to signs of developing pulmonary edema and congestive heart failure, potential complications for the geriatric patient with a myocardial infarction. These and other observations, such as persistent dyspnea, cyanosis, decreasing blood pressure, rising temperature, and arrhythmias, reflect a problem in the patient's recovery and should be promptly brought to the physician's attention.

Acute coronary insufficiency. Arterial narrowing and myocardial damage and increased cardiac stress can result in acute coronary insufficiency. Symptoms of this problem which the nurse can recognize include a low-grade fever and prolonged chest pain. Treatment includes the use of oxygen and analgesics, as well as rest. Areas of necrosis can develop after repeated episodes of this problem, leading to diffuse fibrosis.

Hypertension

The incidence of hypertension increases with advancing age and is a problem which the gerontological nurse commonly encounters in practice. Many aged people have a high blood pressure due to the vasoconstriction associated with aging, which produces peripheral resistance. Hyperthyroidism, parkinsonism, Paget's disease, anemia, and a thiamine deficiency can also be responsible for hypertension. Usually, if the older person's blood pressure is equal to or greater than 200 mmHg systolic and 100 mmHg diastolic, and if the person is symptomatic, treatment is initiated. The nurse should carefully assess the patient's blood pressure by checking it several times with the person in standing, sitting, and lying positions. Anxiety, stress, or activity prior to the blood pressure check should be noted, as these factors may be responsible for a temporary elevation. The anxiety of being examined by a physician or of preparing for and experiencing a visit to a clinic frequently cause an elevated blood pressure in a usually normotensive individual.

Awakening with a dull headache, impaired memory, disorientation, confusion, epistaxis, and a slow tremor may be symptoms of hypertension. The presence of these symptoms with an elevated blood pressure reading usually warrants treatment. Hypertensive older patients are advised to rest, reduce their sodium intake, and if necessary, reduce their weight. Aggressive antihypertensive therapy is discouraged for older persons due to the risk of a sudden dangerous decrease in blood pressure. Nurses should observe for signs indicating a blood pressure which is too low to meet the patient's demands, such as dizziness, confusion, syncope, restlessness, and drowsiness. An elevated blood urea nitrogen level may also be present. These signs should be observed for and communicated to the physician if they appear. In the management of the older person who is hypertensive, it is a challenge to achieve a blood pressure level which is high enough to provide optimum circulation while being low enough to prevent serious related complications.

Arrhythmias

Digitalis toxicity, hypokalemia, acute infections, hemorrhage, anginal syndrome, and coronary insufficiency are some of the many factors which cause an increasing incidence of arrhythmias with age. Of the causes mentioned, digitalis toxicity is the most common.

The basic principles of treatment of arrhythmias do not vary much for older adults. Tranquilizers, digitalis, and potassium supplements are part of the therapy prescribed. Patient education may be warranted to help the individual modify diet, smoking, drinking, and activity patterns. The nurse should be aware that digitalis toxicity can progress in the absence of clinical signs and that the effects can be evident even two weeks after the drug has been discontinued. The aged have a higher mortality rate from cardiac arrest than other segments of the population, emphasizing the necessity for close nursing observation and early problem detection, to prevent this serious complication.

Tachycardia. Tachycardia is one form of conduction disturbance seen in older persons. The most common types are *paroxysmal atrial tachycardia* and *ventricular tachycardia*. With the exception of acute myocardial infarction, ventricular tachycardia—a serious problem for young and old—does not frequently occur. However, ventricular tachycardia has been noted at the time of a person's death and for minutes following clinical death. Decreased blood pressure, impaired cerebral circulation, and congestive heart failure may develop if tachycardia is not corrected.

Premature contractions. Atrial and ventricular premature contractions are cardiac arrhythmias experienced by the aged. Premature contractions can be caused by gastrointestinal disturbances, stress, and agents such as coffee, tea, alcohol, and tobacco. If not corrected, this problem can lead to a serious ventricular arrhythmia.

147

Atrial fibrillation.   As a result of severe cardiovascular disease, hyperthyroidism, high fevers, digitalis intoxication, and pulmonary emboli, atrial fibrillation can occur. If it is prolonged, it encourages the development of an atrial thrombus and thus prompt treatment is important. Signs of·a possible embolus should be observed for. Dyspnea and chest pain may indicate a pulmonary emboli, while an emboli lodged in the mesenteric arteries will cause abdominal pain. Discolored urine may result from a renal emboli, and changes in cerebral function may indicate an emboli there.

Heart block.   Arteriosclerosis, digitalis overdose, quinidine, certain poisons, and changes in the heart structure can cause heart block. Older persons experiencing heart block have a greater risk of suffering cardiac standstill and Stokes-Adams attack—whereby unconsciousness and possible seizures occur as a result of hypoxia from interrupted cerebral circulation.

Bacterial Endocarditis

Subacute bacterial endocarditis.   This may be a potential complication experienced by aged patients with staphylococcal, fungal, and other infections and with collagen disorders, diabetes, and a history of recent surgery; also by patients who have been receiving steroids, cancer chemotherapy, and antibiotics for a long period of time. Diagnosis can be complicated in aged persons because of such nonspecific symptoms as anorexia, fatigue, weight loss, anemia, mental confusion, weakness, pallor, tachycardia, and an elevated sedimentation rate. The difficulty in relating these symptoms to subacute bacterial endocarditis in the aged contributes to the high mortality associated with this problem. As this disease progresses, atrial fibrillation and heart failure may occur. The treatment for this problem in the aged is similar to that employed for younger persons.

Acute bacterial endocarditis. This occurs in the aged to a significantly lesser degree than the subacute form, but with similar difficulty in diagnosis because its symptoms are like those of many other geriatric problems.

Rheumatic Heart Disease

Rheumatic heart disease may occur in aged people who either have had rheumatic fever earlier in life or have had acute episodes during old age. Older individuals who have rheumatic fever suffer moderate joint discomfort, sudden soreness and diffuse redness of the throat, enlarged lymph nodes, and a temperature elevation. Any joint lesions are more disabling to the elderly. It is not unusual for repeated episodes to occur, and the nurse should be alert to symptoms in patients with a history of this disease. With proper therapy, the prognosis for an older person with acute rheumatic fever is favorable, and rheumatic heart disease, which occurs more often in elderly women, can be prevented. Residual valvular deformities from acute rheumatic fever progress differently in each individual. Usually, the mitral and aortic valves are most affected. Some persons have minimal limitations because of adequate compensation by the myocardium; some develop murmurs, hypertension, atrial fibrillation, and congestive heart failure. Aggressive therapy for the disease itself is usually not warranted, and the emphasis is on managing the symptoms and any complications that develop.

Syphilitic Heart Disease

Ten percent of the heart disease in persons 50 years of age or older is a result of syphilis. Aged persons with syphilitic heart disease may have contracted the disease at a time when a definite stigma was attached to venereal diseases, and open discussion and education regarding these diseases was nonexistent or minimal. The individual may have been fearful or felt guilty or may not have noticed or been aware of the significance of the associated symptoms, and therefore may not have sought treatment. Treatment before the 1940s, when penicillin was developed, may have been inadequate and ineffective in eliminating the disease. Older persons who have had recent exposure to syphilis may be reluctant to seek treatment because they are concerned about what others might think of sexual activity in old age.

The first sign of syphilitic heart disease may occur years after the initial infection. The valvular defect most frequently associated with this disease is aortic insufficiency, whereby a leak in the aortic valve during diastole causes blood to be forced back into the left ventricle. The systolic blood pressure is increased, the diastolic blood pressure is reduced, and the pulse pressure is significantly greater. When the heart is no longer able to compensate for these changes, cardiac failure can occur. The most effective treatment may be the replacement of the damaged valve with a ball-valve prosthesis, a procedure viewed with increasing optimism for the aged.

Congenital Heart Disease

Due to the limited medical and surgical correctives for congenital defects that were available when today's aged population was young, people born with serious heart problems most likely did not survive to adulthood. Thus, congenital heart disease is not very common among the aged and is sometimes unrecognized as such. It is believed that

149

some of the arrhythmias, murmurs, and other cardiac diseases found in the geriatric patient are caused by congenital lesions.

Atrial and ventricular septal defects. These are the most common congenital heart defects discovered in the aged. Symptoms of atrial septal defect are similar for all ages, except that older people may have a higher pulse rate, increased blood pressure, dyspnea, recurrent bronchopneunomia, and a greater incidence of coronary artery disease. Most patients with ventricular septal defects are asymptomatic, although they may experience fatigue and episodes of heart failure. Surgery is sometimes effective in improving both these defects in older persons.

NURSING CONSIDERATIONS

The prevention of cardiovascular problems in all age groups should be a primary concern of the nurse. By teaching people of all ages to identify and lower the risk factors related to cardiovascular disease, the nurse will also be contributing to people's optimum health and functioning. The nurse should emphasize the importance of proper nutrition, the relationship of cholesterol and obesity to heart disease, and the benefits of regular exercise. Many Americans today exert minimal physical activity during the workweek and fill the weekend with gardening, swimming, tennis, housecleaning etc., when they should be distributing exercise throughout the entire week. In the absence of a special exercise regimen, one can take advantage of simple daily opportunities, such as using stairs instead of an elevator, walking short distances instead of driving, and making a list of exercises to perform while watching a favorite television show.

Moderation should be recommended in alcohol consumption, and cigarette smoking should be discouraged. The nurse should realize that a smoking habit is difficult to break and should employ methods to educate people regarding the multiple health problems associated with it. Smokers should also be assisted in finding antismoking programs that meet their unique needs. Regarding the association of stress and heart disease, the nurse should review a person's stresses, coping mechanisms, and outlets for stress, promoting insight into factors that can increase the risk and measures that can reduce the risk of heart disease. The nurse should remember that it is much easier to establish good habits early in life than to change long-established practices.

As mentioned throughout this chapter, diagnosis of cardiovascular disease in the aged is often complicated and difficult. Emphysema, hiatus hernia, gall bladder disease and other disorders may mistakenly be assigned responsibility for or mask symptoms of cardiovascular disorders. As the person that probably has the most direct contact with the patient, the nurse should observe closely for even the most subtle clue indicating a possible cardiovascular problem, including those learned in conversations with the patient. Comments such as "My chest felt like it had a butterfly in it while I was mowing the lawn, but it went away" or "Sometimes I wake up from my sleep feeling like someone has a pillow over my face" should be explored further. The same patients who made these comments may have responded negatively when asked by the physician if they had ever experienced chest pain or shortness of breath. It will facilitate diagnosis if such findings are communicated to the physician.

The type of diagnostic measures utilized for older patients with possible cardiovascular disease will not differ greatly from those used with younger patients, and the same nursing measures should be applied. Due to sensory deficits, anxiety, mental confusion or limitations in memory, the older patient may not fully understand or remember the explanations given for the diagnostic measures employed. The nurse should prepare the patient for tests, offer full explanations on a meaningful level, reinforce the teaching provided, and allow the patient to discuss questions and concerns openly. Families should also be part of this process. Commonly, procedures which seem relatively minor to the nurse, such as frequent checks of vital signs, may be alarming to the unprepared patient and family.

Although the basic care of the cardiovascular patient is similar for young and old, there are some specific considerations for the geriatric patient. The edema associated with many cardiovascular diseases may promote skin breakdown, especially in older people who have more fragile skin. Frequent change of position is vital. The body should be supported in proper alignment, and arms and legs should not be allowed to hang off the side of a bed or chair. Clothing and restraints should be checked frequently to make certain that they haven't become constricting due to increased edema. Areas of the body that receive pressure should be protected and should be massaged frequently. If the patient is to be on a stretcher, an examining table, or an operating-room table for a long period of time, the nurse should place protective padding on pressure areas beforehand to provide comfort and prevent skin breakdown. When much edema is present, excessive activity should be avoided. Activity increases the circulation of fluid and also of toxic wastes in the fluid, which can subject the patient to profound intoxication. The nurse should note changes in the patient's edematous state; a tape measure will provide quantitative data.

Accurate observation and documentation of fluid balance is especially important. Within any limitations prescribed by the physician fluid intake should be encouraged, in order to prevent dehydration, to which the aged are more susceptible, and facilitate diuresis (water is effective for this). Fluid loss through any means should be measured; volume, color, odor, and specific gravity of urine should be noted. The patient's weight should be obtained daily. If intravenous fluids are being administered, careful monitoring is essential. Excessive fluid infusion results in hypervolemia, subjecting the aged to the risk of congestive heart failure. It should be remembered that an intravenous glucose solution could stimulate the increased production of insulin, resulting in a hypoglycemic reaction if this solution is abruptly discontinued without an adequate substitute for the intravenous glucose.

Vital signs must be checked frequently, with careful attention to any changes. A temperature elevation can reflect an infection or a myocardial infarction. Remember that the body temperature for the aged may be normally lower and that it is important to have collected data on normal conditions as a basis for comparison. It is advisable to detect and correct temperature changes promptly. A temperature elevation increases metabolism, which in turn increases the body's requirements for oxygen and causes the heart to work harder. A decrease in temperature slows metabolism, which causes less oxygen consumption and thereby less carbon dioxide production and fewer respirations. A rise in blood pressure indicates increased demands on the heart. Headache, dizziness and nosebleed may indicate elevated blood pressure. Chronic hypoxia may be the cause of increased blood pressure, and the nurse should evaluate the patient for this factor. A decreased blood pressure is associated with a reduced cardiac output, vasodilation, and a lower blood volume. Hypotension can result in insufficient circulation to meet the body's needs. Symptoms of mental confusion and dizziness could indicate insufficient cerebral circulation resulting from a reduced blood pressure. Pulse changes are also significant. In addition to cardiac problems, tachycardia could indicate hypoxia due to an obstructed airway. Bradycardia could be associated with digitalis toxicity.

Oxygen is frequently administered in the treatment of cardiovascular diseases, and in aged patients it requires most careful use. Hypoxia should be closely observed for. Patients using a nasal catheter may breathe primarily by mouth and reduce oxygen intake. Although a face mask may remedy this problem, it does not guarantee a sufficient oxygen inspiration. The aged patient may not demonstrate cyanosis as the initial sign of hypoxia; instead he or she might be restless, irritable, and have dyspnea. These signs can also indicate high oxygen concentrations and consequent carbon dioxide narcosis, which is a particular risk to aged patients receiving oxygen therapy. Although blood gas levels will provide data revealing these problems, early correction is facilitated by keen nursing observation.

The nurse may have to help patients fulfill their nutritional needs and encourage older patients to eat if they have cardiovascular disease and suffer from anorexia. Favorite foods attractively served may overcome this, and several smaller meals throughout the entire day rather than a few large ones will compensate for poor appetite and reduce the work of the heart. The cardiovascular patient should be encouraged to maintain a regular intake of glucose, the primary source of cardiac energy. Patient education is frequently necessary regarding low-sodium, low-cholesterol, and/or low-calorie diets. It is not uncommon for the aged to have difficulty accepting a new diet. Ethnic dishes, often an important component of older people's culture, may not be allowed because of prescribed dietary restrictions. This can be a significant sacrifice for the older person, and many choose not to comply at all rather than to forfeit these dietary pleasures. The nurse can offer support to the aged person as these difficult dietary adjustments are made.

Involving patients in setting their own priorities and negotiating compromises in their diet may be worthwhile. A realistic although imperfect diet with which the patient is satisfied is more likely to be complied with than an ideal one that is meaningless to the patient. Older patients may need assistance in developing menus that observe their dietary restrictions. Lists of preferred foods along with notations regarding their sodium, cholesterol, and caloric content should be developed and assessed. It is more meaningful and efficient to focus only on foods commonly eaten by the patient and provide a description of the sodium, cholesterol, or caloric intake, depending on the type of restriction (see Table 8-1). Aged patients should also understand that carbonated drinks, certain analgesic preparations, commercial alkalizers and homemade baking soda mixtures, which they commonly employed for relief of indigestion, also contain sodium.

Reduced activity increases risks of constipation, and to avoid this problem and fecal impaction, ample fluid intake and dietary items that promote bowel elimination should be provided to maintain regular bowel function. Straining due to constipation, enemas, and removal of fecal impactions can cause vagal stimulation and be dangerous to the cardiovascular patient. If the patient is on bed rest, range-of-motion exercises can promote circulation and prevent complications resulting from immobilization; with complete bed rest, passive range-of-motion exercises will cause muscle contractions that compress peripheral veins and thereby facilitate the return of venous blood.

Patients who are weak or who fall asleep while sitting should have their head and neck supported to prevent hyperextension or hyperflexion of the neck. All aged persons, not only cardiovascular patients, can suffer a reduction in cerebral blood flow due to the compression of vessels during this hyperextension and hyperflexion. Those with congestive heart failure need good positioning and support. A semirecumbent position with pillows supporting the entire back maintains good body

TABLE 8-1: PARTIAL LIST SHOWING
SODIUM CONTENT OF PREFERRED FOODS

	Sodium Content	Restriction Required
Meat, Poultry, and Fish		
Ham hock	High	✓
Lean beef	Low	
Oysters	Low	
Corned beef	High	✓
Dairy Group		
Skimmed milk	Low	
Cheddar cheese	High	✓
Fruits and Vegetables		
White turnips	High	✓
Glazed fruits	High	✓
Kale	High	✓
Pickled onions	High	✓
Canned peas	High	✓
Peanut butter	High	✓
Apple	Low	
Breads and Cereals		
Puffed wheat	Low	
Baking powder biscuits	High	✓

alignment, promotes comfort, and also assists in reducing pulmonary congestion. Cardiac strain is reduced by supporting the arms with pillows or armrests. Footboards help prevent foot-drop contracture, and patients should be instructed in how to use them for exercising also.

If hepatic congestion develops, drugs may detoxify more slowly. As the aged may already have a slower rate of drug detoxification, the nurse must be acutely aware of signs indicating an adverse drug reaction. Digitalis toxicity should be especially observed for in older persons. Nausea, vomiting, arrhythmias, and a slow pulse are among the signs which may indicate this problem. Since hypokalemia sensitizes the heart to the effects of digitalis, it should be prevented through proper diet and possibly the use of potassium supplements.

The patient who must manage anginal attacks should be helped to identify factors that precipitate attacks and to review the proper use of nitroglycerin—including its use when an attack is anticipated, such as during a stressful event, rather than after the attack occurs. Since the pain associated with a myocardial infarction may be similar to that of angina, the patient should be instructed to notify the physician or nurse if pain is not relieved by nitroglycerin. The patient's chart should include the factors that precipitate attacks, as well as the nature of the pain and how the patient describes it, the method of management, and the usual number of nitroglycerin tablets used to alleviate the attack.

Relaxation and rest are both important in the treatment of cardiovascular disease, and it is wise to remember that a patient who is at rest is not necessarily relaxed. The stresses from hospitalization, pain, ignorance and fear regarding disability, alteration in life-style, and thoughts about death can cause the aged to become anxious, confused, and irrational. Reassurance and support are needed, including full explanations of diagnostic tests, institutional routines, and other activities. Opportunities should be provided for the patients and their families to discuss questions, concerns, and fears openly. An often unasked question of aged patients relates to the restrictions cardiac disease imposes on sexual activity. Health professionals should not neglect to review any necessary limitations in sexual activity thinking aged patients aren't interested. This may be a serious concern to the geriatric patient, and it requires open discussion. Explanations of any necessary restrictions and changes in life-style should emphasize that the patient need not become a "cardiac cripple" for the remainder of his or her life. Most patients can still live a normal life and should be assured of this.

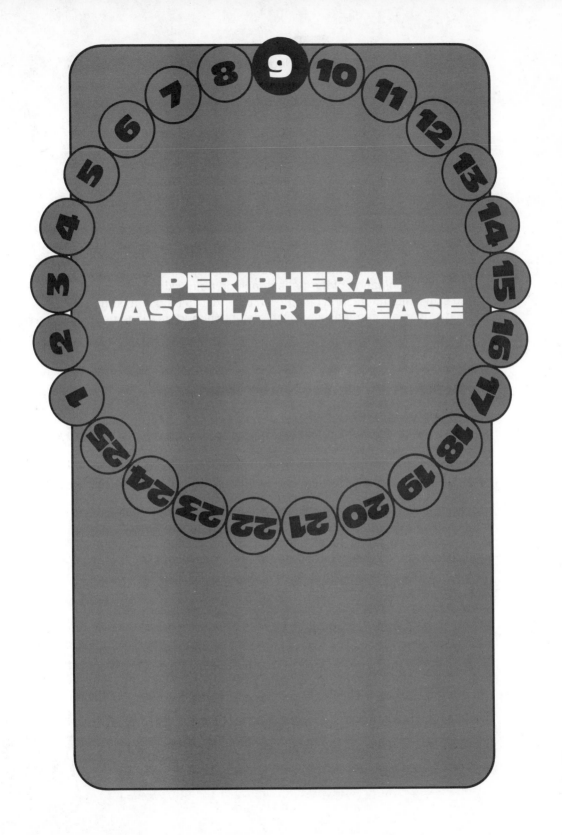

PERIPHERAL
VASCULAR DISEASE

Blood vessels throughout the body undergo changes with age which contribute to a variety of peripheral vascular diseases. A loss of elasticity causes the vessels to dilate and elongate, and the tortuous nature of the vessels can be detected by the naked eye. Greater amounts of calcium, cholesterol, and other lipids are found in arteries, and increased amounts of connective tissue and mucopolysaccharides in the intima. There is also a reduced efficiency in the valves.

Many signs and symptoms of peripheral vascular disease can be noted during the initial assessment of the patient or while assisting with basic care; generalized edema, chills, and pallor, for example, might be suspect. Thick, dry nails and thin, scaling skin are subtle indications of poor circulation, and drowsiness, dizziness, and memory disturbances can be caused by insufficient cerebral circulation. Possible signs revealed by examination of the patient include pain, skin discoloration, altered skin temperature, and changes in the size of a limb or a portion of the body. Nurses can assist in the detection and management of peripheral vascular disease by communicating the development of, or changes in, associated signs and symptoms.

DESCRIPTIVE FEATURES AND TREATMENT

Arteriosclerosis

Arteriosclerosis is a common problem among the aged, especially among diabetics, and unlike atherosclerosis, which more greatly affects the large vessels coming from the heart, it most often affects the smaller vessels farthest from the heart. Arteriography and X-ray can be used to diagnose arteriosclerosis; and oscillometric testing can assess the arterial pulse at different levels. If surface temperature is evaluated, as a diagnostic measure, the nurse should keep the patient in a warm, stable room temperature for at least one hour before testing. Treatment of arteriosclerosis includes bed rest, warmth, Buerger-Allen exercises (see Figure 9-1), and vasodilators. Occasionally, a permanent vasodilation effect is achieved by performing a sympathetic ganglionectomy.

Arteriosclerosis Obliterans

Most of the occlusions that result in the development of ischemic lesions are due to arteriosclerosis. Aortoiliac occlusion, occurring in the terminal abdominal aorta and common iliac arteries, may not produce any difficulty for years. Rest pain and gangrene may be eventual effects as this problem progresses. In the lower extremities the most common site of occlusion is the superficial femoral artery, with the involvement of the popliteal artery tree or the tibial artery tree. Intermittent claudication is the most frequent problem associated with lower-extremity occlusions,

158

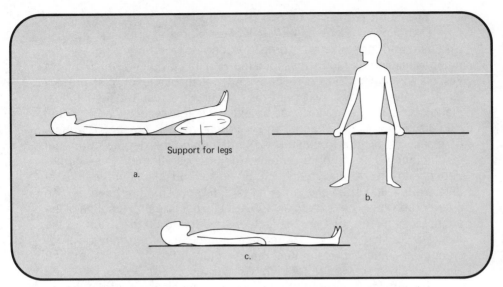

Figure 9-1. Buerger-Allen exercises: (a) Patient lies flat with legs elevated above the level of the heart until blanching occurs (approximately two minutes). (b) Patient lowers legs to fill the vessels and exercises feet until the legs are pink (approximately five minutes). Patient lies flat for approximately 5 minutes before repeating the exercises. Entire procedure is done five times, or as tolerated by the patient, at three different times of the day. The nurse should assist the patient with position changes since postural hypotension can occur. Tolerance and effectiveness of the procedure should be noted.

although some patients do develop ischemic rest pain, neuropathy and, less frequently, ulcers and gangrene. Treatment of arteriosclerosis obliterans depends on the location.

Arterial Embolism

Aneurysms, atrial fibrillation, myocardial infarction, atherosclerosis, and arteriosclerosis are among the problems which give rise to arterial emboli, which lodge primarily in the lower-extremity and brachial arteries. The aged are seriously threatened by gangrene and death from an undetected or untreated embolism, and the nurse should therefore be alert to indicative symptoms and signs. Coldness and numbness below the location of the embolism may prevent the aged from feeling pain until the condition progresses. Any pressure or constriction to the affected part should be avoided. Anticoagulation therapy, which, as discussed in Chapter 22, requires close nursing supervision, and embolectomies have proven beneficial.

159

Special Problems of the Diabetic

Diabetics, who have a high risk of developing peripheral vascular disease and associated complications, commonly display the neuropathies and infections associated with this problem, which affects vessels throughout the entire body. Arterial insufficiency can present itself in several ways: rest pain may occur as a result of intermittent claudication; arterial pulses may be difficult to find or totally absent; and skin discoloration, ulcerations, and gangrene may be present. Diagnostic measures, similar to those used to determine the degree of arterial insufficiency with other problems, include oscillometry, elevation-dependency tests, and palpation of pulse and skin temperature at different levels. Especially when there is the possibility of surgery, an arteriography may be done to establish the exact size and location of the arterial lesion. The treatment selected will depend on the extent of the disease. Walking can promote collateral circulation and may be sufficient management if intermittent claudication is the sole problem, and analgesics can provide relief from rest pain.

Since many of today's older diabetics may have witnessed severe disability and death among other diabetics they have known throughout their lives, they need to be assured that improved methods of medical and surgical management—perhaps not even developed at the time their parents and grandparents had diabetes—increase their chances for a full, independent life. Specific nursing measures used in the care of the older diabetic with peripheral artery disease are provided later in this chapter.

Aneurysms

Advanced arteriosclerosis is usually responsible for the development of aneurysms in aged persons, although they may also result from infection, trauma, syphilis, and other factors. Sometimes they can be seen by the naked eye and are able to be palpated as a pulsating mass; sometimes they can only be detected by X-ray. A thrombosis can develop in the aneurysm, leading to an arterial occlusion or rupture of the aneurysm—the most serious complications associated with this problem.

Aneurysms of the abdominal aorta most frequently occur in older people. Patients with a history of arteriosclerotic lesions, angina pectoris, myocardial infarction, and congestive heart failure more commonly develop aneurysms in this area. A pulsating mass, sometimes painful, in the umbilical region is an indication of an abdominal aorta aneurysm. Prompt correction is essential since if not corrected, rupture can occur. Fewer complications and deaths result from surgical intervention prior to rupture. Among the complications which the aged can develop after surgery for this problem are hemorrhage, myocardial infarction, cerebral vascular accident, and acute renal insufficiency. The nurse should closely observe for signs of postoperative complications.

Aneurysms can also develop in peripheral arteries, the most common sites being the femoral and popliteal arteries. Peripheral aneurysms can usually be palpated, and a diagnosis can be established in this manner. The most serious complication associated with peripheral aneurysms is the formation of a thrombus, which can occlude the vessel and cause loss of the limb. As with abdominal aorta aneurysms, early treatment reduces the risk of complications and death. The lesion may be resected with replacement of the portion of the vessel removed—commonly with a prosthetic material. For certain patients, a lumbar sympathectomy can be performed. The nurse should be aware that these patients can develop a thrombus postoperatively and assist the patient in preventing this complication.

Varicose Veins

Varicosities, a common problem in the aged, can be caused by lack of exercise, jobs entailing a great deal of standing, and losses of elasticity and strength associated with the aging process. Varicosities in all ages can be detected by the dilated, tortuous nature of the vein, especially the veins of the lower extremities. The person may experience dull pain and cramping of the legs, sometimes severe enough to interfere with sleep. Occasionally dizziness may occur as the patient rises from a lying position due to the localization of blood in the lower extremities and reduced cerebral circulation. The effects of the varicosities make the skin more susceptible to trauma and infection, promoting the development of ulcerative lesions, especially if the patient is obese or diabetic.

Treatment of varicose veins is aimed toward reducing venous stasis. The affected limb is elevated and rested to promote venous return. Exercise, particularly walking, will also enhance circulation. The nurse should make sure that elastic stockings and bandages are properly used and not constricting and that the patient is informed of the causes of venous status (e.g., prolonged standing, crossing the legs, wearing constricting clothing), in order to prevent the development of complications and additional varicosities. Ligation and stripping of the veins require the same principles of nursing care which would be used for other age groups undergoing this surgery.

Venous Thromboembolism

An increasing incidence of venous thromboembolism is found among the aged. Patients who have been on bed rest or have had recent surgery or fractures of a lower extremity are high risk candidates. Although the veins in the calf muscles are the most frequently seen sites

161

of this problem, it also occurs in the inferior vena cava, iliofemoral segment, and various superficial veins. The symptoms and signs of venous thromboembolism depend on the vessel involved. Clues which the nurse should be alert for include edema, warmth over the affected area, and pain in the sole of the foot. Edema may be the primary indication of thromboembolism in the veins of the calf muscle since it is not unusual for discoloration and pain to be absent in aged persons with this problem. If the inferior vena cava is involved, there will be bilateral swelling, aching and cyanosis of the lower extremities, engorgement of the superficial veins, and tenderness along the femoral veins. Similar signs will appear with involvement of the iliofemoral segment, but only on the affected extremity.

The location of the thromboembolism will dictate the treatment employed. Elastic stockings or bandages, rest, and elevation of the affected limb may be used to promote venous return. Analgesics may be given to relieve any associated pain. Anticoagulants may be administered and surgery may be performed as well. The nurse should help the patient to avoid situations that cause straining and to remain comfortable and well hydrated.

NURSING CONSIDERATIONS

Preventing problems such as peripheral vascular disease from developing is an important part of nursing. Health education should emphasize the importance of exercise, such as walking to promote circulation, and of not sitting with legs crossed or standing for prolonged periods of time. Obesity, which can interfere with venous return, should be avoided. Clothing that might interfere with circulation should be pointed out, for example, garters, tight-fitting shoes, girdles, and tight slacks. Instruction in such measures can prevent complications from, and avoid the development of, vascular problems. The use of tobacco should be discouraged as it may cause arteriospasms. To prevent thrombus formation, immobility and hypotension should be prevented. The physician may prescribe Buerger-Allen exercises (see Figure 9-1), and the nurse should instruct the patient, and perhaps a family member, in the proper method of doing them, including how to provide comfort for the patient while they are done and how to use any support hose or special elastic stockings correctly.

Persons with peripheral vascular disease must pay special attention to the care of their feet, which should be bathed and inspected daily. To avoid injury, the patient should not walk in bare feet. Any foot lesion or discoloration should promptly be brought to the attention of the nurse or physician. These patients may easily develop fungal infections from the moisture produced by normal foot perspiration. The aged frequently

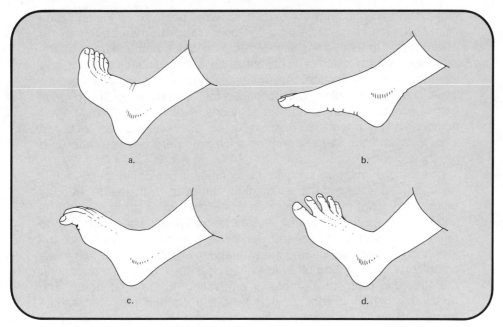

Figure 9-2. Foot and toe exercises: (a) Foot flexion. (b) Foot extension. (c) Curling toes. (d) Moving toes apart.

develop fungal infections under their nails, emphasizing the importance of regular, careful nail inspection. If untreated, a simple fungal infection can lead to gangrene and other serious complications. Placing cotton between the toes and removing shoes several times throughout the day will help keep the feet dry. Shoes should be large enough to avoid any pressure and safe enough to prevent any injuries to the feet, and they should be aired after wearing: patients should be encouraged to have several pairs of shoes, if possible, and rotate their use. Laces should not be tied tightly because they can exert pressure on the feet. Socks should be changed regularly, and to prevent possible irritation from dyes, colored socks should be discouraged. Although the feet should be kept warm, the direct application of heat to the feet, as with heating pads, hot water bottles, and soaks, can increase the metabolism and circulatory demand, thereby compounding the existing problem. Figure 9-2 shows some exercises which may benefit the patient with peripheral vascular disease.

Ischemic foot lesions may be present in patients with peripheral vascular disease. If eschars are present, they should be loosened to allow drainage. Debridement should be performed with care to avoid bleeding and trauma. Chemical debriding agents are sometimes utilized. Systemic antibiotic agents can be helpful in controlling cel-

163

lulitis. Topical antibiotics are usually not used because epithelialization must occur before bacteria flora can be destroyed. Analgesics may be administered to relieve any associated pain. Good nutrition, particularly an adequate protein intake, is essential, as is the maintenance of muscle strength and joint motion. A variety of surgical procedures may be beneficial for the patient with ischemic foot lesions, including bypass grafts, sympathectomies, and amputations. As the proportion of aged persons in the population increases, so does the number of aged amputees, and the serious problems they face are both physical and psychosocial.

Loss of a limb may represent a significant loss of independence to the aged, regardless of the reality of the situation. With an altered body image, new roles may be assumed while other roles are forfeited. The patient and his or her family should be provided the opportunity to openly discuss their fears and concerns. Making them aware of the likelihood of a normal life and the availability of appliances which make ambulation, driving, and other activities possible may help reduce their anxieties and promote a smoother adjustment to the amputation. The rehabilitation period can be long for the aged and may necessitate frequent motivation and encouragement by the nurse. The nurse can be a valuable support person to the patient and the family during this difficult process.

It is hoped that the nurse will explore medical-surgical nursing literature for a complete discussion of general care of the patient with peripheral vascular disease.

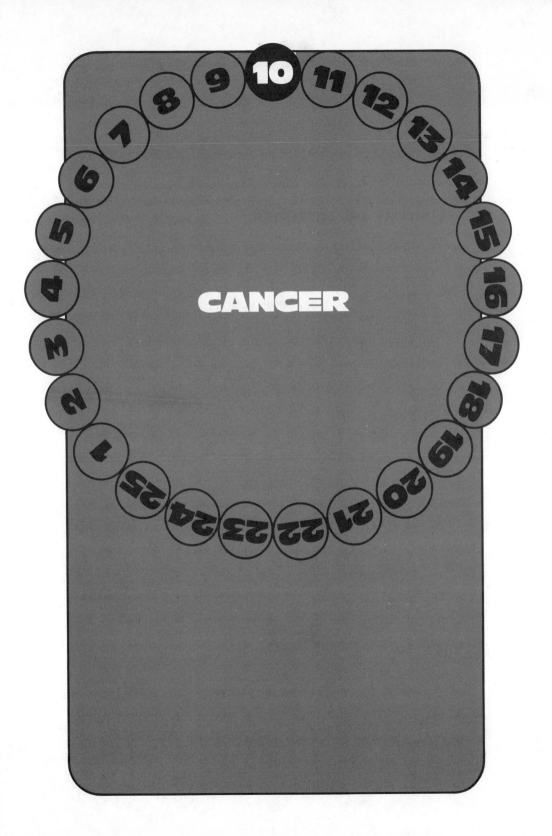

Cancer, a serious problem at any age, is the second leading cause of death among the older population. The incidence of cancer increases with age until the ninth decade, when a tendency for fewer new cases in proportion to that age group is noted. Although the prevalence of most carcinomas is higher among the aged, some forms, such as cervical cancer and sarcomas, are diagnosed less frequently in older persons. Cancer tends to progress more slowly and run a less aggressive course in the aged.

ETIOLOGY AND DETECTION

The exact etiology of cancer is presently unknown, but several factors have been associated with it. Chronic irritation, from pipe smoking for instance, has been known to promote lesions which can become cancerous. Radiation can alter cellular activity and cause abnormal cell growth. Certain agents, such as air pollutants and some food additives, have been found to be carcinogenic. The familial tendency toward certain forms of cancer and the frequent detection of abnormal chromosomal composition of cancer cells raise questions as to the relationship of genes to cancer. Relationships between the incidence of certain forms of cancer in the dietary practices of certain countries also stimulate curiosity. Currently there is speculation as to a viral cause for cancer. Although none of these factors is known to be a definite cause of cancer, gerontological nurses can recognize them as predisposing factors in preventive health practices. The nurse should advise people as follows:

Do not smoke.
Avoid excessive alcohol intake.
Follow a well-balanced diet, avoiding extremes in food temperature and seasoning.
Consult a dentist for poor-fitting dentures or jagged-edged teeth.
Use protection against excessive exposure to sun.
Be alert to signs and symptoms that might indicate cancer: a sore which doesn't heal, unexplained weight loss, a painless mass, increasing digestive problems, blood from any body orifice, or a change in bowel habits.
Receive a complete physical examination, including a rectal and gynecological examination, regularly.

Early detection of cancer improves the potential for a good prognosis. Approximately one-half of the sites that cancer invades can be directly examined—the breast, oral cavity, rectum and skin, for instance—thereby increasing the opportunity for abnormalities to be discovered during a routine physical examination. Unfortunately, people do not always seek regular checkups, waiting, instead, until they feel ill. By the time the disease has progressed to the extent that it causes symptoms, valuable treatment time may be lost and the chances of a good prognosis reduced. Also, symptoms produced by cancer in a particular site may be confused with other problems; for example, constipation associated with cancer of the colon may mistakenly be attributed to poor peristalsis in the aged. If baseline information has been obtained through the nursing assessment, it can provide comparative data for the nurse to use when changes indicating cancer are suspected. An extensive review of cancer facts will not be provided here. Since the general principles of diagnosis and management are similar for old and young, the nurse should consult medical-surgical texts for more information.

FACTORS RELEVANT TO
THE GERONTOLOGICAL NURSE

The gastrointestinal system is frequently the location of cancerous growths. A squamous cell form of cancer may develop on the lip, primarily involving the lower lip. Exposure to sun and irritation from a pipe, teeth, or dentures are among the contributing factors. Cancer of the lip can metastasize to the cervical lymph nodes. Vitamin-B deficiencies, syphilis, excessive smoking, and pressure from jagged edged teeth or dentures can promote cancer of the mouth. Cancer of the tongue can metastasize to local lymph nodes, although it does not usually metastasize to other body organs, and the tonsils can also develop cancer that affects the surrounding lymph nodes. Since bleeding is a symptom that may indicate cancer in this site, and since this symptom can initially be misjudged as hemoptysis, the nurse should carefully examine the mouth and throat when bleeding occurs to more accurately differentiate the cause of the problem. Cancer of the tonsils may be secondary to breast cancer.

There is an increasing incidence of lung cancer, especially among males. A great deal of evidence links a history of smoking to the development of lung cancer. Symptoms of this problem include dyspnea, fever, weakness, cyanosis, and hemoptysis—all of which may be confused with symptoms of other respiratory diseases, thus delaying diagnosis. Without early detection and treatment, metastasis throughout the entire body can occur.

Cancer of the pharynx also requires keen observation and assessment for early detection. Associated symptoms are soreness of and bleeding from the throat and a slight deafness. Cancer of the pharynx may be a result of metastasis from cancer of the esophagus, heart, bronchi, or palate. Tobacco, alcohol, tuberculosis, and irritation from highly seasoned foods may contribute to cancer of the stomach and the

167

esophagus (which is of higher incidence in men). Cancer of the stomach tends to have a poor prognosis due to the difficulty in early diagnosis. Symptoms of stomach cancer—cachexia, weight loss, anemia, hypoalbuminemia, and dyspepsia—are often attributed to other causes, which interferes with early detection. A change in bowel habits, a sign which nurses are often able to detect, should give suspicion as to cancer of the intestines. General symptoms, such as anemia, diarrhea, and weight loss, which can be attributed to other causes, may be indications of cancer of the cecum.

Most persons who develop cancer of the colon and rectum are aged; cancer of the colon occurs more often in females, and cancer of the rectum in males. Cancer of the ascending colon can produce cryptic anemia and a dull pain, which may be easily confused with gallbladder pain. Cancer of the ascending colon can metastasize to the sacral plexus, producing sciatic or back pain. Cancer of the descending colon and rectum can produce anorexia, weight loss, fatigue, weakness, constipation, diarrhea, and bloody, mucus stools. Many masses in this area can be detected through a digital examination; the nurse should make sure the patient is not impacted prior to a digital examination so that a fecal impaction is not confused for a mass. Since cancer in the lower bowel does remain localized for a long time, early surgery is beneficial.

Breast cancer is a serious problem among older women. Any lump in the breast after menopause should give rise to suspicion of breast cancer. Older women should receive instruction regarding the proper method of breast examinations and become familiar with the normal contour of their breasts (Figure 10-1). They should be encouraged to examine their breasts regularly on a specific day of the month, such as their birthday or the day a pension check arrives. Often, a woman will be able to note a change in her breasts more quickly than the physician who examines her several times a year. Any dimpling of the skin or discharge from the nipples should be evaluated. Although cervical cancer does not occur as frequently among older females, they should still be encouraged to receive regular Pap smears and thorough gynecological examinations. Some older women believe that after menopause they needn't be concerned about seeing a gynecologist unless definite symptoms appear; the nurse should be certain to clarify this misconception and encourage regular examinations.

Cancer of the prostate gland is not an uncommon problem for older men, and regular examination of the prostate gland is essential for early detection. A small percentage of benign hypertrophies develop into malignancies, thereby emphasizing the importance of periodic reevaluation of benign prostatic hypertrophy. Cancer at this site is known to metastasize to the pelvis, vertebrae, and brain. Hematuria may be an

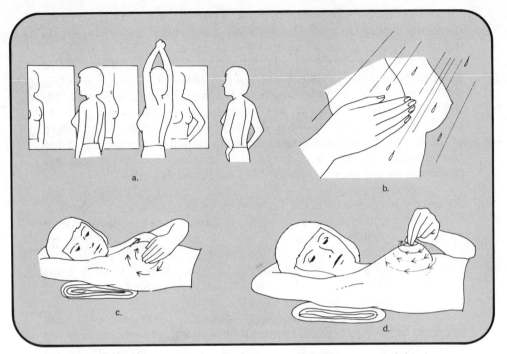

Figure 10-1. Self-examination of breasts: (a) With arms straight at side, arms over head, and hands on hips while flexing chest muscles, inspect breasts before a mirror to detect swelling, changes in contour, dimpling, nipple change, or any other differences. (b) While in tub or shower, run hand over breast with fingers flat to detect thickening or lumps. (c) Inspect breasts while lying down, with folded towel under shoulder of side being examined and arm of that side behind head. (d) With fingers flat, examine outer portion of each breast, progressing in a circular motion around circumference of breast. Move fingers one inch toward center and repeat until entire breast is examined. Then gently squeeze nipple to detect any discharge. (Additional information is available from the American Cancer Society.)

indication of cancer within the genitourinary system and should receive prompt evaluation. Older males tend to have a higher incidence of bladder cancer. Cancer within this system can metastasize to the lungs, liver, lymph nodes, and other organs if not corrected.

Cancer of the pancreas, more prevalent among males, is a difficult problem to diagnose and treat in the aged. Symptoms may include anorexia, weakness, weight loss, dyspepsia, epigastric pain radiating to the back, diarrhea, constipation, obstructive jaundice, and depression and other emotional changes. Sometimes venous thrombosis occurs, believed to be caused by an elevation in serum trypsin. Since these

169

symptoms can be confused with those of pancreatitis and peptic ulcer, diagnosis is often delayed. Unfortunately, surgery and chemotherapy do not offer much success in treatment of pancreatic cancer at this time. Cancer of the gallbladder is also difficult to diagnose and treat. Most persons having this problem are aged. Unlike pancreatic cancer, it tends to have a higher incidence among women. Symptoms of gallbladder cancer include anorexia, weakness, nausea, vomiting, weight loss, pain in the right upper quadrant, jaundice, and constipation. The nature of these symptoms makes early detection difficult. Metastasis to the common duct, peritoneum, lungs, and ovaries can occur, and the prognosis for the patient with gallbladder cancer is poor.

Hoarseness may be an early symptom of cancer of the larynx, and should be evaluated for such. Fortunately, metastasis is rare. Cancer of the thyroid gland is rare among the aged. Skin cancer can develop from excessive exposure to the sun or chronic irritation. Sores which do not heal, new lesions, or changes in the appearance of moles in the aged should arouse suspicion. Depending on location and size, a good prognosis can result from the use of excision, radiation, and electrodesiccation and currettage.

There is a high incidence of leukemia, lymphosarcoma, and myeloma in the aged. Acute leukemia runs an aggressive course in the aged, although chemotherapy is often successful in producing remissions. Chronic lymphocytic leukemia or myeloma, on the other hand, is not an aggressive disease in the aged. Multiple myeloma can be extremely painful and disabling to the aged, but fortunately, the incidence of this disease is lower in older age groups. Hodgkin's disease tends to run a more aggressive course in the aged. Anemia, leukopenia, and thrombocytopenia occur with both multiple myeloma and Hodgkin's disease in the aged.

As mentioned earlier, treatment of cancer in the aged will be basically similar to treatment methods selected for younger adults, striving toward cure with minimal limitation. Surgery may prove beneficial but it should be remembered that the aged are a higher surgical risk. The benefits of chemotherapy must be weighed against the side effects it may cause in the aged. A therapeutic ratio is usually sought whereby the optimum effect is achieved with the least toxicity. Individualized decisions for cancer management are based on the general health status of the person, the form of cancer, the expected outcome, and the preference of the patient. At no time should treatment be discouraged or withheld due to age alone.

The nurse is a key figure in cancer management. It may be the nurse who first detects a symptom of cancer and who can facilitate a prompt diagnosis. The nurse can offer support and explanations during the diagnostic process. Once a positive diagnosis is made, the nurse can help the patient work through the denial, anger, depression, and other reactions frequently associated with a new diagnosis of cancer. While providing hope, the nurse can also guide the patient toward a realistic understanding of the outcomes of his or her disease. If disability and death are to be expected, the patient and his family may need strong nursing support as they learn to accept and plan for these consequences. On the other hand, patients with a good prognosis should be encouraged not to self-impose limitations or become "emotional cripples" as a result of having had a diagnosis of cancer. Within a realistic framework, all patients with cancer should be inspired to maintain a normal life-style and maximize their existing capacities.

When the terminal stage of cancer is reached, additional nursing intervention may be required to compensate for the patient's increasing limitations. The relief of pain is a priority for terminally ill patients. Concern as to the reality of the pain or the risk of narcotic addiction should not prevent the administration of analgesics. A low dosage should be administered initially, with periodic reevaluations as to the need for dosage change. To reduce stress and preserve energy of the terminal patient, analgesics should be given to *prevent* pain and not only *correct* it once it has already occurred. The nurse should observe the nature of the pain as the disease progresses; as death approaches, less pain may be sensed, and consequently less analgesics required to provide relief. Small, frequent feedings of foods enjoyed by the patient may compensate for poor appetite and promote a better food intake. Vitamin and protein supplements may be beneficial. An ample fluid intake should be maintained.

The skin should be kept clean, dry and unbroken. Due to the general debilitated state of the patient, skin breakdown may be a greater risk. Frequent skin care can provide cleanliness, comfort, and prevention of breakdown. Comfort is important, physically and psychologically. Certain forms of cancer produce an unpleasant odor, and the nurse should maintain an attractive appearance of the patient, especially in light of any disfigurement, weight loss, jaundice, or other changes which may be taking place. Positioning should provide optimum comfort. Environmental considerations—such as adequate ventilation, soft lights, and a clean area—mean a great deal to the bedridden patient and the family. Opportunities for conversations should be provided. The terminally ill patient and the family may need to discuss their relationships, feelings, and the impending death. Involvement of the clergy may provide valuable support to them. The skills of the nurse may determine if the patient's death will be an unnecessarily traumatic experience, or one of beauty and dignity.

171

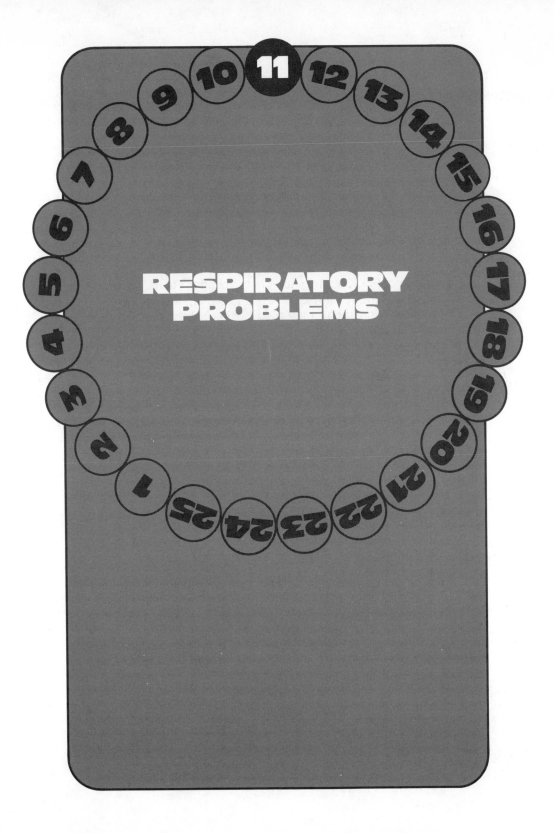

RESPIRATORY
PROBLEMS

Respiratory problems are among the more common and life-threatening disorders the aged experience. Influenza and pneumonia are the fourth leading causes of death, and bronchitis, emphysema, and asthma rank eighth. In addition to the high mortality that results, respiratory diseases impose many limitations that prevent aged people from enjoying an active, full life. Various aging changes, which increase the susceptibility and decrease the capacity of a person to manage these disorders, may explain their high prevalence among the aged. In general, the respiratory system functions less efficiently with advancing age. The lungs lose their elasticity and increase in size, contributing to a higher residual volume and lower vital capacity. The lung capillaries are fewer in number. Bronchioles and alveoli lose elasticity as well. The blood oxygen level (PO_2) may be 75 mmHg instead of 90–95 mmHg, as it is in younger adults; however, the blood carbon dioxide level (PCO_2) tends to remain the same.

Respiratory limitations may also be imposed by other changes associated with aging, such as a more rigid rib cage, ossification of costal cartilage, and a stooped posture which may decrease the chest capacity. To compound these problems, it is not unusual for several respiratory diseases to be present at the same time in an aged individual, thereby complicating the management of any one disease and increasing the risk of developing serious complications. Although most older persons are able to meet ordinary respiratory demands despite these changes to the respiratory system, there is reduced efficiency primarily in the following areas:

1. Meeting respiratory demands under unusual or stressful circumstances
2. Lower resistance to respiratory infections
3. Greater difficulty managing a respiratory problem once one develops

Smoking is the most important factor contributing to respiratory disease. Many of today's older smokers started their habit at a time when the full effects of smoking weren't realized. In fact, when today's aged were young, smoking was considered fashionable, sociable, and a sign of maturity. Like any habit, smoking is not an easy habit to break. Although an individual may be aware of the health hazards associated with smoking, the immediate gratification many times outweighs the potential risks. The effects on the respiratory system may initially be so subtle and gradual that they are not noticed. Unfortunately, by the time respiratory symptoms and signs become serious and uncomfortable enough to stimulate smokers to change their smoking habits, permanent damage may have already been done to the respiratory system.

TABLE 11-1: DEATH RATES FOR
RESPIRATORY DISEASES BY SEX AND AGE

	Influenza and Pneumonia	Emphysema
Male		
15–24	2.4	0
25–44	5.7	0.6
45–64	30.0	22.0
65 and over	266.1	151.4
Female		
15–24	1.6	0
25–44	4.0	0.3
45–64	15.0	6.0
65 and over	171.1	22.3

Source: U.S. Bureau of the Census, *Statistical Abstract of the United States: 1975.* 96th Ed., Washington, D.C., 1975, p. 61, No. 86. Death rates per 100,000 for 1973.

Smoking is the major cause of chronic bronchitis. Smokers have a higher incidence of respiratory disease and a higher incidence of complications with respiratory disease than nonsmokers. Commonly, smokers have a productive cough, episodes of shortness of breath, and a reduced breathing capacity. Also, smokers have twice the incidence of lung cancer. Gerontological nurses should be actively involved with preventing young persons from developing a smoking habit. Education as to the health problems associated with smoking and positive reinforcement to nonsmokers may promote the health of future aged persons. Local health departments and respiratory disease associations provide specific information on various antismoking programs and strategies to help smokers forfeit their habit, and the nurse can help make smokers aware of these programs.

COMMON DISORDERS IN THE AGED

Pneumonia

Pneumonia is common in the aged, especially bronchopneumonia, and as mentioned, it is one of the leading causes of death in this age group. There was a time when pneumonia in an aged person meant death, but fortunately the discovery of antibiotics has significantly reduced the mortality and morbidity associated with this disease. There are several factors contributing to the high incidence. Changes to the respiratory system with age may cause poor chest expansion and more

175

shallow breathing. The aged may have other respiratory diseases which promote mucus formation and bronchial obstruction. Upper respiratory infection is more frequent in the aged, especially since they already have a lowered resistance to infection. The reduced sensitivity of pharyngeal reflexes in many aged persons may promote aspiration of foreign material. Also, the aged are more likely to be debilitated and immobile.

The signs and symptoms of pneumonia may be altered in older persons. A serious pneumonia may exist without symptoms being evident. Pleuritic pain, for instance, may not be as severe as that described by younger patients. Differences in body temperature may cause little or no fever to be present. Symptoms may include a slight cough, fatigue, and rapid respiration. Confusion, restlessness, and behavioral changes may occur as a result of cerebral hypoxia. Nursing care for the geriatric patient with pneumonia is similar to that employed for the younger patient. Close observation for subtle changes is especially important. A complication which the aged patient may develop is paralytic ileus, prevented by mobility.

Asthma

Some aged have been affected with asthma throughout their lives, some develop it during old age. The symptoms and management do not differ much from those of other age groups. Epinephrine, antibiotics, and occasionally adrenocorticosteroids are used in treating older asthmatics. Because of the added stress asthma places on the heart, older asthmatics have a high risk of developing complications such as bronchiectasis and cardiac problems. The nurse should assist in detecting causative factors and should educate the patient regarding early recognition and prompt attention to an asthma attack when it does occur. Careful assessment of the aged asthmatic's use of aerosal nebulizers is advisable. Cardiac arrhythmias leading to sudden death may be risked by the overuse of sympathomimetic bronchodilating nebulizers (Stolley, 1972).

Chronic Bronchitis

Many aged persons demonstrate the persistent, productive cough and wheezing and the recurrent respiratory infections and shortness of breath caused by chronic bronchitis. As with many other chronic respiratory diseases, these symptoms may develop gradually, sometimes taking years for the full impact of the disease to be realized, at which time the patients notice increased difficulty breathing in cold and damp weather due to bronchospasm. They experience more frequent respiratory infections and greater difficulty in managing them. Episodes of hypoxia begin to occur as mucus obstructs the bronchial tree and causes carbon dioxide retention. As the disease progresses, emphysema may develop and death may occur from obstruction. The management of this problem, aimed at removing bronchial secretions and preventing obstruction of the airway, is similar for all age groups. Older patients may need special encouragement to maintain a good fluid intake and expectorate secretions. The nurse can be most effective in preventing the development of chronic bronchitis by discouraging chronic respiratory irritation, such as from smoking, and by helping the aged to prevent respiratory infections.

Emphysema

Of increasing incidence in the aged population is the progressive, chronic, and obstructive lung disease emphysema. Factors causing this destructive disease include asthma, chronic bronchitis, and chronic irritation from dusts or certain air pollutants. Cigarette smoking also plays a major role in the development of emphysema. The symptoms are slow in onset and initially may resemble those of the changes in the respiratory system that come with age, causing many patients to have delayed identification and treatment of this disease. Gradually, increased dyspnea is experienced, which is not relieved by sitting upright as it may have been in the past. A chronic cough develops. As more effort is required for breathing and as hypoxia occurs, fatigue, anorexia, weight loss, and weakness are demonstrated. Recurrent respiratory infections, malnutrition, congestive heart failure, and cardiac arrhythmias are among the more life-threatening complications the aged can experience from emphysema.

Treatment usually includes postural drainage, intermittent positive pressure breathing, bronchodilators, the avoidance of stressful situations and breathing exercises, which are an important part of patient education (Figure 11-1). Cigarette smoking should definitely be stopped. The older patient especially may have a problem with adequate food and fluid intake, requiring special nursing attention. If oxygen is utilized, it must be done with extreme caution and close supervision. It must be remembered that for this patient, a low oxygen level rather than a high carbon dioxide level stimulates respiration. The older patient with emphysema is a high risk candidate for the development of carbon dioxide narcosis. Respiratory infections should be prevented, and any which do occur, regardless of how minor they may seem, should be promptly reported to the physician. Sedatives, hypnotics, and narcotics may be contraindicated because the patient will be more sensitive to these drugs. Patients with emphysema need a great deal of education and support to be able to manage this disease. It is very difficult to adjust to the fact that one has a serious chronic disease requiring special care or even a change in life-style. The patient must learn to pace activities, avoid extremely cold weather, administer medications correctly, and recognize symptoms of infection.

Tuberculosis

The incidence of tuberculosis is increasing among the aged, and a high incidence is found in institutional settings. Rather than a new infection, the aged usually experience a reactivation of an earlier infection which was either asymptomatic or improperly treated. Diagnosis may be delayed, either because the classic symptoms are not demonstrated or because symptoms resemble changes associated with the aging process. For instance, anorexia and weakness may be the primary symptoms. Night sweats may not occur due to reduced diaphoresis with advanced age. Likewise, fever may not be detected due to alterations in the aged's body temperature. These factors emphasize the importance of periodic evaluation for this disease. Screening for tuberculosis should be performed for all patients entering a hospital or facility for geriatric care, and, periodically, groups of aged persons, such as golden age clubs and senior citizen associations, should be checked.

Treatment follows the same principles as for any age group, basically consisting of rest, good nutrition, and medications. Some of the side effects of medications commonly prescribed for tuberculosis have special implications for aged persons. Streptomycin can cause damage to the peripheral and central nervous systems, demonstrated through hearing limitations and disequilibrium. The safety hazards created by these adverse reactions are significant to the aged. Para-aminosalcylic acid can cause irritation to the gastrointestinal tract, anorexia, nausea, vomiting, and diarrhea—predisposing the aged to the risk of malnutrition. In addition, changes in gastric secretions can cause these tablets to pass through the gastrointestinal system without being dissolved, thereby preventing a therapeutic benefit. Stools should be examined for undissolved tablets. Isoniazid, although not as toxic as the other drugs mentioned, can have toxic effects on the peripheral and central nervous systems. The nurse must continuously assess the patient for the appearance of adverse reactions from such medications.

A diagnosis of tuberculosis can be extremely difficult for older persons to accept. Having lived through a time when people with tuberculosis were sent away to sanitariums for long periods of time, they may be unaware of new approaches and fear institutionalization. Believing they might infect family and friends, they may avoid contact with others, promoting social isolation. It is also possible that other people will fear contracting the disease and be reluctant to maintain social contact. Education of patients, their family, and friends is essential in order to clarify these misconceptions, promote a normal life-style.

Two different types of breathing exercises include pursed lip breathing and diaphragm retraining exercises. Since their purpose is to effect a change in the patient's breathing pattern, both should be shown to the patient as a simultaneous effort.

Instruction should include the following:

1. Inhale a normal breath through the nose to the count of one to humidify and cleanse the air.
2. Relax and exhale to the count of three using pursed lips to facilitate CO_2 elimination.
3. Neither gasp for the next breath nor force air out past the count of three. The goal is to develop a slow respiratory rate with an inspiratory-expiratory ratio of 1:3 or 1:4.
4. Place one hand (hand A) below the ribs on the stomach. Place the other hand (hand B) over the middle anterior chest. During exhalation, firmly press hand A inward and upward on the stomach to assist the lungs in expelling air. Concentrate on increasing stomach movement (hand A will rise on expiration and fall on inspiration) and decreasing chest movement (hand B should not move).

By permission of Hilary D. Sigmon, R.N., M.S.N., Clinical Specialist, Johns Hopkins Hospital.

Figure 11-1. Breathing exercises.

Patients should be taught their responsibilities in managing this disease. Medication is essential for the treatment of tuberculosis, and since the aged person may have a problem remembering to take it, nurses should devise a system for helping the patient remember how to administer the medication. For example, medications and denture cream could be placed in the same box so that during daily denture care medications would be remembered; the patient, a family member, or a visiting nurse could fill seven envelopes with medications, labeling them for each day of the week, and devise a chart for recording when medication is taken; a family member or friend could call the patient daily to ask whether medication was taken. With prompt and proper therapy, the aged person can recover from tuberculosis with minimal residual effects.

Lung Cancer

It is uncertain whether the increased incidence of lung cancer in the aged population is due to more cases of lung cancer actually occurring or improved diagnostic tools and greater availability of medical care. Lung cancer occurs more frequently in men, and there is a higher mortality from lung cancer among Caucasions. Cigarette smokers have twice the incidence of nonsmokers. There is also a high incidence among individuals who are chronically exposed to agents such as asbestos, coal gas, radioactive dusts, and chromates. This emphasizes the significance of obtaining thorough information regarding a patient's occupational history as part of the nursing assessment. Although conclusive evidence is presently unavailable, there is some association between the presence of lung scars (such as those resulting from tuberculosis and pneumonitis) and lung cancer.

The individual may have lung cancer long before any symptoms develop. This suggests that individuals at high risk should be regularly screened and should obtain periodic roentgenograms to detect this disease in an early stage. Dyspnea, coughing, chest pain, fatigue, anorexia, wheezing, and recurrent upper respiratory infections are part of the symptomatology seen as the disease progresses. Diagnosis is confirmed through chest roentgenogram, sputum cytology, bronchoscopy, and biopsy. Treatment may consist of surgery, chemotherapy, or radiotherapy, requiring the same type of nursing care for patients of any age with this diagnosis.

Lung Abscess

A lung abscess may result from pneumonia, tuberculosis, a malignancy, or trauma to the lung. Aspiration of foreign material can also cause a lung abscess and this may be a particular risk to aged persons who have decreased pharyngeal reflexes. Symptoms, resembling those of many other respiratory problems, include anorexia, weight loss, fatigue, temperature elevation, and a chronic cough. Sputum production may occur, but this is not always demonstrated in aged persons. Diagnosis and management are the same as for other age groups. Modifications for postural drainage, an important component of the treatment, will be discussed later in this chapter. Since protein can be lost through the sputum, a high-protein, high-caloric diet should be encouraged to maintain and improve the nutritional status of the aged patient.

Bronchiectasis

Bronchiectasis does not occur as frequently in older age groups as it does in the young. Aged persons can develop this problem from chronic bronchitis, asthma, recurrent upper respiratory infections, or aspiration of foreign material. There is also some belief that the weakening of the bronchioles with increased age causes a breakdown of the alveolar and bronchiolar walls. The most outstanding symptoms that older persons demonstrate are a temperature elevation and a chronic cough that produces large amounts of foul-smelling sputum. Diagnostic measures and treatment are similar to those for other age groups. Postural drainage, modified for the aged, and a high-protein high-caloric diet are essential components of the treatment plan.

NURSING CONSIDERATIONS

Respiratory problems are serious for aged individuals. They are at greater risk of developing respiratory complications in association with other diseases and also as a result of changes in the respiratory system with age. Once respiratory diseases have developed, close monitoring of the patient's status is required to minimize disability and prevent mortality. Close nursing observation can prevent and detect respiratory complications. Changes in the rate and volume of respirations can indicate respiratory problems, as can distended neck veins. A sudden increase in pulse can occur with hypoxia. Chronic hypoxia can cause an elevated blood pressure. Changes in mental status may also be associated with hypoxia. The nurse should assist the patient in the removal of secretions and regularly check for the patency of the airway. Body temperature should be frequently checked for elevations, not only to detect an infectious process, but to prevent stress on the cardiovascular and respiratory systems as they attempt to meet the body's increased oxygen demands imposed by an elevated temperature.

Since the aged may have reduced cough efficiency, the nature of the cough and the quality and quantity of sputum production should be observed and documented. To avoid embarrassment, some individuals learn to suppress a chronic cough; the nurse can ascertain this during her assessment by asking the patient to take several deep breaths, which will usually trigger any chronic cough. On the other hand, excessive coughing must be controlled to conserve energy and prevent added stress to the aged heart. The cautious use of medications, especially of diuretics and digitalis, is necessary because drug metabolism can be altered by situations reducing the body's oxygen. For optimum respiratory function the nurse should encourage correct posture, a good diet, the avoidance of obesity, paced activity, prophylactic influenza vaccines, diaphragmatic exercises, protection against and early treatment of upper respiratory infection, regular respiratory examination, and the avoidance of immobility.

One special measure of significance for aged patients with respiratory disorders is the accurate administration of oxygen, which must be used with extreme caution (Figure 11-2). If oxygen is prescribed for home use, the patient and the family must be thoroughly instructed in its safe and correct use. Frequent evaluations of arterial blood gases are essential. The nurse should evaluate the value of one method of oxygen administration over another. Older patients who breathe by mouth or have poor control in keeping their lips sealed most of the time, may not receive the full benefit of a nasal cannula. An emaciated older person whose facial structure does not allow for a tight seal of a face mask may lose a significant portion of oxygen through leakage. A patient who is insecure and anxious inside an oxygen tent may spend oxygen for emotional stress and not gain full therapeutic benefit. When nurses identify problems with the route of oxygen administration, they should make the physician aware of what method would be most effective for the particular patient. The oxygen flow should be checked frequently for any interruption or blockage from an empty oxygen tank, kinked tubing, or any other cause. The patient should be evaluated for hypoxia and suctioned when necessary. The nasal passages should be regularly cleaned to maintain patency. It must be remembered that some aged patients will not become cyanotic when hypoxic, thus close nursing observation for insufficient oxygenation is essential.

Postural drainage is commonly prescribed for the removal of bronchial secretions in certain respiratory diseases. The general procedure is the same for the aged, with some modifications. If aerosal medications are prescribed, they should be administered preceding the postural drainage. The position for postural drainage depends on the individual patient and on the portion of the lung involved. The older patient should change positions slowly and have a few minutes rest between position changes to allow for accommodation to the new position. The usual last position for postural drainage—lying face down across the bed with the head at floor level—may be stressful for the aged and cause adverse effects. The nurse can consult with the physician as to the advisability of this particular position and possible alterations to meet the needs of the individual patient. Cupping and vibration facilitate drainage of secretions; it should be remembered that old tissues and bones are more fragile and may more easily become injured. The nurse should discontinue the procedure and inform the physician if dyspnea, palpitation, chest pain, diaphoresis, apprehension, or any other signs of distress occur. Thorough oral hygiene and a period of rest should follow postural drainage. Documentation of the tolerance of the procedure and the amount and characteristic of the mucus drained is essential.

Coughing to remove secretions is important in the management of respiratory problems; however nonproductive coughing may be a useless expenditure of energy and stressful to the older patient. A variety of measures can be employed to promote effective coughing. Hard candy and other sweets increase secretions, thereby loosening the cough. Breathing exercises, as shown in Figure 11-1 will promote a productive cough. The patient can be instructed to take slow, full respirations, forcefully exhaling with pursed lips. The focus should be on relaxing abdominal muscles during inspiration and contracting them during

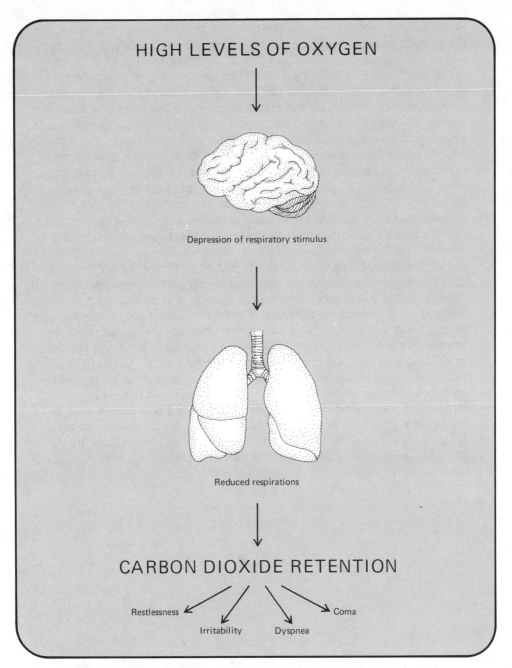

HIGH LEVELS OF OXYGEN

Depression of respiratory stimulus

Reduced respirations

CARBON DIOXIDE RETENTION

Restlessness   Irritability   Dyspnea   Coma

Figure 11-2. Oxygen must be administered to the aged with caution. High levels of oxygen can depress the respiratory stimulus in the brain, thereby reducing respiration and promoting carbon dioxide retention.

183

expiration. An intermittent positive-pressure breathing machine may be prescribed, proving especially beneficial to a weak patient or one who will not comply with breathing exercises. Bronchodilators may or may not be used with this machine. The IPPB machine may be prescribed for home use; the patient should be fully instructed in its use and must understand not to readjust the pressure gauge without the physician's advice. A variety of humidifiers, which may be purchased without a physician's prescription, are available; the nurse should ensure that the patient understands the safe, correct use of such apparatus. Expectorants may also be prescribed to loosen secretions and make coughing more productive. A good fluid intake will be helpful in liquifying secretions. Patients should be advised to use paper tissues, not cloth handkerchiefs, for sputum expectoration. Paper bags within easy reach of the patient should be used for tissue disposal; careful disposal of sputum must be emphasized. Frequent hand washing and oral hygiene are essential, having several physical and psychological benefits.

Respiratory problems are very frightening and anxiety producing. These patients will need psychological support and reassurance, especially during periods of dyspnea. Patients should have a complete understanding of their disease and its management to help reduce their anxiety. Repeated encouragement may be required to assist the patient in meeting the demands of a chronic respiratory disease. Some patients may find it necessary to spend most of their time indoors to avoid extremes of hot and cold weather; some may move to a different climate for relief. These changes in life-style may have a significant impact on the aged's total life. As with any chronic disease, patients and their families can benefit from nursing intervention as they adjust to the physical, emotional, and social adjustments associated with the disease.

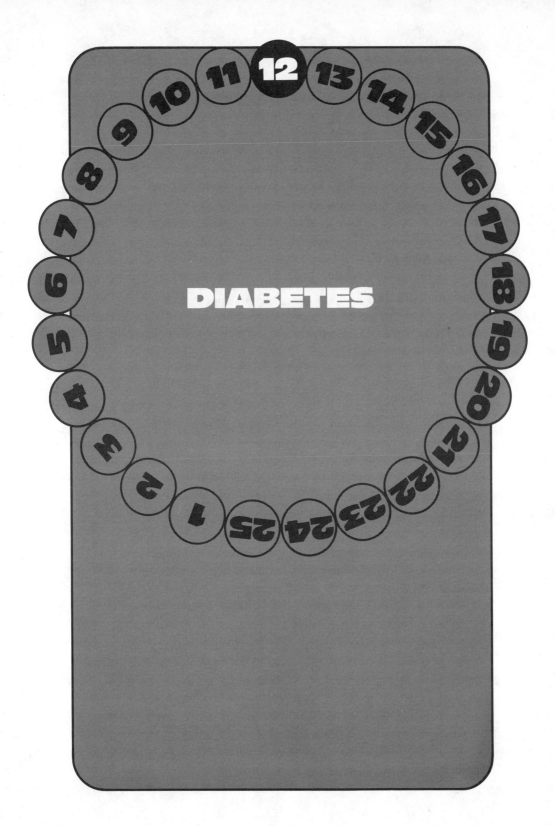

A proficient blend of various kinds of knowledge and skills is required in nursing diabetics, and older diabetics, with their unique set of problems, present an even greater challenge. Diabetes, the seventh leading cause of death among the aged, has a particularly high prevalence among blacks and among persons 65 to 74 years of age. Consequently, nurses have to be adequately informed of how the detection and management of diabetes in aged persons differs from that in others. The increasing number of individuals achieving old age, and the expanding health care services for the aged further emphasize the necessity for nurses to become prepared in meeting the needs of older diabetics.

DIAGNOSIS

Several explanations are offered for the high prevalence of hyperglycemia among the aged. Some researchers claim that a physiologic deterioration of glucose tolerance occurs with increasing age (Andres, 1967). Others believe that the high prevalence of glucose intolerance is a result of an increase in the incidence of diabetes throughout the general population. Regardless of the reason behind glucose intolerance in the aged, it is agreed that different standards must be applied in evaluating their glucose tolerance.

Early diagnosis of diabetes in older persons is often quite difficult. The classic symptoms of diabetes may be absent, leaving nonspecific symptoms as the only clues. Some indications of diabetes are orthostatic hypotension, stroke, gastric hypotony, impotence, neuropathy, glaucoma, dupuytren's contracture, and infection. Laboratory tests, as well as symptoms, may be misleading. Since the renal threshold for glucose increases with age, older individuals can be hyperglycemic without evidence of glycosuria, thus limiting the validity of urine testing for glucose. Fasting blood sugar testing is not a dependable diagnostic measure since some aged individuals may have a normal fasting blood sugar level while experiencing significant hyperglycemic levels after meals (Rifkin and Ross, 1971a).

Of all the diagnostic measures, the glucose tolerance test is the most effective, and to avoid a false positive diagnosis, it is recommended that more than one test be performed (McDonald, Fisher, and Burnham, 1965). The American Diabetes Association recommends that a minimum of 150 grams of carbohydrate be ingested daily for several days prior to the test; older malnourished individuals may be prescribed 300 grams. Recent periods of inactivity, stressful illness, and inadequate dietary intake should be communicated to the physician, since these situations can contribute to glucose intolerance. In such circumstances, more accurate results can be obtained if the test is postponed to one month after the episode. Nicotinic acid, ethacrynic acid, estrogen,

186

TABLE 12-1: AGE-RELATED
GRADIENTS FOR GLUCOSE TOLERANCE TESTS

U.S.P.H.S. Standard Values*		Age-Related Gradients Based on U.S.P.H.S. Values		
Sample Time	Point Values (2 points = Diabetes)	55–64 Years	65–74 Years	75–85+ Years
Fasting 110	1	110	110	110
1 Hour 170	½	180	190	200
2 Hour 120	½	130	140	150
3 Hour 110	1	120	130	140

Source: Charles R. Shuman, *Special Problems of the Older Diabetic,* scientific exhibit at the AMA Clinical Convention, Cincinnati, Ohio, November 26–29, 1972.
Note: Increments of 10 mg/% added to one- two- and three-hour values in standard curve for each decade; fasting values remain unchanged.
* Values given for venous whole blood in mg/%-plasma values are 15% higher.

furosemide, and diuretics can decrease glucose tolerance and should not be administered prior to testing. Monoamine-oxidase inhibitors, propranolol, and high dosages of salicylates may lower blood sugar and also interfere with testing.

The usual nursing measures are applied during glucose tolerance testing of the aged. If unusual symptoms develop during the test, such as mental confusion, it is important to tell the physician. Those interpreting the glucose tolerance test may find it beneficial to utilize age-related gradients (Table 12-1). For each decade after age 55, 10 mg/% are added to the standard values at the first, second, and third hours. Thus, a glucose level which would be significantly elevated for a 35-year-old may be within normal limits for an 85-year-old.

MANAGEMENT

Although the basic principles of diabetic management are applicable to all age groups, special considerations and adjustments must be made for the older diabetic. It is impractical and unrealistic to expect that individuals who have established specific practices over the past six or seven decades will drastically alter their life-style when diagnosed as diabetics. Many compromises may be required by the diabetic individual *and* the professionals managing his or her care.

Educating the Older Diabetic

Once the diagnosis has been confirmed, a teaching plan should be established by the nurse. Diabetes is known as a serious and chronic

187

problem to most lay individuals, and it is frightening to have it diagnosed in oneself. Fear and anxiety can interfere with the learning process for newly diagnosed older diabetics, who may have witnessed the crippling or fatal effects of diabetes in others and associate them with themselves. Having lived through a period in which diabetes was not able to be successfully managed and was always severely disabling or fatal, the older individual may not be aware of the advancements in diabetic management. Insulin was isolated in 1921, when many of today's elderly were children and young adults.

Elderly persons may be depressed or angry that this disease further threatens the short period of their remaining life; they may question the "trade-off" value in exchanging an unrestricted life-style for a potentially longer but restricted life. Concerns may arise as to how a special diet and medications will be afforded on an already limited budget. Social isolation may develop from fear of becoming ill in public or facing restrictions that make diabetics different from their peers. They may question their ability to manage their diabetes independently and worry that institutionalization will be necessary. These and a multitude of other concerns which the older diabetic may have must be recognized and dealt with by the nurse to reduce the risk of other limitations and to promote the individual's self-care capacities. Reassurance, support, and information can reduce barriers to learning about and managing diabetes. The following steps, helpful in any patient education situation, may offer guidance in teaching the older diabetic.

1. **Assessment of Readiness to Learn.** Discomfort, anxiety and depression may block learning and the retention of knowledge. Relieving these symptoms and allowing time for patients to develop to the point where they desire and can cope with information may be necessary.
2. **Assessment of Learning Capacities and Limitations.** This would include consideration of educational level, language problems, literacy, present knowledge, willingness to learn, cultural background, previous experience with the illness, memory, vision, hearing, speech, and mental status.
3. **Outline of What to Teach.** Your outline should not only be specific and clear, but should also consider learning priorities. Nurses sometimes feel obligated to teach every last detail about an illness, compacting a multitude of new facts and procedures into a short time frame. Most people need time to receive, absorb, sort, and translate new information into behavioral changes; the elderly are no different. Altered brain function or slower responses may further interfere with learning

in the aged. Patients and their families should have a role in setting teaching priorities; the most vital information should be given first, followed by other relevant material. Visiting nurses and other resources should be used after hospital discharge to continue the teaching plan if the proposed outline is not completed during the hospitalization.

4. *Altering the Teaching Plan in View of Capacities and Limitations.* The nurse may feel that an explanation of the physiological effects of diabetes is significant for new diabetics. However, the older person who tends to be confused or has a poor memory may not have long-range benefit from this type of information. It may be better to use that time to reinforce diet information or to make sure the most significant information required for self-care is retained.

5. *Preparing the Patient for the Teaching-Learning Session.* Patients should understand that education is an integral part of care and not just icing on the cake. Whenever possible, a specific time should be arranged in advance to avoid conflict with other activities and to allow the family to be present if desired.

6. *Providing an Environment Conducive to Learning.* An area that is quiet, clean, relaxing, and free from odors and interference will help to create a good atmosphere for learning. Distraction should be minimal, especially in view of the aged's reduced capacity to manage multiple stimuli.

7. *Using the Most Effective Individualized Educational Method.* The nurse must recognize the limitations of standard teaching aids and the importance of individualized methods. An aid that was successful for one person may not be effective for another. The variety of sophisticated audio-visual aids that are commercially prepared and available in many agencies as resources for nurses are impressive; but they may not necessarily be effective for the given patient. The quality of an audio cassette may be excellent, but it is of little benefit to the older person with a hearing problem. A slide presentation, even slowly paced, may present facts more rapidly than can be absorbed by an older person with delayed response time. The print on a commercial pamphlet may appear minute to older eyes. The language used in many commercial materials may not be one to which the person is accustomed. Original handmade aids suited for the individual's unique needs may have a value equal to or greater than commercially prepared ones. Selectivity in methodology is essential.

189

8. **_Using Several Approaches to the Same Body of Knowledge._** The greater number of different exposures to new material, the higher the probability that the material will be learned. Combine verbal explanation with flipcharts, diagrams, pamphlets, demonstrations, discussions with other patients, and audio-visual resources.

9. **_Leaving Material with the Patient for Later Review._** It is often helpful to summarize the teaching session in writing, using language familiar to the patient. This provides concrete material which the patient can independently review later and also share with the family.

10. **_Reinforcing Key Points._** Reinforcement should be regular and consistent, with all staff members supporting the teaching plan. For example, if the objective of the nurse caring for the patient has been to increase competency in self-injection of insulin, then the person substituting on the nurse's day off should comply with the established objectives rather than administering the insulin for the individual. Informal reinforcement of information during other daily activities should also be planned.

11. **_Obtaining Feedback._** Evaluate whether the patient and family have accurately received and understood the information communicated. This can be done by observing return demonstrations, asking questions, and listening to discussions among patients.

12. **_Periodic Reevaluating._** To ascertain retention and effectiveness of the teaching sessions, informally reevaluate at a later time. Remember that retention of information may be especially difficult for the older individual.

13. **_Documentation._** Describe specifically what was taught, when, who was involved, what methodology was used, the patient's reaction and understanding, and future plans for remaining learning needs. This assists the staff caring for patients during their hospitalization and also serves as a guide for those providing continued care after discharge.

Care and Health Supervision

One factor which must be considered in the management of the older diabetic is that the ability to handle a syringe and vial of insulin may be decreased due to arthritic fingers. Several return demonstrations of this skill should be performed during the hospitalization, especially on days in which arthritis discomfort is actively present. As most elderly persons have some degree of visual impairment, the ability to read the

TABLE 12-2: INSULINS USED IN
THE MANAGEMENT OF DIABETES MELLITUS

Types of Insulin	Onset of Action	Peak	Duration
Fast-acting			
Injection: Regular, unmodified	20–30 min	1–2 hr	5–8 hr
Zinc suspension: prompt, crystalline (Semi-Lente)	50–60 min	2–3 hr	6–8 hr
Medium-acting			
Globin, with zinc	1–2 hr	8–16 hr	18–24 hr
Isophane suspension (NPH)	1–2 hr	10–20 hr	28–30 hr
Zinc suspension (Lente)	1–2 hr	10–20 hr	20–32 hr
Long-acting			
Zinc suspension, extended (Ultra-Lente)	4–6 hr	16–24 hr	24–36 hr
Protamine zinc suspension (Protamine Zinc)	4–6 hr	16–24 hr	24–36 hr

calibrations on an insulin syringe must be evaluated. The yellowing of the lens with age tends to filter out low-tone colors, such as blues and greens; since these colors are frequently used to identify various levels of glycosuria in urine testing kits, it is important to assess the older individual's ability to discriminate these shades. Older individuals may also be limited in their ability to purchase and prepare adequate meals due to financial, energy, or social limitations. Since this can interfere with management of the illness, Meals on Wheels, food stamps, the assistance of a neighbor, and other appropriate resources should be utilized to assist the individual.

Altered tubule reabsorption of glucose may lead to inaccurate results from urine testing. As mentioned, the older individual can be hyperglycemic without being glycosuric. On the other hand, higher blood glucose levels are common in the aged, and minimal or mild glycosuria is not usually treated with insulin (Rifkin and Ross, 1971b). Although nurses aren't responsible for prescribing the insulin coverage, they need to be aware that the insulin requirements of the older diabetic are individualized. Responses to various insulin levels are to be carefully observed and communicated to the physician. Table 12-2 reviews the various insulins that may be prescribed. As insulins are selected not only for their timing but for their specific tolerance by the patient, the nurse must be careful to administer the correct type of insulin prescribed. The patients must understand that they cannot borrow a vial of insulin from a friend if their supply should become exhausted.

Attempts should be made to maintain a consistent daily food

intake, as the insulin dosage is prescribed to cover a specific amount of food. This may be a problem if the elderly person has a minimal food intake during the week when alone but an increased intake when visiting with family on weekends or if he or she skimps on meals when the budget is thinning. Sociological and psychological factors can influence consistent food intake as much as physical factors. The nurse and physician must carefully assess, plan, and manage insulin needs in view of the individual's unique problems and life-style. Special attention must also be paid to the aged in a hosptial or nursing home setting to ensure that food intake is regular and adequate.

At times, oral agents are prescribed for the elderly diabetic. Chlorpropamide (Diabinese) is an oral hypoglycemic agent with approximately six times the potency of tolbutamide. It is readily absorbed in the gastrointestinal tract, reaching its maximum level in 2 to 4 hours, and is slowly excreted in the urine. The biological half-life of chlorpropamide is normally 36 hours, with most of the dose excreted within 96 hours. Chlorpropamide is contraindicated in individuals having severe impairment of hepatic, renal, or thyroid function. This drug can prolong the action of barbiturates, a consideration for gerontological nurses since elderly patients may be receiving both medications. Close nursing observation is essential when patients receiving oral hypoglycemic agents are prescribed antibacterial sulfonamides, phenylbutazone, salicylates, probenecid, dicoumarol or MAO (monoamine oxidase) inhibitors, since these drugs can potentiate a hypoglycemic reaction. Chlorpropamide may cause an exaggerated hypoglycemic effect in individuals with Addison's disease.

If hypoglycemia occurs in the patient receiving chlorpropamide it could be prolonged. A slightly higher blood glucose level is considered acceptable for adequate functioning in the aged, and therefore the nurse should note and communicate to the physician observations indicating dysfunction from a reduced blood sugar level; perhaps a higher than "normal" glucose level will promote optimum function in a given individual. Adverse reactions to chlorpropamide include pruritus, rash, jaundice, dark urine, light-colored stools, diarrhea, low-grade fever, and sore throat. Tolbutamide, acetohexamide, tolazamide and phenformin are among the other oral hypoglycemic agents which may be prescribed. Suggestions, special precautions, and adverse reactions for these drugs resemble those mentioned with chlorpropamide.

Some individuals only need oral hypoglycemic agents to control their diabetes. Those on insulin therapy who have lost weight or have not been ketoacidotic may have their insulin substituted by oral hypoglycemic agents. Still others will need periodic changes in their insulin dosages to meet changing demands. These factors, combined with other management difficulties in the older diabetic, necessitate frequent reevaluation of the patient's status. The continuation of health supervision is an essential part of diabetic management.

Complications

The elderly are subject to a long list of complications from diabetes and have a greater risk of developing these complications than younger adults. Hypoglycemia seems to be a greater threat to older diabetics than ketoacidosis, and this is especially problematic due to the possible presentation of a different set of symptoms. The classic tachycardia, restlessness, perspiration, and anxiety may be totally absent in the older individual with hypoglycemia. Instead, any of the following may be the first indication of the problem: behavior disorders, convulsions, somnolence, confusion, disorientation, poor sleep patterns, nocturnal headache, slurred speech, and unconsciousness. The nurse must be careful not to mistake signs of hypoglycemia with "senility" as this may delay detection and correction of this serious problem. Uncorrected hypoglycemia can cause tachycardia, arrhythmias, myocardial infarctions, cerebrovascular accident, and death.

Peripheral vascular disease is a common complication in the older diabetic, influenced by the poorer circulation and atherosclerosis often associated with increased age. Symptoms may range from numbness and weak pulses to infection and gangrene. The nurse should identify and promptly communicate symptoms of peripheral vascular disease. Education of the patient in proper foot care can help reduce the risk of this problem. Another significant vascular problem of older diabetics is retinopathy with consequent blindness. Individuals who are hypertensive or who have had diabetes for a long period of time have a greater risk of developing this complication. Hemorrhage, pigmentory disturbances, edema, and visual problems are manifested with this problem.

A variety of additional complications face older diabetics. They may develop neuropathies, demonstrated through tingling sensations, pain, paresthesias, nocturnal diarrhea, tachycardia, and postural hypotension. They have twice the mortality rate from coronary artery disease, twice the mortality rate from cerebral arteriosclerosis, and a higher incidence of urinary tract infections. There is a higher risk of problems developing with virtually every body system. Early detection of complications is essential and can be facilitated by nursing intervention and patient education. Competent management of the older diabetic is an extremely skillful and vital activity, posing a great challenge and responsibility to the practice of nursing. The recognition of differences in symptomatology, diagnosis, management, and complications is crucial.

REFERENCES

Andres, R. "Diabetes and Aging." *Hospital Practice,* 2:63, 1967.

McDonald, G. W., Fisher, G. F., and Burnham, C. "Reproducibility of the Oral Glucose Tolerance Test." *Diabetes,* 14:473, 1965.

Rifkin, H., and Ross, H. "Diabetes in the Elderly." In Rossman, I. (ed.), *Clinical Geriatrics.* Lippincott, Philadelphia, 1971. (a) p. 391; (b) p. 400.

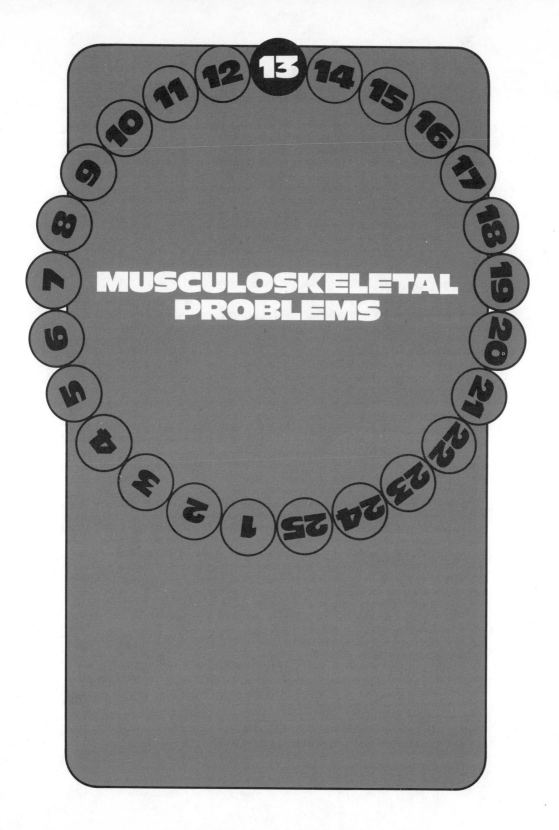

MUSCULOSKELETAL
PROBLEMS

t is the rare older individual who does not experience some degree of discomfort, disability, or deformity from musculoskeletal disorders. In addition to the influence of diet, heredity, stress, and hormonal balances on the status of the musculoskeletal system, changes associated with the aging process also contribute to these problems. With age, there is a reduction in the number of muscle fibers and in muscle strength and endurance. Some wasting of the skeletal muscle occurs, and a loss of bone minerals causes the bones to become more brittle. Muscle movements and tendon jerks are decreased. Some joints become more mobile due to stretching of the ligaments; others stiffen and lose some range of motion. Hip and knee flexion, kyphosis of the dorsal spine, and shortening of the vertebral column can be evidenced by a reduction in height as an individual ages.

Pain frequently accompanies musculoskeletal problems. Degenerative changes in the tendons and arthritis are often responsible for painful shoulders, elbows, hands, hips, knees, and spine, and cramps, especially during the night, are commonly experienced in calves, feet, hands, hips, and thighs. Joint strain and damp weather more frequently cause musculoskeletal pain in the aged than in the young. The gerontological nurse should assess the musculoskeletal pain and note in the documentation the location, nature, duration, severity, precipitating factors, and relief measures used by the patient. This information can provide the baseline data by which changes in the characteristics of the pain can be measured. Also, the nurse can help the patient avoid situations that cause pain and to seek prompt relief once pain has developed.

A variety of nursing measures can be implemented to assist the patient with musculoskeletal pain. Heat often will relieve muscle spasms, and a warm bath at bedtime accompanied by blankets or clothing to keep the extremities warm can reduce spasms and cramps throughout the night and promote uninterrupted sleep. Passive stretching of the extremity also may be helpful in controlling muscle cramps. Excessive exercise and musculoskeletal stress should be avoided. Pain in the weight-bearing joints can be helped by resting those joints; supporting the parts under the painful joint when moving and lifting the patient can be beneficial, as can the assistance of a walker or cane (Figure 13-1). Correct positioning, whereby all body parts are in proper alignment, can help prevent and manage pain. Accidental bumping against the patient's bed or chair, and rough handling of the patient during routine care activities must be prevented. The nurse may have to emphasize to other care providers the need for gentleness in turning and lifting the patient while providing support to all limbs.

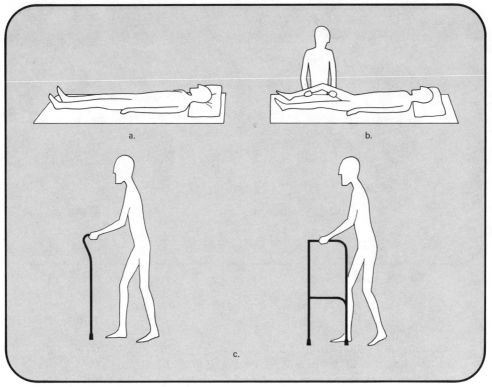

Figure 13-1. Methods for reducing musculoskeletal pain: (a) Good body alignment. (b) Support of parts of limb adjacent to painful joint when moving or lifting. (c) Use of walker or cane.

DISORDERS AND RELATED NURSING CARE

Fractures

Trauma, cancer metastasis to the bone, osteoporosis, and other skeletal diseases contribute to fractures in aged persons. The neck of the femur is a common site for fractures in the aged, especially in older females (Habermann, 1971). Not only do the more brittle bones of the aged fracture more easily, but their rate of healing is longer than in younger persons, potentially predisposing the aged to the many complications associated with immobility. Knowing that the risk of fracture and its multiple complications is high among the aged, the gerontological nurse must aim toward prevention, drawing on the effectiveness of basic commonsense measures. Since their coordination and equilibrium are poorer, the aged should be advised against climbing on ladders or chairs to reach high places and similarly risky activities. To prevent

197

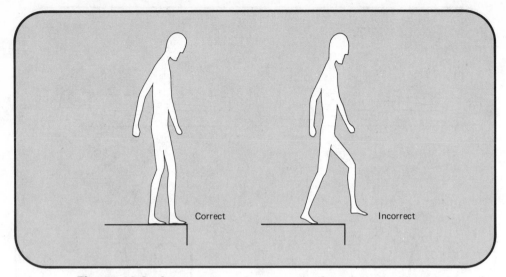

Figure 13-2. Stepping to or from a curb: Correct method is to place both feet near edge of curb before stepping up or down. Incorrect method is to stretch legs apart before stepping.

dizziness and falls resulting from postural hypotension, the older individual should rise from a kneeling or sitting position slowly. Safe, proper-fitting shoes with a low, broad heel can prevent stumbling and loss of balance, and handrails for climbing stairs or rising from the bathtub provide support and balance.

Placing both feet near the edge of a curb or bus before stepping up or down is safer than a poorly balanced stretch of the legs (Figures 13-2). The aged person should be reminded to carefully notice where he or she is walking to avoid tripping in holes and damaged sidewalks or slipping on pieces of ice. Since older eyes are more sensitive to glare, sunglasses may be helpful for improving vision outdoors. A nightlight is extremely valuable in preventing falls during night visits to the bathroom. Loose rugs and clutter on floors and stairs should be removed. Since even the most healthy aged person can experience some confusion when waking during the night, bedrails can be used to prevent falls from bed and attempts at sleepwalking, whether at home or away. Putting the bed against a wall with a straight chair at the other side is an effective substitute.

As mentioned, fractures heal more slowly in the aged, and the risk of complications is great. Pneumonia, thrombus formation, decubiti, renal calculi, fecal impaction, and contractures are among the complications that special nursing attention can help prevent. Activity, within the limits determined by the physician, should be promoted, including deep-breathing and coughing exercises, isometric and range-of-motion exercises, and frequent turning and position changes. Fluids should be encouraged, and the characteristics of the urine output noted. Good nutrition will facilitate healing and increase the resistance to infection and other complications. Joint exercises and proper positioning can prevent contractures. Correct body alignment can be maintained with the use of footboards, trochanter rolls, and sandbags. Keeping the skin dry and clean, preventing pressure, stimulating circulation through massage, and frequent turning may reduce the risk of decubiti. Sheepskin, water beds, and alternating-pressure mattresses are beneficial, but they do not substitute for good skin care and frequent position changes.

As early as possible, the patient should be mobilized. It is not unusual for the patient to fear using the fractured limb and avoid doing so. Explanations and reassurance are required to help the patient understand that the healed limb is safe to use. Since progress in small steps may be easier for the patient to tolerate physically and psychologically, the first attempt at ambulation may be to stand at the bedside, the next to walking to a nearby chair, and the next to walk to the bathroom. Initially, it may be helpful for two people to assist the patient with ambulation, especially since weakness and dizziness are not uncommon. The principles of nursing management for specific types of fractures are available in medical-surgical nursing textbooks and the reader is advised to explore that literature for more detailed information.

Osteoarthritis

Osteoarthritis is the deterioration and abrasion of joint cartilage, with the formation of new bone at the joint surfaces. This problem is increasingly seen with advanced age, affecting women more than men. Unlike rheumatoid arthritis, osteoarthritis arthritis does not cause inflammation, deformity, and crippling—a fact that is reassuring to the affected individual who fears the severe disability he has seen in persons with rheumatoid arthritis. The wear and tear of the joints as an individual ages is thought to have a major role in the development of osteoarthritis. Excessive use of the joint, trauma, obesity, and genetic factors may also predispose an individual to this problem. There is a high incidence of osteoarthritis in patients with acromegaly. Usually osteoarthritis affects several joints rather than a single one. Weight-bearing joints are those most affected, the common sites being the knees, hips, vertebrae, and fingers, and the classic symptoms associated with arthritis are present—aching, stiffness, and limited motion of the joint.

Systemic symptoms do not accompany osteoarthritis. Crepitation on joint motion may be noted, and the distal joints may develop bony nodules (Heberden's nodes). The patient may notice that the joints are more uncomfortable during damp weather and periods of extended use. Rest will help relieve the joint aching, as will heat and gentle massage. Although isometric and mild exercises are beneficial, excessive exercise will cause more pain and degeneration. Analgesics may be prescribed to control pain, and splints, braces, and canes offer support and rest to the joints. The importance of maintaining proper body alignment and using good body mechanics should be emphasized in educating the patient. Weight reduction may improve the obese patient's status and should be encouraged. It is beneficial if a homemaker's service or other household assistance relieves the patient of strenuous activities that cause the joints to bear weight. Occupational and physical therapists can be consulted for assistive devices to promote independence in self-care activities.

Rheumatoid Arthritis

Rheumatoid arthritis affects many persons, young and old; it is commonly seen among the aged. The deformities and disability associated with this disease primarily begin during early adulthood, peaking during middle age; in old age, greater systemic involvement occurs. This disease occurs more frequently in women and in persons with a family history of this problem (Habermann, 1971). The joints affected by rheumatoid arthritis are extremely painful, stiff, swollen, red, and warm to the touch. Joint pain is present during rest or activity. Subcutaneous nodules over bony prominences and bursae may be present, as may deforming flexion contractures. Systemic symptoms include fatigue, malaise, weakness, weight loss, wasting, fever, and anemia.

Encouraging patients to rest and thus providing support to the affected limbs is helpful. Limb support should be such that decubiti and contractures are prevented. Splints are commonly made for the patient in an effort to prevent deformities. Range-of-motion exercises are vital to maintain musculoskeletal function; the nurse may have to assist the patient with active exercises. Physical and occupational therapists can provide assistive devices to promote independence in self-care activities, and heat, gentle massage, and analgesics can help to control pain. In addition, patients with rheumatoid arthritis may be prescribed antiinflammatory agents, corticosteroids, antimalarial agents, gold salts, and immunosuppressive drugs. The nurse should be familiar with the many toxic effects of these drugs and detect them early.

The patient with rheumatoid arthritis and the family need considerable education to be able to manage this condition. Patient education should include a knowledge of the disease, treatments, administration of medications and identification of side effects, exercise regimen, use of

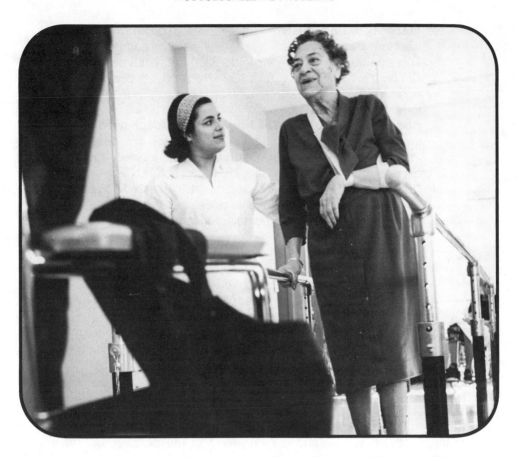

assistive devices, methods to avoid and reduce pain, and an understanding of the need for continued medical supervision. Accepting this chronic disease is not an easy task, either for the patient or the family. The patient may be a prime target for a salesperson offering a quick "cure" or "relief" for arthritis and should be advised to consult the nurse or physician before investing many dollars of an already limited budget on useless fads.

Osteoporosis

Osteoporosis is the most prevalent metabolic disease of the bone, primarily affecting adults in middle to late life. Demineralization of the bone occurs, evidenced by a decrease in the mass and density of the skeleton. Any problem in which there is inadequate calcium intake, excessive calcium loss, or poor calcium absorption can cause osteoporosis. Many of the potential causes listed below are problems commonly found among aged persons.

1. *Inactivity or Immobility.* A lack of muscle pull on the bone can lead to a loss of minerals, especially calcium and phosphorus. This particularly may be a problem for limbs in a cast.
2. *Cushing's Syndrome.* An excessive production of glucocorticosteroids by the adrenal gland is thought to inhibit the formation of bone matrix.
3. *Reduction in Anabolic Sex Hormones.* A decreased production or loss of estrogens and androgens may be responsible for insufficient bone calcium. Postmenopausal women, therefore, may be at high risk of developing this problem.
4. *Diverticulitis.* Excessive diverticulitis can interfere with the absorption of sufficient amounts of calcium.
5. *Hyperthyroidism.* This increased metabolic activity causes a more rapid bone turnover. Bone resorption occurs at a rate faster than bone formation, causing osteoporosis.
6. *Poor Diet.* An insufficient amount of calcium, protein, and other nutrients in the diet can cause osteoporosis.
7. *Heparin.* Prolonged use of heparin can increase bone resorption and inhibit bone formation.
8. *Diabetes Mellitus.* Although the direct relationship is uncertain at this time, diabetes can contribute to the development of osteoporosis.

Osteoporosis may cause kyphosis and a reduction in height. Spinal pain can be experienced, especially in the lumbar region. There may be a tendency for the bones to fracture more easily. Some patients may be asymptomatic, however, and not be aware of the problem until it is detected on X-ray. Treatment depends on the underlying cause and may include calcium supplements, vitamin D supplements, hormones, anabolic agents, fluoride, or phosphate. A diet rich in protein and calcium is encouraged. Braces may be used to provide support and reduce spasms. A bedboard is also beneficial and should be recommended. The patient must be advised to avoid heavy lifting, jumping or other activities that could result in a fracture. Persons providing care to the patient must remember to be gentle when moving, exercising, or lifting these patients since fractures can occur easily. (Compression fractures of the vertebrae are a potential complication of osteoporosis). Range-of-motion exercises and ambulation are important to maintain function and prevent greater damage.

Osteitis Deformans (Paget's Disease)

Osteitis deformans is a metabolic disease of the bone which produces excessive bone resorption and deposits. Although the exact cause is unknown, developmental defects, chronic inflammation of the bone, and wear and tear to the skeletal system throughout the years are thought to be contributing factors. This disease primarily involves middle-aged and aged males. The common sites affected are the skull, lumbar vertebrae, sacrum, pelvis, and long bones. The deformities most commonly displayed include enlargement and thickening of the skull, kyphosis, and bowing of the femur and tibia. Bone pain is usually present, as is the tendency for the bones to fracture easily. Complications to other organs may result, such as paraplegia due to pressure on the spinal cord and blindness due to pressure on the optic nerve. Symptomatic treatment is usually employed. Pain control and the prevention of complications are the major goals. Since osteitis deformans predisposes the individual to bone sarcoma, close observation and periodic evaluation are needed to identify this problem. In general, the prognosis associated with this disease is very poor.

NURSING CONSIDERATIONS

A good diet is important in preventing and managing musculoskeletal problems. A well-balanced diet, rich in proteins and minerals, will help maintain the structure and function of the bones and muscles. In addition to the quality of the diet, attention also must be paid to the quantity. Obesity places strain on the joints which aggravates conditions like arthritis. Weight reduction will frequently ease musculoskeletal discomforts and reduce limitations, and it should be stressed when gerontological nurses counsel individuals of all ages on intelligent aging.

Pain relief is essential in promoting optimum physical, mental, and social function. Aching joints may prevent aged persons from properly caring for their basic needs, managing their household, and maintaining social contact. To enrich the quality of an older person's life, every effort should be made to minimize or eliminate pain—whether by proper positioning, gentle massage, heat, analgesics, or passive stretching to relieve muscle cramps. Situations which are known to cause pain—such as heavy lifting and damp weather—should be avoided whenever possible. Diversional activities can prevent the patient's preoccupation with pain. The family may need support and education in learning to understand and assist the patient during episodes of pain. The patient should be helped to achieve a balance between the maximum level of activity and the least degree of pain.

Activity promotes optimum musculoskeletal function and reduces the many complications associated with immobility. Fear of reinjuring a healing bone or causing pain, however, may cause the patient to limit his or her activities unnecessarily. Realistic explanations describing the healing process or the benefit of exercise to aching joints are most

203

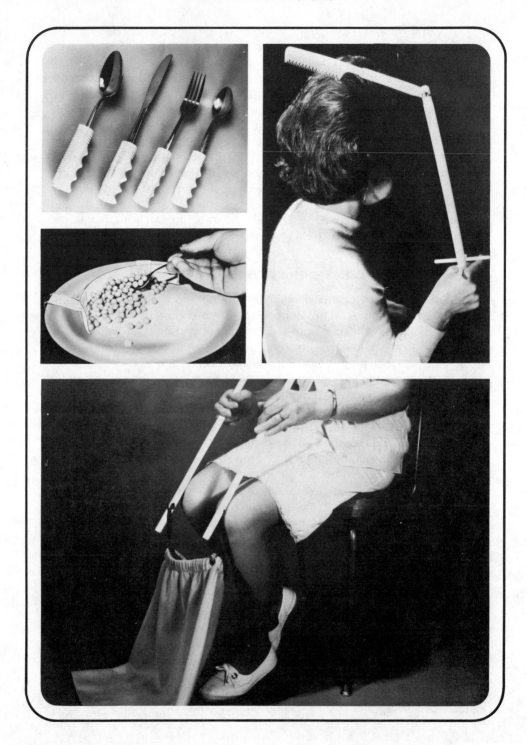

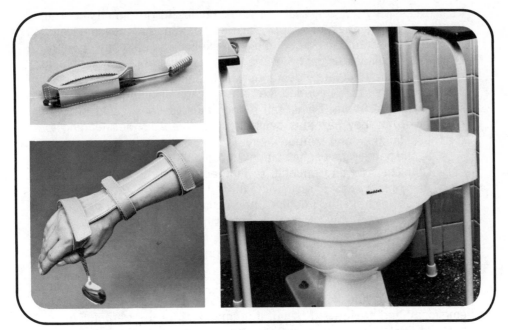

Figure 13-3. Self-care devices can help the patient achieve maximum independence: (a) Set of 4 built-up hand utensils. (b) Long-handled comb. (c) Food-bumper. (d) Dressing sticks with carter clips. (e) Universal ADL cuff. (f) Dorsal wrist splint. (g) Tall-Ette with safety bars. (Courtesy of Maddak Inc. Subsidiary of Bel-Air Products, Pequannock, N.J.)

important. Patients and families can benefit from an understanding of the hazards arising from immobility; sympathetic family members who believe they are helping the patient by allowing him or her to remain inactive may be more willing to encourage activity if they are aware of the harm immobility can cause. Continued support, encouragement, and positive reinforcement by the gerontological nurse can help the patient considerably.

Safety considerations are essential for all aged persons due to the high incidence of accidents and musculoskeletal injuries and the prolonged healing period. Prevention includes paying attention to the area where one is walking, climbing stairs and curbs slowly, using both feet for support as much as possible (Figure 13-2), using railings and canes for added balance, wearing properly fitting, safe shoes for good support, and avoiding trousers, nightgowns, or robes that are long enough to get caught by a shoe or slipper. Since heat is frequently used by aged persons to relieve joint pain or muscle spasm, attention must be paid to its safety hazards. Altered cutaneous sensations may allow burns

205

from excessively hot soaks or hot water bottles to go unnoticed. The patient should be advised to apply heat with care and to measure water temperature (with a dairy thermometer). Patients who also have peripheral vascular disease must be warned that the local application of heat can cause extra circulatory demands which their body will be unable to meet; they should be informed that other means of pain relief may be more beneficial. Warm baths can reduce muscle spasm and provide pain relief, but they can also cause hypotensive episodes leading to dizziness, fainting, and serious injury.

Gentle handling must be emphasized in instructing those providing care. Carelessly turning patients so that legs hit the bedrail or "dropping" them into a chair or restraining them in an unaligned position can lead to muscle strain and fractures. Attempting to use force to straighten a contracture or roughly handling a limb without support can also result in fractures. Gentle handling will prevent unnecessary musculoskeletal discomfort and injury. Limbs should be supported below and above the joint for safety and comfort.

Since any loss of independence associated with the limitations imposed by musculoskeletal problems has a serious impact on physical, emotional, and social well-being, it is important for the gerontological nurse to explore all avenues to help patients minimize limitations and strengthen capacities, thus promoting the highest possible level of independence. Canes and walkers can enhance independence in ambulation, and self-care devices can often be obtained through physical and occupational therapists to help patients eat, bathe, and care for themselves (Figure 13-3).

REFERENCES

Habermann, E. T. "Orthopaedic Aspects of the Lower Extremities." In Rossman, I. (ed.), *Clinical Geriatrics.* Lippincott, Philadelphia, 1971, p. 311.

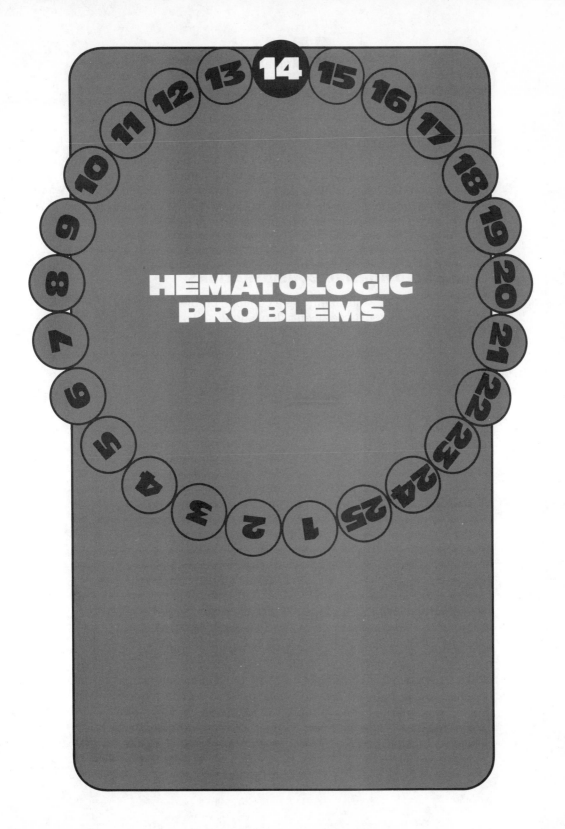

HEMATOLOGIC PROBLEMS

Hematologic problems are not uncommon in the aged, and lymphosarcoma, chronic lymphocytic leukemia, reticulum cell sarcoma, macroglobulinemia, and multiple myeloma are of high incidence. Anemia occurs with such frequency in aged persons that it is often mistakenly considered a normal consequence of growing old. These and other hematologic diseases which reduce the aged person's capacity to deal with stress are believed to be a result of several aging factors, including atrophy of the thymus and lymph nodes, impaired cutaneous hyper-reactivity, decreased immunoglobulin production in response to stress, increased lymphocytes in the bone marrow, and a reduction in the circulating red cell mass.

TYPES OF ANEMIA AND
RELATED NURSING CONSIDERATIONS

As mentioned, while anemia is a common problem in the aged, it is not a normal condition. In addition to the fatigue and pallor which usually accompany this problem, the aged may demonstrate a greater susceptibility to infection, mental confusion, angina attacks, and episodes of congestive heart failure. Certain problems are associated with the various types of anemia in the aged.

Poor diet
Rheumatoid arthritis
Uremia
Chronic hepatitis
Cirrhosis
Prostatic hypertrophy
Diabetes

Cancer, especially of the
   hematopoietic organs
   and digestive tract
Peptic ulcers
Chronic bronchitis
Tuberculosis
Urinary-tract infections and
   other chronic or subacute
   infections

In addition to treatment, a thorough evaluation of the patient is needed to detect any underlying disease causing the anemia.

Iron Deficiency Anemia

Iron deficiency anemia is the most common form of anemia in all age groups. In addition to poor dietary intake of iron, the aged can develop this anemia as a result of hemorrhoidal bleeding, peptic ulcers, or impaired absorption of iron. The clinical manifestations of this imparied tissue nutrition are dry inelastic skin, headache, dizziness, fatigue, thin and brittle hair, atrophy of the tongue, and thin, brittle, and easily breakable fingernails. Blood tests confirm the diagnosis of iron deficiency anemia, and a misdiagnosis can result if problems that reduce iron-binding capacity and serum iron are also present—such as rheumatoid arthritis and chronic infection. Because anemia in the presence of an adequate iron intake can indicate poor absorption, bleeding, or other problems, a complete review of the older person's diet is essential. Theurapeutic measures, similar to those used with younger patients, include correcting any underlying cause, maintaining good nutrition, and using iron preparations. The patient should be instructed to administer the iron after meals and preferably not with dairy products.

It is important for the nurse to assist in the *prevention* of iron deficiency anemia through the encouragement of a well-balanced diet and a good nutritional status. Helping the aged patient obtain food stamps, introducing the patient to lunch programs, encouraging the correction of dental problems, teaching about diet, and providing guidance in the purchase of the best quality foods within limited budgets can be beneficial. The nurse can also discuss with the physician the value of iron supplements as a prophylactic measure.

Pernicious Anemia

Pernicious anemia is found mostly in aged patients (Maekawa, 1976), where it is usually accompanied by a reduced platelet and white blood cell count. A vitamin B-12 deficiency is the cause of pernicious anemia, which is frequently associated with cancer of the stomach. Accompanying the usual symptoms of anemia are premature graying or whitening of the hair; atrophy of the tongue, with a flattening of the papillae; and leg edema. Gastrointestinal changes contributing to this disease may cause anorexia, weight loss, diarrhea, constipation, and other related symptoms. The central nervous system may also be involved, depending on the extent of the problem. The treatment plan is the same at all ages. The patient needs to understand that monthly vitamin B-12 injections will be required for the remainder of his or her lifetime. Since gastric cancer is of greater incidence in patients with pernicious anemia, close follow-up and periodic stool examination are essential.

Folic Acid Deficiency

Folic acid deficiency is one of the major causes of nutritional anemia. Persons with limited fruit and vegetable intake are more likely to develop this form of anemia. Although folic acid deficiency is most commonly found in alcoholics, it is wise to realize that many aged persons risk developing this problem because a limited budget prevents them from including fruits and vegetables in their diet. Treatment consists of folic acid therapy, which, fortunately, can be replaced by good nutrition once the serum folic acid level has returned to normal.

OTHER HEMOTOLOGIC DISEASES

Hodgkin's Disease and Multiple Myeloma

Hodgkin's disease in the aged and multiple myeloma are associated with anemia, leukopenia, or thrombocytopenia. Since symptomatology, diagnostic measures, and therapy for Hodgkin's disease are similar to those described for other age groups, the reader is advised to explore medical-surgical nursing literature for a complete review of this disease, which runs a more rapid and aggressive clinical course in the aged.

Multiple myeloma, more frequently diagnosed in middle-aged persons, has a decreasing incidence with age. Pathological fractures are a particular risk in aged people with multiple myeloma. Not only are these problems disabling in themselves, but they can pose serious threats to the aged as a result of emboli, pneumonia, and complications resulting from immobility. Mental confusion, behavioral changes, and coma are threats resulting from hypercalcemia associated with this disease. Many supportive measures to control pain and close observation for signs of complications are required of the nurse.

Leukemias

Leukemias have a higher incidence in aged people, where they (1) have an insidious onset; (2) manifest nonspecific symptoms which interfere with early diagnosis; (3) are difficult to manage; and (4) have a complicated course. A review of leukemias, readily available in medical-surgical literature, will not be presented here. However, there are some factors that are unique to the aged. *Acute leukemia* runs an aggressive course in the aged, is difficult to manage, and has a poor prognosis. *Chronic lymphoctic leukemia,* which is the most common leukemia in the aged, progresses slowly. With *chronic myeloid leukemia,* the associated spleen and liver enlargement may not develop in the aged.

Special nursing considerations.

Although aged patients with leukemia require the same general care as younger patients, the gerontological nurse must be especially alert to complications. The aged are already at higher risk of infection than the young, and a disease like leukemia compounds that risk. Infections must be prevented and promptly treated if they occur. Since the aged do not manage the stress of hemorrhage well, this complication should be prevented; if it should occur, it should be readily detected and promptly treated. Radiation therapy and chemotherapy may cause nausea, vomiting, stomatitis, anorexia, and other problems which threaten the nutritional status of the patient. Careful attention to the prevention of mouth trauma, avoidance of extremes in the temperature and seasoning of food, and the encouragement of a good diet are beneficial. The patient's psychological state may be affected by changes in body image resulting from chemotherapy, radiation, or surgery. Maintaining the best possible appearance, through wigs and attractive clothing, for instance, and allowing patients to vent their reactions openly and discuss their disease may help them cope with these difficult adjustments.

REFERENCES

Maekawa, T. "Hematologic Diseases." In Steinberg, F. U. (ed.), *Cowdry's, The Care of the Geriatric Patient,* 5th ed. Mosby, St. Louis, 1976, p. 159.

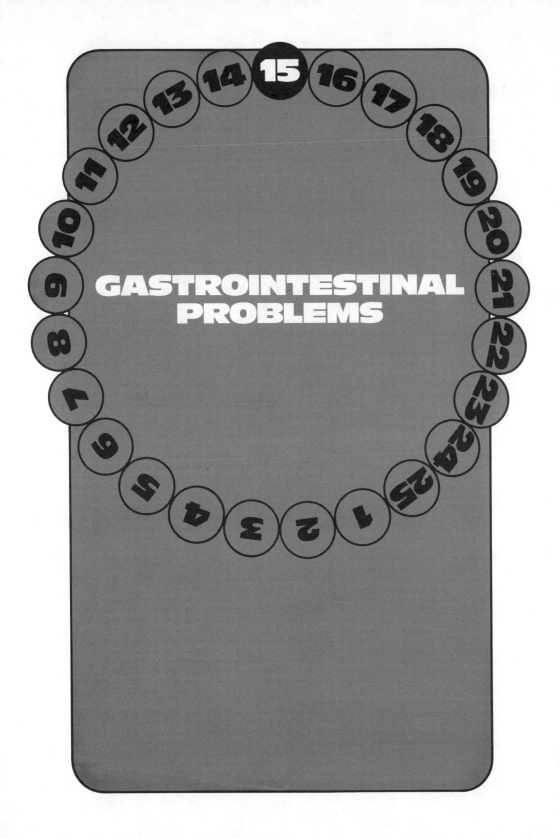

GASTROINTESTINAL PROBLEMS

The gastrointestinal system becomes the most problematic body system with age and is the frequent cause of many complaints voiced by older persons. All gastrointestinal symptoms increase with advancing age. Problems that occur in the absence of any organic cause include indigestion, belching, diarrhea, constipation, nausea, vomiting, anorexia, weight loss, and flatulence. The aged have a higher incidence of cancer throughout the gastrointestinal tract, and also of high incidence are biliary tract disease, intestinal obstruction, and peptic ulcer. Gallbladder disease with cholelithiasis is a frequently diagnosed condition in older persons. In the absence of disease, there is no significant change in the functions of the liver, gallbladder, and pancreas.

A variety of factors related to the aging process contribute to the high incidence of gastrointestinal problems. A majority of the aged have lost most or all of their teeth, often needlessly. There is a reduction in taste sensation, particularly affecting the taste buds for sweet and salt, and poor appetite is not uncommon. Less gastric acid is secreted, and the stomach mucosa becomes thinner. The stomach takes a longer period of time to empty, and hunger contractions are reduced. Although supporting scientific data is inadequate, there is believed to be some atrophy throughout the intestines, colon, and rectum. Absorption is reduced by fewer absorbing cells on the walls of the intestines. Peristalsis becomes slower throughout the entire system. Secretory activity is altered, and salivary amylase secretion is lower. There is a decrease in pepsin secretion, and pancreatic enzymes. The changes in secretory function affect the absorption of all nutrients—protein absorption being affected more than fat and carbohydrate absorption.

The diagnosis of gastrointestinal problems is difficult due to an atypical symptomatology, which easily causes confusion with other problems. Among the tests frequently used to diagnosis these problems are barium swallow, esophagoscopy, gastroscopy, gastric analysis, barium enema, cholecystogram, sigmoidoscopy, and proctoscopy. A great deal of education, reassurance, and comfort should be provided for the aged during these procedures, many of which demand uncomfortable introductions of equipment into body orifices and awkward positioning on hard examination tables. Since the aged patient may become dehydrated or hypoglycemic if kept NPO for diagnostic procedures, prolonged or repeated periods of restricted nourishment intake necessitate close nursing observation and assessment to detect development of these problems.

COMMON DISORDERS AND REQUIREMENTS FOR CARE

Dental Problems

Continued dental care is important throughout an individual's lifetime. Dental examination can be instrumental in the early detection

214

and prevention of many problems that affect other body systems. Poor teeth can restrict food intake, which can cause constipation and malnourishment; they also detract from appearance, which can affect socialization, and this in turn can result in a poor appetite, which can also lead to malnourishment. Periodontal disease can predispose the aged to systemic infection. Although dental care is important in preventing these problems, financial limitations prevent many aged persons from seeking dental attention. Some aged persons have the misconception that dentures eliminate the need for regular visits to the dentist. Others, like many younger persons, fear the dentist. The nurse should encourage regular dental examination and promote dental care, explaining that serious diseases can be detected by the dentist and helping patients find free or inexpensive dental clinics. Understanding how modern dental techniques minimize pain can alleviate fears. Although older persons may not have had the benefit of fluoridated water or fluoride treatments when younger, topical fluoride treatments are as beneficial to the teeth of the aged as they are to younger teeth. Patients should be instructed to inform their dentists about health problems and medications they are taking to help them determine how procedures need to be modified, what healing rate to expect, and which medications cannot be administered.

Dental problems can be caused by altered taste sensation, a poor diet, or a low-budget carbohydrate diet with excessive intake of sweets, which can cause tooth decay. Deficiencies of the vitamin B complex, hormonal imbalances, hyperparathyroidism, diabetes, osteomalacia, Cushing's disease, and syphilis can be underlying causes of dental problems in the aged, and certain drugs, such as aspirin and dilantin, can also play a part. The aging process itself takes its toll on teeth, surfaces are commonly worn down from many years of use, varying degrees of root absorption take place, and loss of tooth enamel increases the risk of irritation to deeper dental tissue (Goldman, 1971; Rowe, 1976). While benign neoplastic lesions occur more frequently than malignant ones, cancer of the oral cavity, especially in males, is of increasing incidence with age, as is moniliasis, which is often associated with more serious problems, such as diabetes or leukemia. It should not be assumed that all white lesions found in the mouth are moniliasis—biopsy is important to make sure they are not cancerous. Periodontal disease, damaging the soft tissue surrounding teeth and supporting bones, is of high incidence among the aged, and although they occur less frequently in older people, dental caries are a problem as well.

Good oral hygiene is especially important to the aged, who already may be having problems with anorexia or food distaste. Teeth, gums, and tongue can be helped by regular brushing using a soft toothbrush, which can also be used in gentle gum massage for people with dentures.

215

Daily flossing of natural teeth should be performed, and brushing may be better than using swabs, even for the teeth of unconscious patients. Since the buccal mucosa is thinner and less vascular with age, trauma to the oral cavity should be avoided. The nurse should notify the dentist and physician of an atonic or atrophic tongue, lesions, mucosa discoloration, loose teeth, soreness, bleeding, or any other problem identified during inspection and care of the oral cavity.

Esophageal Diverticulum

Dysphagia, gagging, and the regurgitation of undigested food are among the clues indicating esophageal diverticulum. The accumulation and decomposition of food in the diverticulum may cause the breath to have an extremely foul odor. A particularly dangerous complication of this disorder for older people is aspiration, which leads to many serious respiratory problems. A barium swallow confirms the diagnosis, and surgical intervention usually follows. Close nursing observation is important postoperatively to detect leakage from the esophagus, which could cause the formation of a fistula. Nasogastric feedings, discussed at the end of this chapter, are employed until the patient can progress to oral feedings.

Hiatus Hernia

The incidence of hiatus hernia increases with age and tends to affect females more than males (Straus, 1971a; Hodkinson, 1975a). It is estimated that over 50 percent of all aged persons are affected by this disease. Heartburn, dysphagia, belching, vomiting, and regurgitation are common symptoms associated with hiatus hernia. These symptoms are especially problematic when the patient is in a recumbent position. Pain, sometimes mistaken for a coronary, and bleeding may also occur. Diagnosis is confirmed by a barium swallow and esophagoscopy. A majority of patients are managed medically. If the patient is obese, weight reduction can minimize the problems. A bland diet may be recommended, as may the use of milk and antacids for symptomatic relief. Several small meals rather than three large ones are of extreme benefit in bringing about improvement, and may also be advantageous to the aged in coping with other age-related gastrointestinal problems. Eating before bedtime should be discouraged. Some patients may find it beneficial to sleep in a partly recumbent position.

Cancer of the Esophagus

Most persons affected by cancer of the esophagus are aged. This disease commonly strikes between the ages of 60 and 65 years and is of higher incidence in males, blacks, and alcoholics (Straus, 1971a; Ber-

216

man and Kirsner, 1976b). Poor oral hygiene and chronic irritation from tobacco, alcohol, and other agents contribute to the development of this problem. Dysphagia, excessive salivation, thirst, hiccups, anemia, and chronic bleeding are symptoms of this disease. Barium swallow, esophagoscopy, and biopsy are performed as diagnostic measures. Treatment consists of an esophagectomy, and a poor prognosis is not uncommon among aged patients. Benign tumors of the esophagus are rare in the aged.

Peptic Ulcer

Although peptic ulcers occur most frequently at younger ages, the incidence of this problem is on the rise for the aged (Straus, 1971b). Older females develop ulcers more often than older males, and most frequently, these ulcers are gastric rather than duodenal (Berman and Kirsner, 1976b). In addition to stress, diet, and genetic predisposition as causes, particular factors are believed to account for the increased incidence of ulcers in the aged, including longevity, more precise diagnostic evaluation, and the fact that ulcers can be a complication of the increasingly prevalent disorder chronic obstructive pulmonary disease. Drugs commonly prescribed for the aged that can increase gastric secretions and reduce the resistance of the mucosa include aspirin, reserpine, tolbutamide, phenylbutazone, colchicine, and adrenal corticosteroids.

Early symptoms commonly associated with peptic ulcer may not occur in the aged patient, and pain, bleeding and perforation may be the only indication of this problem. Diagnostic and therapeutic measures resemble those employed for younger adults. The nurse should be alert to complications associated with peptic ulcer, which may be especially threatening to the geriatric patient. Constipation or diarrhea can be caused by antacid therapy, and pyloric obstruction can result in dehydration, peritonitis, hemorrhage, and shock.

Cancer of the Stomach

Although stomach cancer is of lower incidence in the aged, it is not uncommon. The incidence is greater among men, in patients with pernicious anemia or atrophy of the gastric mucosa, and in persons between the ages of 75 and 85 years (Straus, 1971c; Berman and Kirsner, 1976c). Anorexia, epigastric pain, weight loss, and anemia are symptoms of gastric cancer. Bleeding may occur, as can enlargement of the liver. Symptoms related to pelvic metastasis may also develop. Diagnosis is confirmed by barium swallow and gastroscopy with biopsy. Surgical treatment consisting of a partial or total gastrectomy is preferred. Unfortunately, the aged have a poor prognosis with gastric cancer.

217

Superior Mesenteric Vascular Occlusion

The aged, especially aged males, experience superior mesenteric vascular occlusion more frequently than younger adults do (Straus, 1971d). This occlusion usually involves the jejunum and ileum. Congestion, obstruction, peritonitis, and ischemic necrosis can result from this problem, seriously threatening the aged person's life. Pain, vomiting, abdominal distention, and bloody diarrhea are symptoms associated with superior mesenteric vascular occlusion. Surgical intervention, possibly a bowel resection, is employed, and the prognosis is not favorable for the aged.

Abdominal Angina

Arterial insufficiency may cause the aged patient to experience abdominal angina. Upper abdominal pain after meals and while walking (relieved by a recumbent position) are manifestations of this problem. Back pain also may be a symptom. Aortography is used to diagnose abdominal angina. Medical management is preferred and will include a feeding schedule of several small meals instead of three large ones. Sometimes surgical intervention is employed to replace the involved artery.

Diverticulosis and Diverticulitis

Multiple pouches of intestinal mucosa in the weakened muscular wall of the large bowel, known as *diverticulosis,* are common among the aged. Chronic constipation, obesity, hiatus hernia, and an atrophy of the intestinal wall muscles with aging contribute to this problem. Slight bleeding may occur with diverticulosis, and usually a barium enema identifies the problem. Surgery is not performed unless severe bleeding develops. Medical management is most common and includes a bland diet, weight reduction, and avoidance of constipation. Bowel contents can accumulate in the diverticuli and decompose, causing inflammation and infection. This is known as *diverticulitis.* Although less than half the patients with diverticulosis develop diverticulitis, most patients who do are aged. Older men tend to experience this problem more than any other group (Straus, 1971e).

Overeating, straining during a bowel movement, alcohol, and irritating foods may contribute to diverticulitis in the patient with diverticulosis. Pain in the left lower quadrant, similar to that of appendicitis but over the sigmoid area, is a symptom of this problem. Nausea, vomiting, constipation, diarrhea, low-grade fever, and blood or mucus in the stool may also occur. These attacks can be severely acute or slowly progressing; while the former can cause peritonitis, the latter can also be serious due to the possibility of lower-bowel obstruction resulting from scarring and abscess formation. In addition to the mentioned complica-

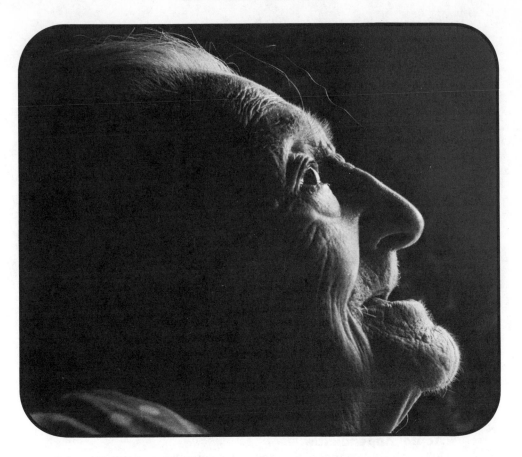

tions, fistulas to the bladder, vagina, colon, and intestines can develop. During the acute phase, efforts are focused on reducing infection, providing nutrition, relieving discomfort, and promoting rest. Usually nothing is ingested by mouth and intravenous therapy is employed. When the acute episode subsides, the patient is taught a low-residue diet. Surgery, performed if medical management is unsuccessful or if serious complications occur, may consist of a resection or temporary colostomy. Continued follow-up should be encouraged.

Cancer of the Colon

Cancer at any site along the large intestine is common in the aged and affects both sexes equally. The sigmoid colon and rectum tend to be frequent sites for carcinoma. Bloody stools, a change in bowel function, epigastric pain, jaundice, anorexia, and nausea may be symptoms of this problem, although the pattern of symptoms frequently varies for each person. Some older patients ignore bowel symptoms, believing them

219

to be from constipation, poor diet, or hemorrhoids. The patient's description of his bowel problems is less reliable than a digital rectal examination, which detects half of all carcinomas of the large bowel and rectum (Straus, 1971f; Hodkinson, 1975b). The standard diagnostic tests, including barium enema and sigmoidoscopy with biopsy, are used to confirm the diagnosis. Surgical resection, with anastomosis or the formation of a colostomy, is usually performed. Medical-surgical nursing textbooks can provide information on this surgery, and nurses should consult them for specific guidance on caring for patients in this condition.

It is important to realize that a colostomy can present many problems for the aged. In addition to having to adjust to many bodily changes with age, a colostomy presents a major adjustment and a threat to a good self-concept. The aged may feel that a colostomy further separates them from society's view of normal. Socialization may be impaired by the patient's concern over the reactions of others, or by his fear of embarrassing episodes. Reduced energy reserves, arthritic fingers, slower movement, and poorer eyesight are among the problems which may hamper the aged's ability to care for a colostomy, thus causing dependency on others to assist with this procedure. This need for assistance may be perceived as a significant loss of independence for the aged. Tactful, skilled nursing intervention can promote a psychological as well as physical adjustment to a colostomy. Continued follow-up is beneficial to assess the aged patient's changing ability to engage in this self-care activity, identify problems, and provide ongoing support and reassurance.

Acute Appendicitis

Although acute appendicitis does not frequently occur in aged persons, it is important to note that it can occur and that it may present altered signs and symptoms in the aged. The severe pain which occurs in younger persons is absent in aged persons, whose pain may be minimal and referred. Fever may also be minimal, and leukocytosis may be absent. These differences often cause a delayed diagnosis. Prompt surgery will increase the patient's prognosis. Unfortunately, delayed or missed diagnosis and the inability to improve the general status of the patient before this emergency surgery can lead to greater complications and mortality in aged persons with appendicitis.

Chronic Constipation

It is not uncommon for the aged to be bothered by and concerned about constipation. An inactive life-style, less bulk and fluids in the diet, depression, and laxative abuse contribute to this problem. Certain medications will promote constipation, such as opiates, sedatives, and aluminum hydroxide gels. Dulled sensations may cause the signal for bowel elimination to be unnoticed, leading to constipation. Not allowing sufficient time for complete emptying of the bowel can also cause constipation. (It should be remembered that the aged may not fully empty the bowel at one sitting and it is not unusual for a second bowel movement to be required one-half hour after the initial one.) A diet high in bulk and fluid and regular activity can promote bowel elimination, and particular foods that patients find effective—prunes, chocolate pudding, etc.—can be incorporated into the regular diet. Providing a regular time for bowel elimination is often helpful; the mornings tend to be the best time for the aged to empty their bowels. Sometimes rocking the trunk from side to side, and back and forth while sitting on the toilet will stimulate a bowel movement. Only after these other measures have failed should medications be considered.

Older persons may need education concerning bowel elimination. The misconception that daily bowel movements are necessary must be corrected with realistic explanations. Safe use of laxatives should be emphasized to prevent laxative abuse. The patient should be aware that diarrhea resulting from laxative abuse may cause dehydration and be a serious threat to life. The aged in a hospital or nursing home setting may benefit from a stool chart which reflects the time, amount, and characteristics of bowel movements. This chart can help the nurse prevent constipation and impaction by providing easily accessible data regarding bowel function. Even aged persons in the community can benefit from the use of a stool chart which they can maintain.

Chronic constipation which does not improve with the usual measures may require medical evaluation, including anal, rectal, and sigmoid examinations to determine the presence of any underlying cause.

Fecal Impaction

Constipation frequently leads to fecal impaction in the aged. The absence or an insufficient amount of stool should create suspicion regarding an impaction. What may appear to be diarrhea may occur as a result of oozing of liquid feces around the impaction. While taking a rectal temperature the nurse may detect a resistance to the thermometer and find feces on the thermometer when it is withdrawn. A movable mass may be palpated by digital examination. The best approach to fecal impactions is to prevent them from developing; the preventive measures discussed with constipation should be exercised. Once the impaction has developed it must be softened, broken, and removed.

Since policies may vary, the nurse is advised to review the permissive procedures of her employing agency to ensure that removal of a fecal impaction is an acceptable nursing action. An enema, usually oil retention, may be prescribed to assist in the softening and elimination process. Manual breaking and removal of feces with a lubricated gloved

221

finger will promote removal of the impaction. Sometimes, injecting 50 ml of hydrogen peroxide through a rectal tube will cause breakage of the impaction as the hydrogen peroxide foams. Care should be taken not to traumatize or exert the patient during these procedures.

Cancer of the Pancreas

Pancreatic cancer, which occurs most frequently in thin aged men, is a difficult disease to detect until it has reached an advanced stage (Straus, 1971g; Hodkinson, 1975c). Anorexia, weakness, weight loss, and wasting are generalized symptoms, which are easily attributed to other causes. Dyspepsia, belching, nausea, vomiting, diarrhea, constipation, and obstructive jaundice may occur as well. Fever may or may not be present. Epigastric pain radiating to the back may be experienced. This pain is relieved when the patient leans forward and is worsened when a recumbent position is assumed. Surgery is performed to treat this problem. Unfortunately, the disease is so advanced by the time diagnosis is made that the prognosis is usually poor.

Biliary Tract Disease

The incidence of gallstones increases with age and affects women more frequently than men (Hodkinson, 1975d; Straus, 1971h). Pain is the primary symptom associated with this problem. Diagnostic and treatment measures include the standard ones prescribed for adults of any age. Obstruction, inflammation, and infection are potential outcomes of gallstones and should be observed for. Cancer of the gallbladder primarily affects older persons, especially aged females (Straus, 1971i). Fortunately, this disease does not occur very frequently. Pain in the right upper quadrant, anorexia, nausea, vomiting, weight loss, jaundice, weakness, and constipation are the usual symptoms. Although surgery may be performed, the prognosis for the patient with cancer of the gallbladder is poor.

NURSING CONSIDERATIONS

Preventive measures that should be incorporated into the care of geriatric patients in an effort to avoid many of the gastrointestinal problems they commonly experience include the following:

Good dental hygiene
Regular physical and dental examinations
Weight control
A diet of the proper quantity and quality
Avoidance of constipation

222

Through teaching, supporting, and guiding, the nurse can help the aged comply with these measures and enhance gastrointestinal function.

Gavage feedings may be required to supply nutrition for some aged patients. When feeding the patient in this manner and instructing others how to gavage feed, certain points must be remembered. The patient should be placed in a sitting or high Fowler's position during the feeding to prevent aspiration. Prior to instilling the solution, the Levin tube must be checked to make sure it is in the stomach and has not slipped out of place. This is done as follows:

1. Using a 20-ml syringe and aspirating stomach contents
2. Injectioning 5 ml of air into the tube and listening with a stethoscope for a swishing sound as the air enters the stomach
3. Placing the end of the Levin tube in a glass of water so that the absence of regular air bubbles and coughing indicate that the tube is in the stomach

When it has been established that the Levine tube is in the stomach, the feeding can be given. The flow of the solution is not to be fast or forceful. For the geriatric patient, the solution reservoir may achieve a good flow if held at the level of the patient's nose. Rapid feeding can cause discomfort and regurgitation. The nurse or some other care provider should remain with the patient during the feeding; attaching the reservoir to a pole and allowing the feeding to flow in unattended could lead to serious complications and death. Dyspnea, coughing, cyanosis, or any other unusual sign necessitates that the feeding be discontinued and that a physician be notified. Because the time required for stomach emptying is greater in older persons, they should remain in an upright position for at least one-half hour after the feeding. To prevent the entry of air into the stomach, the tube is clamped, except during instillation of solution.

Figure 15-1 demonstrates the proper way to anchor the tube to the patient's face. The tube is not to be pulled and taped to the side of the nose; this causes the tube within the nasal passage to place pressure on the nasal mucosa, predisposing the aged's fragile skin to breakdown in that area. Sometimes, applying a small amount of lubricant in the nostril will prevent irritation. The nostrils are to be cleansed and kept patent. Gentle manipulation with a cotton-tipped applicator can be effective in removing dried crusts and preventing any interference with breathing. Frequent oral hygiene is also essential: It is the policy of some agencies to irrigate the Levine tube at intervals to maintain patency; the nurse is advised to review the standard gastric feeding procedure of her agency and learn the recommended practices.

223

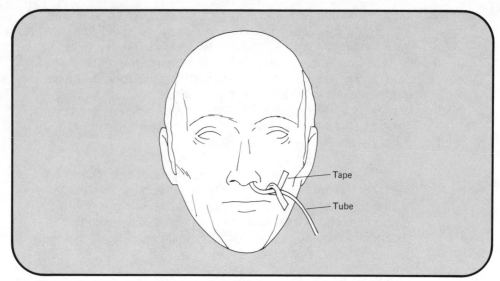

Tape

Tube

Figure 15-1. Proper anchoring of nasogastric tube to prevent irritation and breakdown of the nasal mucosa.

In some chronic care settings, the aged patient may be receiving gastric feedings over a long period of time. If this is the situation, special attention must be paid to the development of complications associated with prolonged use of a nasogastric tube, including respiratory infection, ulceration anywhere along the area in which the Levine tube is located (especially the nasal and gastric mucosa), sinusitis, and esophagitis. Regular assessment is required by the gerontological nurse to determine the continued need for gastric feeding. These feedings should be used only if the patient is unable to ingest food orally. At no time is tube feeding to be employed only because it is a faster and easier way to feed an older patient.

Since aged persons may have poor appetites, every effort should be made to promote an adequate food intake. A variety of foods that the older person can easily cut, manage, chew, and digest and that are attractively served will facilitate eating. A pleasant, colorful, odor-free environment, an opportunity for socialization, and ample time to allow for the slower movements of the older person should be provided. For many aged persons, a nutritional diet of the right quality and quantity will promote and maintain a high enough level of physiological and mental functioning to prevent the development of gastrointestinal disorders.

REFERENCES

Berman, P. M., and Kirsner, J. B. "Gastrointestinal Problems." In Steinberg, F. U. (ed.), *Cowdry's, The Care of the Geriatric Patient,* 5th ed. Mosby, St. Louis, 1976. (a) p. 95; (b) p. 96; (c) p. 97.

Goldman, R. "Decline in Organ Function with Aging." In Rossman, I. (ed.), *Clinical Geriatrics.* Lippincott, Philadelphia, 1971, p. 30.

Hodkinson, H. M. *An Outline of Geriatrics.* Academic Press, New York, 1975. (a) p. 108; (b) p. 113; (c) pp. 110–111; (d) p. 111.

Rowe, N. H. "Dental Surgery." In Steinberg, F. U. (ed.), *Cowdry's, The Care of the Geriatric Patient,* 5th ed. Mosby, St. Louis, 1976, p. 301.

Straus, B. "Disorders of the Digestive System." In Rossman, I. (ed.), *Clinical Geriatrics.* Lippincott, Philadelphia, 1971. (a) p. 186; (b) p. 187; (c) p. 188; (d) p. 190; (e) p. 194; (f) p. 196; (g) p. 198; (h) p. 199; (i) p. 200.

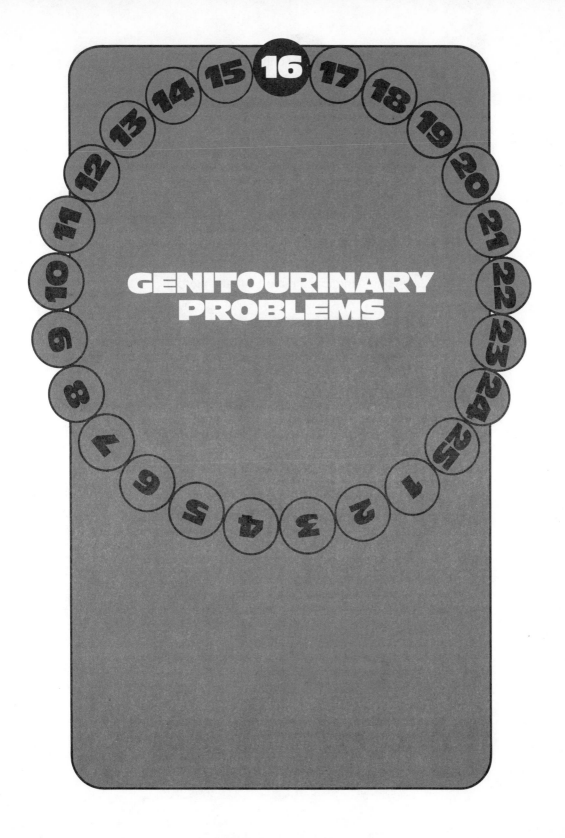

16

GENITOURINARY PROBLEMS

Genitourinary problems in older adults, while bothersome, potentially life threatening, and frequently occurring, are disorders which the aged are often reluctant to discuss. Some feel embarrassment or distaste at making others aware of these problems. Others fear societal reactions to an older person's concern about sexual function or believe symptoms of genitourinary disorders are merely a result of changes with age. Occasionally, the aged may associate genitourinary problems with sexual "wrongdoing" and feel guilty over the development of these disorders. These factors, along with reluctance to obtain gynecological and urologic examinations, often delay early detection and treatment. The nurse is in a position to develop a close relationship with the geriatric patient and can be a key person in identifying problems of the urinary tract and reproductive system. By demonstrating sensitivity, acceptance, and an understanding of the patient's problems, the nurse can facilitate medical attention.

URINARY TRACT PROBLEMS

The urinary tract undergoes many changes with age. Muscles lose their elasticity, and the supportive structures lose some of their tone. Arteriosclerotic changes reduce this system's resistance to injury and infection. There is a reduced bladder capacity and often residual urine. Bladder diverticulae, rare in older women, are common in older men (Brocklehurst, 1971a). There is a reduction in renal plasma flow and the glomerular filtration rate. The kidneys become much more sensitive to changes in the acid-base balance. Decreased tubular function reduces the kidneys' ability to concentrate urine. The renal threshold for glucose increases, so that an older person can be hyperglycemic without evidence of glycosuria. Although proteinuria with an abnormal sedimentation rate may be an early indication of chronic renal disease, a 1+ proteinuria may be present in older adults, usually being of no significance if the sedimentation rate is normal. The blood urea nitrogen level for a 70-year-old may be 21.2 mg% whereas it averages 12.9 mg% during the third decade of life (Kahn and Snapper, 1974a). These changes manifest themselves in a variety of ways, producing the common urologic symptoms observed in many aged persons.

Frequency, Urgency, and Retention

Frequency and urgency are common complaints among the aged. These bothersome problems can interfere with rest, social activities, and other normal functions. The affected individual may avoid bus trips, club meetings, and long walks due to the fear of not having a bathroom available when the need arises. If fluid intake is restricted to reduce the frequency of voiding, there is a threat to adequate hydration. Frequent night trips to the bathroom, a problem shared by most aged persons, are disruptive to sleep and can result in falls due to poor vision in dimly lit areas, blood pressure changes when rising from a lying position, disorientation, and reduced coordination. Limiting fluids at bedtime may be helpful, but this should be counterbalanced by adequate fluid intake during the entire day. Diuretics should be administered so that their peak is not reached during sleeping hours. Good lighting throughout the night and a bedside commode may also prove valuable. Since nocturia, urgency, and frequency can indicate infection or a variety of disease processes, thorough medical evaluation should be encouraged.

Urinary retention may be another problem, and the most common causes of this in the aged are fecal impactions in older women and prostatic hypertrophy in older men (Brocklehurst, 1971b). Urinary retention is also associated with a neurogenic bladder.

Urinary Incontinence

A common and bothersome problem of the aged that requires sensitive and skillful nursing attention is urinary incontinence. Changes that cause sphincter relaxation, altered bladder reflexes, and missed signals to void contribute to this problem. Urinary tract infections can cause temporary periods of incontinence. Tabes dorsalis, diabetic neuropathy, myasthenia gravis, and cerebral cortex lesions are responsible for incontinence as a result of neurogenic bladder. Certain medications used in the management of Parkinson's disease can exaggerate existing urinary tract lesions (Jaffe, 1974a). Incontinence also can be a result of mechanical causes, such as prostatic enlargement, calculi, and tumors. Incontinence can be quite problematic since irritation and breakdown of the aged patient's fragile skin is risked and the patient is subject to the development of urinary tract infection. In addition, odors, embarrassment, and fear of social inacceptance cause the aged to avoid active socialization.

The initial nursing action in caring for the incontinent patient is to arrange for a medical evaluation—to determine the cause of the problem, ensure treatment if possible, and provide a realistic assessment for use in rehabilitation. While specific nursing interventions are determined by the cause of the incontinence, there are some general measures that can prove beneficial. Observing and recording incidents of incontinence can reveal a pattern for scheduling bathroom trips and use of bedpans. Regularly asking patients whether they need to void and promptly answering calls for assistance can often prevent unnecessary episodes of bedwetting. Since concentrated urine can irritate the bladder and cause incontinence, fluids should be forced, unless another condition contraindicates this measure. Incontinence can be diminished by upright positioning during voiding (including while using the bedpan), which reduces the amount of urine retained, and by staying at the

229

commode or urinal for several minutes after voiding to ensure complete emptying. Exercises to tighten the perineum while sitting, and interrupting the flow of urine midstream can improve sphincter control.

For dribbling or stress incontinence, women may find it helpful to wear sanitary pads, and men may benefit from the use of a condom catheter. Thorough, frequent cleansing of the perineal area and genitalia are essential. If an indwelling catheter is utilized, the patient should be observed closely for signs of infection. There are differences of opinion about how frequently an indwelling catheter should be changed and the nurse is encouraged to consult with the physician or review the policy of her agency. Intermittent catherterization is gaining popularity, and patients and their families may need to be instructed in this technique. In some geriatric settings it has been found that incontinence is reduced when patients wear their own clothing—a strategy with multiple benefits.

The nurse can assist patients in the development of a program for bladder training. The success of this program depends upon the patients' physical capacity to regain bladder control, their comprehension of the program, and their motivation. Therefore, a complete assessment of capacities and limitations and joint planning with the patient are prerequisites to the initiation of this regimen. When the patient is fully prepared to begin the program, a schedule is developed indicating the times for voiding. Usually, two hour intervals are planned first, with increased intervals as the patient's progress indicates and reduced intervals during the night. Approximately one-half hour prior to the time scheduled, the patient should drink a full glass of fluid and make a conscious effort to retain urine. At the scheduled time, the patient should attempt to void; if there is difficulty, massaging the bladder area or rocking forward and backward may facilitate voiding (Figure 16-1). It is important to keep an accurate record of intake and output and of the patient's responses to the training program and its effectiveness. The essential role for the nursing staff in this procedure is to make sure the schedule is strictly adhered to by all. Inconsistency on the part of the nursing staff will be destructive to the progress of patients and denigrating to their efforts. Conversely, positive reinforcement and encouragement are most beneficial to the patient during this difficult program.

Urinary Tract Infections

Infections of the urinary tract are not uncommon in the aged, especially in institutional settings. They are second to pulmonary disorders as the most frequent cause of fever in older persons (Jaffe, 1974b). Primarily responsible for urinary tract infections are escherichia coli in wcmen and B. proteus in men. The presence of any foreign body in the urinary tract or anything that slows or obstructs the flow of urine—such as immobilization, urethral strictures, neoplasms, or a clogged indwelling

230

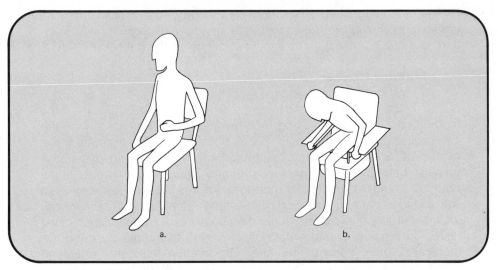

Figure 16-1. Measures to facilitate voiding: (a) Massaging bladder area. (b) Rocking back and forth.

catheter—predisposes the individual to these infections. They can result from poor hygienic practices or improper cleansing after bowel elimination, from a predisposition created by low fluid intake and excessive fluid loss, and from hormonal changes, which reduce the body's resistance. Persons in a debilitated state or who have neurogenic bladders, arteriosclerosis, or diabetes also have a high risk of developing infections.

The gerontological nurse should be alert to the signs and symptoms. Early indicators include burning, urgency, and fever. Awareness of the patient's *normal* body temperature helps the nurse recognize the presence of fever, for instance, 99° F in a patient whose normal temperature is 96.8° F. Some urologists believe that many urinary tract infections in the aged seem asymptomatic due to unawareness of elevations in normal temperature. The gerontological nurse can significantly facilitate diagnoses by informing the physician of temperature increases.

As a urinary tract infection progresses, retention, incontinence, and hematuria may occur. Treatment is aimed at establishing adequate urinary drainage and controlling the infection through antibiotic therapy. The nurse should carefully note the fluid intake and output. Forcing fluids is advisable, providing the patient's cardiac status doesn't contraindicate this action. If an indwelling catheter is utilized, attention should be paid to preventing infection and maintaining an unobstructed urinary flow. Regular meatus care for the patient with an indwelling catheter may

231

consist of thorough cleansing followed by the application of an antibiotic cream. Observation for new symptoms, bladder distension, skin irritation, and other unusual signs should continue as the patient recovers.

Bladder Cancer

Neoplasms of the bladder reach their peak incidence of occurrence in the sixth decade (Bowles, 1976a). Chronic irritation of the bladder and cigarette smoking, both avoidable factors, are among the main causes of bladder tumors. Some of the symptoms resemble those of a bladder infection, such as frequency, urgency, and dysuria. A painless hematuria is the primary sign and characterizes cancer of the bladder. Standard diagnostic measures for this disease are employed with the aged patient, including cystoscopic examination. Treatment can include surgery or radiation, depending on the extent and location of the lesion. The nurse should employ the nursing measures described in medical-surgical nursing literature. Observation for signs indicating metastasis, such as pelvic or back pain, is part of the nursing care for these patients.

Bladder Diverticula

Bladder diverticula, usually occurring in numbers rather than singularly, may be present in aged individuals. Since they predispose the individual to infection, antibiotic therapy and surgical correction are typically major parts of the treatment plan.

Renal calculi

Renal calculi occur most frequently in middle-aged adults. In the aged, the formation of stones can be caused by immobilization, infection, changes in the pH or concentration of urine, chronic diarrhea, dehydration, excessive elimination of uric acid, and hypercalcemia. Pain, hematuria, and symptoms of urinary tract infection are commonly associated with this problem, and gastrointestinal upset may also occur. Standard diagnostic and treatment measures are used for the aged, and the nurse can assist by preventing urinary stasis, by providing ample fluids, and by facilitating prompt treatment of urinary tract infections.

Glomerulonephritis

Most frequently, chronic glomerulonephritis already exists in aged persons who develop an acute condition. It is possible for the symptoms of this disease to be so subtle and mild that they are initially unnoticed. Clinical manifestations include fever, fatigue, nausea, vomiting, anorexia, abdominal pain, anemia, edema, elevated blood pressure, and an increased sedimentation rate. Oliguria may occur, as can proteinuria and hematuria. Headache, convulsions, paralysis, aphasia, coma, and an altered mental status may be a consequence of cerebral edema associated with this disease. Diagnostic and treatment measures do not differ significantly from those used with the young. The use of antibiotics, a restricted sodium and protein diet, and close attention to fluid intake and output are basic parts of the treatment plan. If the aged person is receiving digitalis, diuretics, or antihypertensive drugs, close observation for cumulative toxic effects resulting from compromised kidney function must be observed for. The patient should be evaluated periodically after the acute illness is resolved for detection of exacerbations of chronic glomerulonephritis and signs of renal failure.

Pyelonephritis

Pyelonephritis is the most commonly diagnosed renal problem in the aged female. Although urinary obstruction is the primary cause of this disease in older persons, there is some thought that autoimmune reactions may have some relationship as well. Symptoms of this problem vary from mild to severe. Dull back pain, fever, gastrointestinal upset, frequency, dysuria, burning, bacteriuria, and pyuria are usually present with acute pyelonephritis. As the chronic form develops, progressive kidney damage leads to polyuria, anorexia, weight loss, fatigue and the classic symptoms associated with uremia. Aged patients have been found to have no fever and no voiding difficulty, however, even when high bacterial counts have been present (Kahn and Snapper, 1974b). The treatment depends on the causative factor and usually includes antibiotic therapy to eliminate the causative organism, correct the obstruction, and strengthen the patient's resistance. As with glomerulonephritis, periodic evaluation for the recurrence of infection and close follow-up are essential.

PROBLEMS IN THE FEMALE REPRODUCTIVE SYSTEM

Changes and disease processes common in old age contribute toward various problems in the female reproductive tract, many of which could be corrected or more easily managed through early detection. Unfortunately, older women do not always get regular gynecologic examinations, and by the time the symptoms produce enough discomfort to motivate them to do so, chances for a good prognosis can be significantly reduced. Some older women, having delivered their children at home, never had a gynecologic examination in their entire lifetime. Others mistakenly think that this procedure is not necessary for women over childbearing age. Some find it an embarrassing and uncomfortable procedure, and some have limited finances that must be spent attending to more disturbing medical problems.

Inquiry into the frequency of gynecologic examinations is an

233

essential component of nursing assessment, and education should be provided regarding the continued importance of such examinations in old age. Health departments that offer examinations free or inexpensively to women attending family planning and prenatal clinics would provide a valuable service by extending their availability to the older woman, especially since she is more likely to be living on a lower income. Long-term care facilities should also recognize their importance and provide for them.

Infections and Tumors of the Vulva

The vulva loses hair and subcutaneous fat with age, and this is accompanied by a flattening and folding of the labia. A general atrophy occurs as well. These changes cause the vulva to be more fragile and more easily susceptible to irritation and infection. *Senile vulvitis* is the term used to describe vulvar infection associated with hypertrophy or atrophy. Vulvar problems in the aged may reflect serious disease processes such as diabetes, hepatitis, leukemia, and pernicious anemia. Incontinence and poor hygienic practices can also be underlying causes of vulvitis. Pruritis is the primary symptom associated with vulvitis. Patients who are confused and noncommunicative may display restlessness, and the nurse may discover that they are suffering from irritation and thickening of the vulvar tissue as a result of scratching. Initially, treatment is aimed at finding and managing any underlying cause. A good nutritional status assists in improving the condition, as does special attention to cleanliness. Sitz baths and local applications of saline compresses or steroid creams may be included in the treatment plan. Special attention is required to keep the incontinent patient clean and dry as much as possible. Sometimes alcohol is injected into the subcutaneous tissue of the perineum to provide relief.

Although pruritis is commonly associated with vulvitis, it may be a symptom of a *vulvar tumor*. Pain and irritation also may be associated with this problem. Any mass or lesion in this area should receive prompt attention and be biopsied. The clitoris is commonly the site of a vulvar malignancy. Cancer of the vulva may be manifested by large, painful, and foul-smelling fungating or ulcerating tumors. The adjacent tissues may also be affected. A radical vulvectomy is usually the treatment of choice and tends to be well tolerated by the aged female. Less commonly used is radiation therapy, which is not tolerated as well as surgery. Early treatment, prior to metastasis to inguinal lymph nodes, promotes a good prognosis.

Problems of the Vagina

Vaginitis. With advancing age, the vaginal epithelium thins, and this is accompanied by a loss of tissue elasticity. Secretions become alkaline and of lesser quantity. The flora changes, affecting the natural protection the vagina normally provides. These changes predispose the older female to the common infection, *senile vaginitis*. Soreness, pruritis, burning, and a reddened vagina are symptoms, and the accompanying vaginal discharge is clear, brown, or white. As it progresses, this vaginitis can cause bleeding and adhesions.

Local estrogens in suppository or cream form are usually effective in treating senile vaginitis. Nurses should make sure that patients understand the proper utilization of these topical medications and do not attempt to administer them orally. Acid douches may also be prescribed, and if the patient is to administer a douche at home, it is important to emphasize the need to measure the solution's temperature with a dairy thermometer. Altered receptors for hot and cold temperatures and reduced pain sensation in many aged persons predispose the patient to burns from solutions excessively hot for fragile vaginal tissue. Good hygienic practices are beneficial, not only in the treatment but also in the prevention of vaginitis.

Cancer of the vagina. Cancer of the vagina is rare in older females, resulting more frequently from metastasis than from the vaginal area as a primary site (Birnbaum, 1974). All vaginal ulcers and masses detected in aged females should be viewed with suspicion of malignancy and be biopsied. Since chronic irritation can predispose women to vaginal cancer, those who have chronic vaginitis and or who wear a pessary should obtain Pap smears frequently. Treatment is similar to that used for younger women and may consist of radiation or surgery, depending on the extent of the carcinoma.

Problems of the Cervix

With age, the cervix becomes smaller, and this is accompanied by an atrophy of the endocervical epithelium. Occasionally the endocervical glands can seal over, causing the formation of nabothian cysts. As secretions associated with these cysts accumulate, fever and a palpable tender mass may be evident. It is important, therefore, for the aged female to receive regular gynecologic examinations in which the patency of the cervix can be checked.

Cancer of the cervix. The incidence of cervical cancer decreases with age. Although most endocervical polyps are benign in older females, they should be viewed with suspicion until biopsy confirms a benign diagnosis. Vaginal bleeding and leukorrhea are signs of cervical cancer in aged females. Pain does not commonly occur. As the disease progresses, the patient can develop urinary retention or

235

incontinence, fecal incontinence, and uremia. Treatment of cervical cancer can include radium or surgery.

Problems of the Uterus

The uterus decreases in size with age, becoming so small in some older women that it cannot be palpated on examination. It is important to note that the endometrium does continue to respond to hormonal stimulation.

Cancer of the endometrium. Cancer of the endometrium is not uncommon in the aged and is of higher incidence in obese, diabetic and hypertensive women. Any postmenopausal bleeding should give rise immediately to suspicion of this disease. Dilation and curettage usually are done to confirm the diagnosis since not all cases are detected through Pap smears alone. Treatment consists of surgery, radiation, or a combination of both. Early treatment can prevent metastasis to the vagina and cervix. Endometrial polyps can also cause bleeding and should receive serious attention since they could be indicative of early cancer.

Problems of the Fallopian Tubes and Ovaries

Although masses are occasionally detected in the fallopian tubes, they rarely present any significant problem to the aged female. The primary changes the fallopian tubes undergo with age are shortening, straightening, and atrophy. The ovaries also atrophy with age, becoming smaller and thicker. It is possible for them not to be palpable during the gynecologic examination, due to their decreased size. *Ovarian cancer* is occasionally diagnosed in the aged female. The clinical manifestations of this disease include bleeding, ascites, and the presence of multiple masses. Treatment may consist of surgery or radiation. Benign ovarian tumors commonly occur in the aged and surgery is usually required to differentiate them from malignant ones.

Perineal Herniation

As a result of the stretching and tearing of muscles during childbirth and of the muscle weakness associated with advanced age, perineal herniation is a common problem among older women. Cystocele, rectocele, and prolapse of the uterus are the types most likely to occur. Associated with this problem are lower back pain and pelvic heaviness and a pulling sensation, classic symptoms. Urinary and fecal incontinence, retention, and constipation may also occur. Sometimes the female is able to feel pressure or palpate a mass in her vagina. These herniations can make intercourse difficult and uncomfortable. Although rectoceles do not tend to worsen with age, the opposite is true for cystoceles, which will cause increased problems with time. Surgical repair is the treatment of choice and can be successful in relieving these problems. If surgery cannot be performed, the patient is usually fitted for a pessary, although this method is discouraged since the pessary can cause ulceration and infection.

Dyspareunia

Dyspareunia is a common problem among aged females but is not necessarily a normal consequence of aging. Nulliparous women experience this problem more frequently than women who have had children. Since vulvitis, vaginitis, and other gynecologic problems can contribute to dyspareunia, a thorough gynecologic examination is important, and any lesions or infections should be corrected to alleviate the problem. All effort should be made to help the aged female achieve a satisfactory sexual life. A more detailed discussion of sexual problems is offered in Chapter 23.

Breast Problems

The breasts atrophy with age, sagging more and hanging at a lower level. Some retraction of the nipples may occur as a result of shrinkage and fibrotic changes. Linear firm strands may develop on the breasts due to fibrosis and calcification of the terminal ducts.

Cancer of the breast.   Due to the visual manifestations of decreased fat tissue and atrophy in aged women's breasts, it is not unusual for tumors, possibly present for many years, to become more evident. Since breast cancer is a leading cause of cancer deaths in aged as well as younger women, regular breast examinations should be encouraged. A more detailed explanation of breast examination is presented in Chapter 10. Diagnostic and treatment measures for women with breast cancer are the same at any age.

PROBLEMS OF THE MALE REPRODUCTIVE SYSTEM

Benign Prostatic Hypertrophy

A majority of aged men have some degree of benign prostatic hypertrophy (Howell, 1970; Jaffee, 1974c). Symptoms of this problem progress slowly but continuously; they include hesitancy, decreased force of urinary stream, frequency, and nocturia. As the condition progresses, dribbling, poor control, overflow incontinence, and bleeding may occur. Unfortunately, some men are reluctant or embarrassed to seek prompt medical attention and may develop kidney damage by the time symptoms are severe enough to motivate them to be evaluated.

237

Treatment can include prostatic massage and the use of urinary antiseptics. The most common prostatectomy approach used for aged men with prostatism is transurethral surgery. The patient should be reassured that this surgery will not cause impotence. On the other hand, realistic explanations are needed so that the patient understands that this surgery will not guarantee a sudden rejuvenation of sexual performance.

Cancer of the Prostate

Prostatic cancer is of increasing incidence with age. Although this disease can be asymptomatic, a majority of prostatic cancers can be detected by rectal examination—emphasizing the importance of regular physical examinations. Benign hypertrophy should be followed closely since it is thought to be associated with prostatic cancer, the symptoms of which can be similar (Hodkinson, 1975). In addition, symptoms such as back pain, anemia, weakness, and weight loss can develop as a result of metastasis. If metastasis has not occurred, treatment may consist of radiation or a radical prostatectomy; the latter procedure will result in impotency. Estrogens may be used to prevent tumor dissemination. Palliative treatment, employed if the cancer has metastasized, includes radiation, transurethral surgery, orchiectomy, and estrogens. General principles associated with these therapeutic measures are applicable to the aged patient. Many men are able to continue sexual performance after orchiectomy and during estrogen therapy; the physician should be consulted for specific advice concerning the expected outcomes for individual patients.

Tumors of the Penis, Testes, and Scrotum

Cancer of the penis is rare and tends to occur more frequently in men who have not been circumcised (Bowles, 1976b). It appears as a painless lesion or wartlike growth on the prepuce or glans. The resemblance of this growth to a chancre can cause a misdiagnosis or a reluctance on the part of the patient to seek treatment. A biopsy should be done of any penile lesion. Treatment may consist of radiation and local excision for small lesions and partial or total penile amputation for extensive lesions. Uncommon in the aged but usually malignant when they do occur are testicular tumors; testicular enlargement and pain and enlargement of the breasts are suspicious symptoms. Chemotherapy, radiation, and orchiectomy are among the treatment measures. Scrotal masses, usually benign, can be caused by conditions such as hydrocele, spermatocele, varicocele, and hernia. Symptoms and treatment depend on the underlying cause and are the same as for younger males.

NURSING CONSIDERATIONS

A basic nursing action for early detection of genitourinary problems is to encourage regular physical examinations for every aged person, including examination of the reproductive organs. Subtle clues of disturbances, such as nocturia and problems in sexual performance, should not be considered a result of aging without thorough medical evaluation. The nurse must understand that genitourinary problems may not be easy for geriatric patients to discuss; they require a great deal of sensitivity and respect from the nurse involved. Related to this is the need for respecting the dignity and privacy of the individual during urologic and gynecologic examinations. In overcoming patients' embarrassment at having others care for urinary drainage or perform treatments on their genitalia, a matter-of-fact but respectful approach and an understanding attitude on the part of the nurse are valuable assets. Exposure should be prevented, and this holds true for disoriented and unconscious patients as well. In addition, the nurse should be certain that ancillary staff and others working with aged patients demonstrate an understanding that few patients are intentionally incontinent, that few are not bothered or embarrassed by their incontinence, and that making an incident over it usually serves no therapeutic value and can be quite demeaning. A review of information regarding the genitourinary system is also useful for the aged patient. Some may believe that a particular sexual event caused their problem; others may believe that a urinary problem will alter their sexual performance. Realistic explanations help alleviate anxiety, fear, and guilt, and increased patient understanding can increase compliance. It is useful to include the spouse in such educational sessions.

REFERENCES

Birnbaum, S. J. "Geriatric Gynecology." In Chinn, A. B. (ed.), *Working with Older People,* Vol. IV. U.S. Dept. of Health, Education, and Welfare, 1974, p. 150.
Bowles, W. T. "Urologic Surgery." In Steinberg, F. U. (ed.), *Cowdry's, The Care of the Geriatric Patient,* 5th ed. Mosby, 1976. (a) p. 278; (b) p. 282.
Brocklehurst, J. C. "The Urinary Tract." In Rossman, I. (ed.), *Clinical Geriatrics.* Lippincott, Philadelphia, 1971. (a) p. 222; (b) p. 226.
Hodkinson, H. M. *An Outline of Geriatrics.* Academic Press, New York, 1975, p. 129.
Howell, T. H. *A Student's Guide to Geriatrics.* Staples, London, 1970, p. 173.
Jaffe, J. W. "Common Lower Urinary Tract Problems in Older Persons." In Chinn, A. B. (ed.), *Working with Older People,* Vol. IV. U.S. Dept. of Health, Education, and Welfare, 1974. (a) p. 144; (b) p. 141; (c) p. 142.
Kahn, A. I., and Snapper, I. "Medical Renal Diseases in the Aged." In Chinn, A. B. (ed.), *Working with Older People,* Vol. IV. U.S. Dept. of Health, Education, and Welfare, 1974. (a) p. 131; (b) p. 133.

239

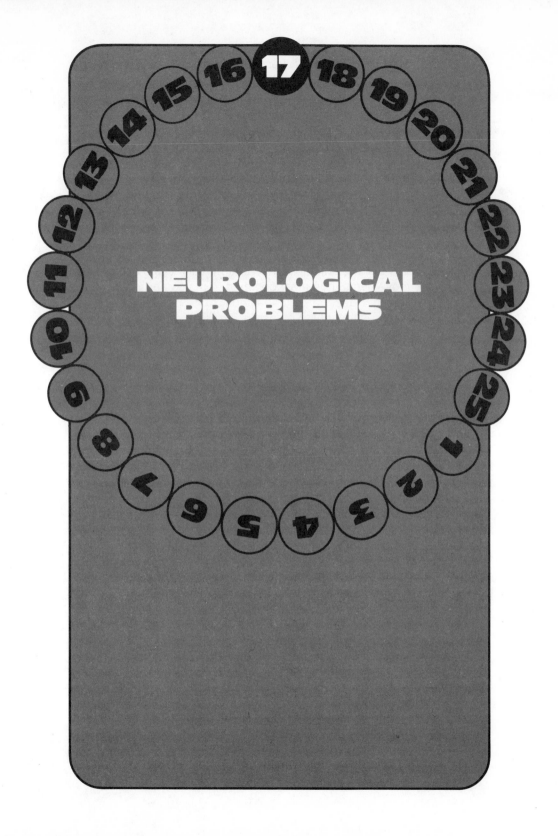

NEUROLOGICAL PROBLEMS

After age 25, there is a gradual but steady loss of neurons, manifested in various ways in each individual. Interestingly, the nervous system does not always demonstrate a correlation between the anatomic changes that occur as an individual ages and the signs and symptoms he or she manifests. Persons with reduced brain substances may be capable of unimpaired performance while those with severe limitations may have no alteration in brain substance. In addition to the aging process, the status of the circulatory system and nutritional factors can also affect neurologic functioning.

DISORDERS AND RELATED CARE PROCEDURES

Parkinson's Disease

Parkinson's disease affects the central nervous system's ability to control body movements. It is most common in males and occurs most frequently in the fifth decade of life. Although the exact cause is unknown, this disease is thought to be associated with a history of metallic poisoning, encephalitis, and cerebrovascular disease—especially arteriosclerosis in aged persons. A faint tremor that progresses over a long period of time may be the first clue. The tremor is reduced when the patient attempts a purposeful movement. Muscle rigidity and weakness develop, witnessed by drooling, difficulty in swallowing, slow speech and a monotone. The face of the patient has a masklike appearance and the skin is moist. Appetite frequently increases and emotional instability may be demonstrated. A characteristic sign is the shuffling gait with the trunk leaning forward. The rate of the patient's gait increases as he walks and may not be able to be stopped voluntarily. As the disease progresses, the patient may be unable to ambulate.

A variety of measures are used to control the tremors and maintain the highest possible level of independence. Levodopa or anticholinergics may be prescribed to decrease the patient's symptoms. Joint mobility is maintained and improved by active and passive range-of-motion exercises; warm baths and massage may facilitate these exercises and relieve muscle spasms caused by rigidity. Contractures are a particular risk to the aged person with Parkinson's disease. Physical and occupational therapists should be actively involved in the exercise program, assisting the patient to find devices that increase self-care ability. Surgical intervention is rare for aged patients since they do not tend to respond as well (Carman, 1968; Carter, 1971; Hodkinson, 1975).

Since tension and frustration will aggravate the symptoms, the nurse should attempt to offer psychological support and minimize emotional upsets. Teaching is beneficial in helping patients and their families gain a realistic insight into the disease. The nurse should emphasize that the disease progresses slowly and that therapy can minimize disability. Although intellectual functioning is not impaired by this disease, the speech problems and helpless appearance of patients may cause others to underestimate their mental ability; this can be extremely frustrating and degrading to the patient, who may react by becoming depressed or irritable. Continuing support by the nurse can help the family maximize the patient's mental capacity and understand personality changes that may occur. Communication and mental stimulation should be encouraged on a level which the patient always enjoyed. As the disease progresses, increased assistance is required by the patient. Skillful nursing assessment is essential to ensure that the demands for assistance are met while the maximum level of patient independence is preserved.

Transient Ischemic Attacks

Transient ischemic attacks, or temporary episodes of central nervous system dysfunction, can be caused by any situation which reduces cerebral circulation. Hyperextension and flexion of the head, such as that which occurs when an individual falls asleep in a chair, can impair cerebral blood flow. Reduced blood pressure resulting from anemia and certain drugs (diuretics and antihypertensives, for example) and cigarette smoking, due to its vasoconstrictive effect, will also decrease cerebral circulation. Hemiparesis, hemianesthesia, aphasia, unilateral loss of vision, diplopia, vertigo, nausea, vomiting, and dysphagia are among the signs which may be manifested with a transient ischemic attack, depending on the location of the ischemic area. These signs can last from minutes to hours, and complete recovery is usual within a day. Treatment may consist of correction of the underlying cause, anticoagulant therapy, or vascular reconstruction. A significant concern regarding transient ischemic attacks is that they increase the patient's risk of cerebral vascular accident.

Cerebral Vascular Accident

Aged persons with hypertension, severe arteriosclerosis, diabetes, gout, anemia, hypothyroidism, silent myocardial infarction, transient ischemic attacks, and dehydration are among the high risk candidates for a cerebral vascular accident, the third leading cause of death in the aged according to the U.S. Bureau of the Census, 1975. Although a ruptured cerebral blood vessel could be responsible for this problem, most cerebral vascular accidents in the aged are caused by partial or complete cerebral thrombosis. Lightheadedness, dizziness, headache, drop attack, and memory and behavioral changes are some of the warning signs of a cerebral vascular accident. A drop attack is a fall caused by a complete muscular flaccidity in the legs but with no alteration in consciousness (Agate, 1971). Patients describing or demonstrating these symptoms should be referred for prompt medical evaluation. Since the

243

nurse is in a key position to learn of these signs, she can be instrumental in helping the patient avoid disability or death from a stroke.

Although the aged have a higher mortality from cerebral vascular accident than the young, those who do survive have a good chance of recovery. Good nursing care can improve the patient's chances of survival and minimize the limitations that impair a full recovery. In the acute phase, nursing efforts have several aims:

1. Maintaining a patent airway
2. Providing adequate nutrition and hydration
3. Monitoring neurologic and vital signs
4. Preventing complications associated with immobility

In addition, unconscious patients need good skin care and frequent turning since they are more susceptible to decubiti formation. If an indwelling catheter is not being utilized, it is important for the nurse to examine the patient for indications of an overdistended bladder and promptly remedy the situation if it should occur. The eyes of the unconscious patient may remain open for a long period of time, risking drying, irritation, and ulceration of the cornea. Corneal damage can be prevented by eye irrigations with a sterile saline solution followed by the use of eyedrops of sterile mineral oil. Eye pads may be used to aid in keeping the lids closed; these are changed daily and frequently checked to make sure the lids are actually closed. Regular mouth care and range-of-motion exercises are also standard measures.

When consciousness is regained and the patient's condition stabilizes, more active efforts can focus on rehabilitation. It may be extremely difficult for patients to understand and participate in their rehabilitation due to speech, behavior, and memory problems. Although these problems vary depending on what side of the brain is affected, some general observations can be noted. Retention span is reduced, and long, complicated directions may be confusing. Memory for old events may be intact, while recent events or explanations are forgotten (a characteristic demonstrated by many aged persons without a history of cerebral vascular accident). Patients may have difficulty transferring information from one situation to another. For example, they may be able to remember the steps in lifting from the bed to the wheelchair but be unable to apply the same principles in moving from the wheelchair to an armchair. Confusion, restlessness, and irritability may be present due to sensory deprivation. Emotional lability may also be a problem.

To minimize the limitations imposed by these problems, the nurse may find the following helpful:

1. Talk to the patient during routine care activities.

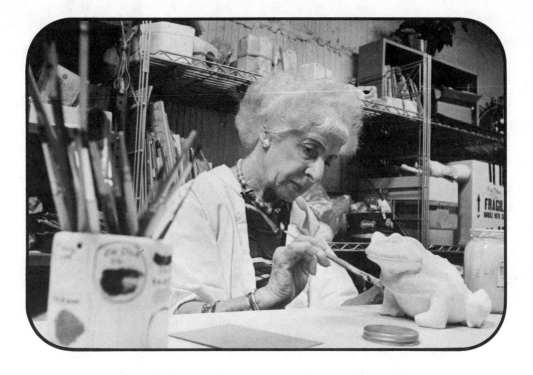

2. Explain in brief form the basics of what has occurred, the procedures being performed, and the activities to expect.
3. Speak distinctly but do not shout.
4. Devise an easy means of communication, such as a picture chart to which one can point.
5. Minimize environmental confusion, noise, and clutter.
6. Aim toward consistency—of those providing care and of the activities.
7. Use objects familiar to patients—their own clothing, clock, etc.
8. Keep a calendar and/or sign in the room showing the day and date.
9. Supply sensory stimulation through conversation, radio, television, wall decorations, and objects for patients to handle.
10. Provide frequent positive feedback; even a minor task may be a major achievement for the patient.
11. Expect and accept errors and failures.

The reader is advised to consult general medical-surgical textbooks for more detailed guidance in the care of patients with stroke. Local chapters of the American Heart Association also provide much useful material for the nurse, the patient, and the family on the topic of stroke.

245

Brain Tumors

Although brain tumors are not of high incidence in the aged, the resemblance of their symptoms to those commonly attributed to senility often results in delayed diagnoses. For instance, poor memory, confusion, personality change, headache, visual difficulties, poor coordination, and sensory-motor changes may be associated with arteriosclerosis or a multitude of other age-related problems. If these signs are not evaluated thoroughly in an early stage, valuable and potentially successful treatment time may be lost. It is important for the nurse to be aware of the general course of the patient's symptoms and facilitate their prompt evaluation.

NURSING CONSIDERATIONS

A few general statements can be added to the nursing considerations already presented throughout this chapter. The aged patient with a neurological problem may have a greater problem maintaining independence, not only due to the limitations imposed by the disease, but also as a result of those related to the aging process. Skillful and creative nursing assistance can help the patient achieve a maximum level of independence. Some of the self-help devices mentioned—rails in hallways and bathrooms and numerous other household modifications—can promote independent living in the individual's home environment. It is reassuring for the patient to know that assistance is available should the need arise. Periodic home visits by the nurse, regular contact with a family member or friend, and a daily call from a local telephone reassurance program can help the patient feel confident and protected, which also encourages independence. Although patients may perform tasks slowly and awkwardly, family members need to understand that allowing them to function independently is physically and psychologically more beneficial then doing the tasks for them. Continuing patience, reassurance, and encouragement are essential in maximizing the patient's capacity for independence.

Personality changes frequently accompany neurological problems. Patients may become depressed as the realization of their limitations is experienced or frustrated by their need to be dependent on others. Their reactions may be displaced and evidenced as irritability to others. Family members and those caring for the patient may need help in understanding the reasons for the patient's reactions and in learning ways to deal therapeutically with such behavior. Getting offended or angry at such patients may upset or frustrate them further. Understanding, patience, and tolerance are needed to accept any personality changes.

Protecting the patient from hazards is particularly important in nursing the neurologic patient. Uncoordinated movements, weakness, and dizziness are among the problems that cause these patients to have a high risk of accidents. Whether in an institutional setting or a home, the nurse should actively scrutinize the environment for potential sources of mishaps, such as loose carpeting, poorly lit stairwells, clutter, ill-functioning appliances, and for a lack of safeguards such as fire warning systems, fire escapes, and rails and a slip-proof surface in bathtubs. Safety considerations should also include prevention of contractures, decubiti, and other hazards to the structure and function of the body which neurologic patients are more prone to develop. It is an injustice to the patient for preventable complications to hamper progress and compound disability.

REFERENCES

Agate, J. "Common Symptoms and Complaints." In Rossman, I., *Clinical Geriatrics*. Lippincott, Philadelphia, 1971, p. 365.

Carman, J. B. "Anatomic Basis of Surgical Treatment of Parkinson's Disease." *New England Journal of Medicine,* 279:919, 1968.

Carter, A. B. "The Neurologic Aspects of Aging." In Rossman, I. (ed.), *Clinical Geriatrics.* Lippincott, Philadelphia, 1971, p. 138.

Hodkinson, H. M. *An Outline of Geriatrics.* Academic Press, New York, 1975, p. 123.

U.S. Bureau of the Census: *Statistical Abstract of the United States: 1975,* 96th ed., Washington, D.C., 1975, p. 61, No. 86.

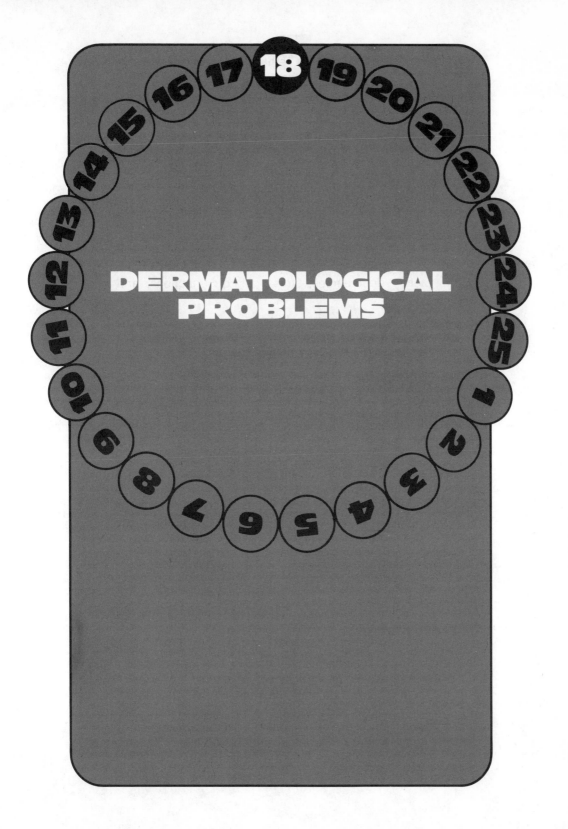

DERMATOLOGICAL
PROBLEMS

Perhaps the most obvious and most scorned effects of the aging process are those involving the integumentary system. Wrinkles, lines, and drooping eyelids gradually develop due to a loss of elasticity; the skin may appear a gray or pale yellow color; skin pigmentation occurs on hands and other frequently exposed areas; skin resistance is lessened as the skin becomes more dry and thin; the nails become dry and brittle, occasionally to the extent that they may peel. The rate of these changes varies according to the person's activity and to individual nutritional, emotional, biochemical, environmental, and genetic factors. Although the aged can experience the dermatological problems of any other age group, normal aging changes in the integumentary system, impaired circulation, and a generally greater susceptibility to infection contribute to dermatological problems in the older adult. These disorders can also result from irritation, poor hygiene, dietary deficiencies, stress, allergic reactions, and certain diseases.

COMMON PROBLEMS IN THE AGED AND RELATED CARE

Senile Pruritus

The most common dermatological problem in the aged is pruritus. Although atrophic changes alone may be responsible for this problem, senile pruritus can be precipitated by any circumstance which dries the person's skin, such as excessive bathing and dry heat. Diabetes, arteriosclerosis, uremia, liver disease, cancer, pernicious anemia, and certain psychiatric problems can also contribute to pruritus. If not corrected, the itching may cause traumatizing scratching, leading to breakage and infection of the skin. Prompt recognition of this problem and implementation of corrective measures are therefore essential. If possible, the underlying cause should be corrected. Bath oils, moisturizing lotions, and massage are beneficial in treating and preventing pruritus. Vitamin supplements may be recommended, as may a high quality, vitamin-rich diet. Antihistamines and topical steroids may be prescribed for relief.

Senile Keratoses

Senile keratoses, also referred to as actinic or solar keratoses, are small, light-colored lesions (usually gray or brown) found on exposed areas of the skin. Keratin may be accumulated in these lesions, causing the formation of a cutaneous horn with a slightly reddened and swollen base. Freezing agents and acids can be employed to destroy the keratotic lesions, but electrodesiccation or surgical excision ensures a more thorough removal. Close nursing observation for changes in keratotic lesions is vital since they are precancerous.

Seborrheic Keratoses

It is not uncommon for aged persons to have several dark, wartlike projections on various parts of their bodies. These lesions, called seborrheic keratoses, may be as small as a pinhead or as large as a quarter. They tend to increase in size and number with age. In the sebaceous areas of the trunk, face, and neck and in persons with oily skin, these lesions appear dark and oily; in less sebaceous areas they are dry in appearance and of a light color. Normally, seborrheic keratoses will not have swelling or redness around their base. Sometimes abrasive activity with a gauze pad containing oil will remove small seborrheic keratoses. Larger, raised lesions can be removed by freezing agents or by a currettage and cauterization procedure. Although these lesions are benign, medical evaluation is important in order to differentiate them from precancerous lesions. In addition, the cosmetic benefit of removing them should not be overlooked for the aged patient.

Stasis Dermatitis

Poor venous return can cause edema of the lower extremities, which leads to poor tissue nutrition. As the poorly nourished legs accumulate debris, inadequately carried away with the venous return, the legs gain a pigmented, cracked, and exudative appearance. Subsequent scratching, irritation, or other trauma can then easily result in the formation of a leg ulcer. Stasis ulcers need special attention to facilitate healing. Infection must be controlled, and necrotic tissue removed, before healing will take place. Good nutrition is an important component of the therapy, and a diet high in vitamins and protein is recommended. Once healing has occurred, concern should be given to avoiding situations that promote stasis dermatitis. The patient may need instruction regarding a diet for weight reduction or the planning of high-quality meals. Venous return can be enhanced by elevating the legs several times a day and by preventing interferences to circulation such as standing for long periods of time, sitting with legs crossed, and wearing garters. Some patients may require ligation and stripping of the veins to prevent further episodes of stasis dermatitis.

Decubitus Ulcers

Tissue anoxia and ischemia resulting from pressure can cause the necrosis, sloughing, and ulceration of tissue commonly known as a decubitus ulcer. Any part of the body can develop a decubitus ulcer, but the most common sites are the sacrum, greater trochanter, and ischial tuberosities. The aged are high risk candidates for several reasons:

1. Their skin is more fragile and is damaged more easily.
2. They often are in a poor nutritional state.

251

3. They have reduced sensation of pressure and pain.
4. They are more frequently affected by immobile and edematous conditions, which contribute to skin breakdown.

Prevention. In addition to developing more easily in the aged, decubitus ulcers require a longer period to heal in older persons. As mentioned earlier, it has been estimated that wounds taking 31 days to heal in a 20-year-old, take 55 days in a 40-year-old and 100 days in a 60-year-old (Manney, 1975). Therefore, the most important nursing measure is to prevent their formation, and to do this, it is essential to prevent pressure. Encouraging activity or turning the patient who can't move independently at least every two hours is necessary. Shearing forces which cause two layers of tissue to move across each other should be prevented by not elevating the head of the bed more than 30 degrees, by not allowing patients to slide in bed, and by lifting instead of pulling patients when moving them. Pillows, flotation pads, alternating pressure mattresses, and water beds can be used to disperse pressure from bony prominences. It must be emphasized that these devices do not eliminate the need for frequent position changes. While sitting in a chair, patients should be urged and assisted with shifting their weight at certain intervals. Lamb's wool and heel protectors are useful in preventing irritation to bony prominences. Sheets should be kept wrinkle free and the bed should be checked frequently for foreign objects such as syringes and utensils which the patient may be lying on unknowingly.

A high-protein, vitamin-rich diet to maintain and improve tissue health is essential in avoiding decubitus ulcer formation. Good skin care is another essential ingredient in decubiti prevention. Skin should be kept clean and dry, and blotting the patient dry will avoid irritation from rubbing the skin with a towel. Bath oils and lotions, used prophylactically, will help keep the skin soft and intact. Massage of bony prominences and range-of-motion exercises promote circulation and assist in keeping the tissue well nourished. The incontinent patient should be thoroughly cleansed with soap and water and dried after each episode to avoid skin breakdown from irritating excreta.

Techniques to treat decubiti. Special nursing attention is warranted to promote healing and prevent complications. A variety of techniques are employed in treating the ulcer, including the topical application of granulated sugar, Karaya, antacids, chemical debriding agents, and wet to dry dressings. Cleansing of the ulcer and debriding of necrotic tissue are required for the regeneration of epithelium. Gentle massage to the tissue around the decubitus ulcer will promote circulation and decrease edema. Topical antibiotics may be used to control infection. The nursing measures discussed above regarding decubiti prevention will also benefit the patient who has developed an ulcer. For severe ulcers, surgery may be required. The various techniques used to treat decutiti are described below. More detail regarding these procedures can be obtained by exploring some of the literature cited in the bibliography.

Chemical debriding: Elase (a fibrinolytic enzyme) or Santyl (a collagenase) can be applied to a cleansed wound and dressed with a dry bandage or gauze. Specific instructions and frequency vary according to the agent. These agents facilitate the removal of necrotic tissue, allowing granulation and epithelization of tissue to occur.

Gelfoam with flotation therapy: The compressed or powder form of Gelfoam is implanted in the tissue of a clean wound to promote the growth of new cells. The dressing is left undisturbed for from three to seven days; tissue granulation is better when the dressing is allowed to remain in place longer. A nonpurulent discharge may occur, but it is no cause for alarm. Flotation pads are used to displace weight.

Insulin: After cleansing and irrigation of the wound, ten units of U-40 regular insulin are dropped on the wound. The ulcer is then exposed to air to dry, with no dressing applied. This procedure is performed twice daily.

Karaya: After cleansing the wound with pHisohex and irrigation with a hydrogen peroxide solution, the edges of the wound are massaged. A Karaya ring is then fitted around the wound and Karaya powder sprinkled directly into the wound. Reston is sometimes used to relieve pressure on the wound. A piece of plastic wrap is attached to the Reston to cover the wound while allowing view of it. This window is changed and additional powder added every eight hours.

Maalox or sugar: After cleansing and irrigation of the wound, Maalox or sugar is applied to promote granulation. Irrigation and reapplication of the substance is repeated every eight hours.

Surgical debriding: Necrotic tissue can be removed surgically to promote faster debridment and new tissue growth.

Wet to dry dressings: Following cleansing of the ulcer, gauze dressing soaked in normal saline or other prescribed solutions is placed on the wound for from six to eight hours (or as specified) and allowed to dry. Some debridment occurs as the dry dressing is removed.

General measures: Techniques to treat decubiti including the following general procedures: (1) frequent turning to prevent

253

reduced circulation from blocked capillaries; (2) the use of flotation pads, alternating pressure matresses, water beds, and heel protectors to displace body weight; (3) the use of sheepskin to prevent irritation to the skin and to promote evaporation of skin moisture; (4) using a turn sheet to allow greater weight distribution when lifting or turning the patient and to prevent friction to the skin during these activities; (5) providing a high-protein, high-vitamin diet to promote a positive nitrogen balance and tissue growth.

NURSING CONSIDERATIONS

Some general measures are employed to prevent and manage dermatological problems in the aged. It is important to avoid drying agents, rough clothing, highly starched linens, and other items irritating to the skin. Good skin nutrition and hydration can be promoted by activity, bath oils, lotions, and massages. Although skin cleanliness is important, excessive bathing may be hazardous to the skin; daily partial sponge baths and complete baths every third or fourth day are sufficient for the average aged person. Early attention to and treatment of pruritus and skin lesions is advisable in preventing irritation, infection, and other problems.

Psychological support can be especially important to the patient with a dermatological problem. Unlike respiratory, cardiac, and other disorders, dermatological problems are often visibly unpleasant—to the patient and others. Visitors and staff may unnecessarily avoid touching and being with the patient in reaction to the skin problems they see. The nurse can reassure visitors regarding the safety of contact with the patient and provide instruction for any special precautions that must be followed. The most important fact to emphasize is that the patient is still normal, with normal needs and feelings, and will appreciate normal interactions and contact.

All persons should be encouraged to look their best and make the most of their appearance. However, efforts to avoid the normal outcomes of the aging process are for the most part fruitless and frustrating. Money which could be applied to more basic needs is sometimes invested on attempts to defy reality. The nurse should emphasize to persons young and old that no cream, lotion, or miracle drug will remove wrinkles and lines or return youthful skin. While clarifying misconceptions regarding rejuvenating products, the nurse can encourage cosmetic use for the purpose of protecting the skin and maintaining an attractive appearance—from which many benefits may be derived. Perhaps, as society achieves a greater acceptance and understanding of the aging process, cosmetic use will be replaced by an appreciation for the natural beauty of age.

REFERENCE

Manney, J. R. *Aging in American Society*. Univ. of Michigan Press, Wayne State University, Ann Arbor, Mich., 1975, p. 27.

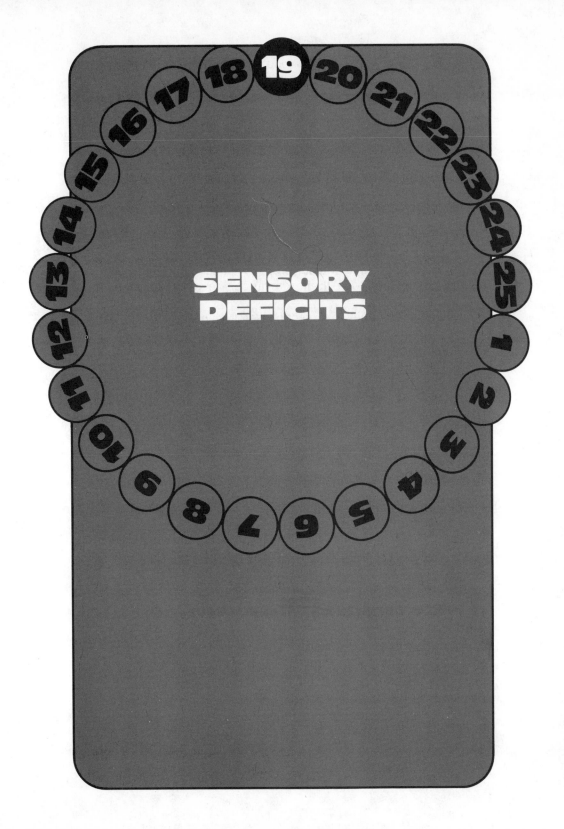

SENSORY DEFICITS

Good sensory function is an extremely valuable asset, one which is often taken for granted. Intact senses facilitate accurate perception of the environment. People are better able to protect themselves from harm when they can see, hear, smell, touch, and verbalize danger; and the beauties of the earth are more fully appreciated when the senses are functioning at their optimum level. In addition, communication, the sharing of experiences, and the exchange of feelings are more complete when all the senses can participate. Imagine with what distortion the environment is perceived when sensory function is impaired. People might suspect they are being talked about if they are unable to hear the conversation of those around them. Common everyday experiences, such as reading the newspaper and recognizing a familiar face on the street, can be hampered by poor eyesight. Food tastes bland without properly functioning taste buds; and freshly cut flowers lose their fragrances to poor olfactory functioning.

The reduced ability to protect oneself from hazards due to sensory deficits can result in serious falls from unseen obstacles; missed alarms and warnings; ingestion of hazardous substances from not recognizing their taste; an inability to detect the odor of smoke or gas; and burns and skin breakdown because of decreased cutaneous sensation of excessive temperature and pressure. And as though the multiple problems which affect the elderly aren't enough, they are also the most frequent victims of these sensory deficits. Alterations during the aging process, excessive use and abuse, and the disease processes that affect all age groups contribute to their problems. Sensory deficits compound the other problems which threaten the health and well-being of the aged—their increased vulnerability to accidents, their social isolation and declining physical function, and their many other limitations regarding self-care activities. Since it is the rare older individual who does not also suffer from sensory deficit, it behooves the nurse working with the aged to have a sound knowledge of the sensory problems affecting them and of the associated assistive techniques.

VISUAL DEFICITS AND RELATED CARE

As the eye undergoes a variety of structural and functional changes with age, the lids become thinner and wrinkled, displaying skin folds commonly known as "bags" (Figure 19-1). Ptosis, inversion, and eversion of the lid are common. The conjunctiva, easily irritated by dust particles and air pollutants, is thinner and more fragile. The cornea gains a smoky appearance, being less translucent and more spherical. Deposits of fat over the cornea and grayish plaques on the sclera may be detected. The pupil decreases in size, becoming less responsive to light, and there is sclerosis of the pupil sphincter. Peripheral vision is

258

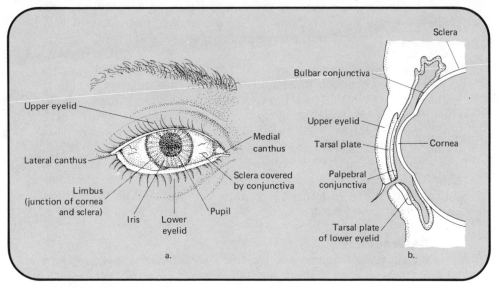

Figure 19-1. Gross anatomy of the eye. (a) Anterior view. (b) Cross-sectional view. (Source: Barbara Bates, *A Guide to Physical Examination,* Lippincott, Philadelphia, 1974.)

more difficult as the visual field narrows, and vision at night and in dimly lit areas is a greater problem due to the increase in the threshold of light perception. Yellowing of the lens makes vision for low-tone colors (blues and greens) more difficult. Visual acuity is reduced, and there is a slower adaptation to dark. Defective accommodation due to loss of elasticity in the lens of the eye (presbyopia) is common. The eyes have slower responses, fewer secretions, and a lower tissue resistance, predisposing the aged person to eye irritation and trauma. There may be a liquefaction of vitreous humor, accompanied by the release of supporting tissue, and cholesterol crystals may develop, causing bothersome but harmless spots before the aged individual's eyes.

In spite of these changes, a majority of older persons have sufficient visual capacity to meet normal self-care demands with the assistance of corrective lenses. Serious visual problems can develop, however, and should be recognized early to prevent significant visual damage. Routine eye examinations by an *ophthalmologist* are important in detecting and treating eye problems early. Frequently, people postpone eye examinations because their present corrective lenses are still functional or because there seems to be no apparent need or because they have limited finances. The gerontological nurse can be instrumental in ensuring appropriate visual care by emphasizing that beyond the need for corrective lenses, eye examinations are important in detecting

259

other problems. It is important to inform people that while an *optician* prepares lenses and an *optometrist* fits the lenses to the visual deficit, only the *opthalmologist* diagnoses and treats the full range of eye diseases.

In addition to annual eye examinations, prompt evaluation is required for any symptom that could indicate a visual problem, including burning or pain in the eye, blurred or double vision, redness of the conjunctiva, spots, headaches, and any other change in vision. There are a variety of disorders that can threaten the aged's vision. For instance, arteriosclerosis and diabetes can cause damage to the retina, and nutritional deficiencies and hypertension can result in visual impairment. The reader is advised to refer to the sections of this book discussing these diseases to gain an understanding of the pathophysiology involved.

Cataracts

A cataract is a clouding of the lens or its capsule whereby the lens loses its transparency. Cataracts are common in the aged and it is said that everyone would develop cataracts if they lived long enough. Most aged persons do have some degree of lens opacity with or without the presence of other eye disorders. There is no discomfort or pain associated with cataracts. At first, vision is distorted and objects appear blurred. The opacification continues, and eventually there is complete lens opacity and complete loss of vision. Glare from sunlight and bright lights is extremely bothersome to the affected person. Nuclear sclerosis develops; with this the lens of the eye becomes yellow or yellow-brown, and eventually the color of the pupil changes from black to a cloudy white.

Surgery to remove the lens is the only cure for a cataract. Patients with a single cataract may not necessarily undergo surgery if vision in the other eye is good, and these individuals should concentrate on strengthening their existing visual capacity, reducing their limitations, and employing the safety measures applicable to any visually impaired person (Figure 19-2). Sunglasses, sheer curtains over windows, furniture placed away from bright light, and several soft lights instead of a single

Figure 19-2. Compensating for visual deficits in the aged: (a) Face person when speaking. (b) Use several soft indirect lights instead of a single glaring one. (c) Avoid glare from windows by using sheer curtains or stained windows. (d) Use large-print reading material. (e) Have frequently used items within visual field. (f) Avoid use of low-tone colors and attempt to use bright ones. (g) Use contrasting colors on doorways, stairs, and for changes in levels. (h) Identify personal belongings and differentiate room and wheelchair with a unique design rather than by letters or numbers.

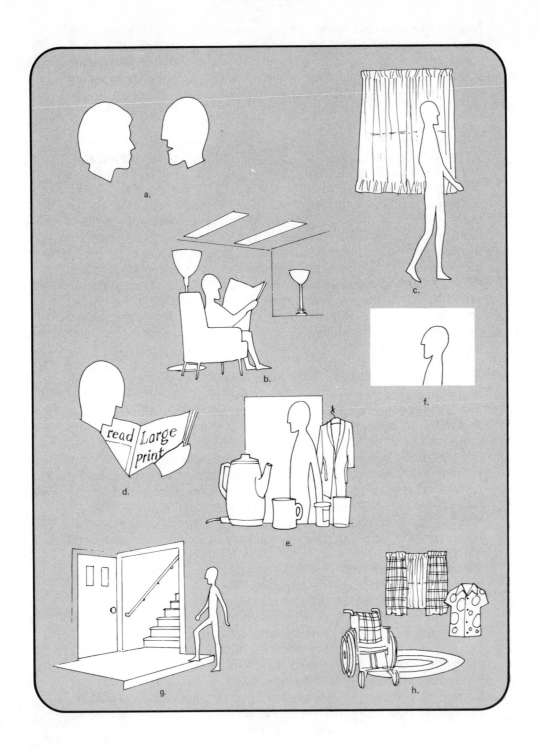

a.

b.

c.

d.

read Large print

e.

f.

g.

h.

261

bright light minimize annoyance from glare. It is beneficial to place items within the visual field of the unaffected eye, a consideration when preparing a food tray and arranging furniture and frequently used objects. Regular reevaluations of the patient by an opthalmologist are essential in order to detect changes or a new problem in the unaffected eye.

Surgery. For most patients, surgery is successful in improving vision. Cataract surgery is not a complicated procedure and the aged withstand it quite well. Gerontological nurses are in a position to reassure older patients and their families that age is no deterrent to cataract surgery. The simple surgical procedure and several weeks of rehabilitation can result in years of improved vision and, consequently, a life of higher quality. There are two types of surgical procedures for removing the lens. *Intracapsular extraction* is the surgical procedure of choice for the aged patient with cataracts, and consists of removing the lens and the capsule. *Extracapsular extraction* is a simple surgical procedure in which the lens is removed and the posterior capsule is left in place. A not uncommon problem with this type of surgery is that a secondary membrane may form, requiring an additional procedure for discission of the membrane.

Regardless of the surgical approach used to remove the lens, some general nursing measures are applicable. Preoperatively, it is vital to orient patients to their environment and offer clear descriptions of what they can expect. Explanations of even the most minor procedures are important. Telling patients that bed rails can assist in orientation and prevent falls and responding promptly to their requests for assistance in using bedrails may reduce their anxiety or resistance regarding this procedure. Explaining the procedures they will be experiencing and the routines of the hospital, such as changes of shift, meal times, and visiting hours helps patients feel more secure. The staff caring for the visually impaired patient should make an effort to achieve consistency. Call lights, bedside tables, and other necessary objects should be placed within easy reach and kept in the same location. Orientation can be enhanced by radios, chiming clocks, and personal communication of the date, time, weather, current events, etc. The patient should be accompanied during ambulation and in transfers between bed and chair.

Postoperative care can be explained to patients during the preoperative phase. They must understand that rapid movements, bending, and strain from coughing, sneezing, lifting, and bowel movements are to be avoided. They should be informed that their eyes will be bandaged. Ambulation is usually allowed within a few days after surgery, depending on the preference of the individual physician. Because of poor vision and weakness, assistance is necessary for all

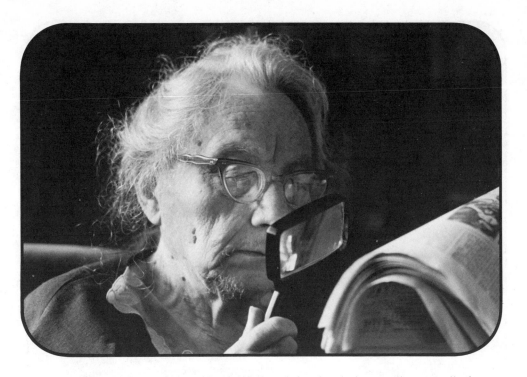

activities performed out of bed. While minimal pain is usually controlled by analgesics, severe pain indicates a complication requiring the immediate attention of the surgeon. After several weeks, the patient will receive temporary corrective lenses. A true adjustment to these requires time and practice. Permanent lenses are usually prescribed two months after surgery. Contact lenses are being used increasingly for patients who have had cataract surgery. Some patients are unable to use them but those who can tend to make a more rapid adjustment to their new vision.

Glaucoma

Glaucoma ranks after cataracts as a major eye problem in the aged, tending to have a high incidence between the ages of 40 and 65 and declining in incidence in old age. Ten percent of all blindness in the United States is a result of glaucoma. Although the exact cause is unknown, glaucoma can be associated with an increased size of the lens and with iritis, allergy, endocrine imbalance, emotional instability, and a family history of this disorder. An increase in intraocular pressure occurs rapidly in acute glaucoma and gradually in chronic glaucoma.

Acute glaucoma. With acute glaucoma, the patient experiences severe eye pain, nausea, and vomiting. In addition to the increased

263

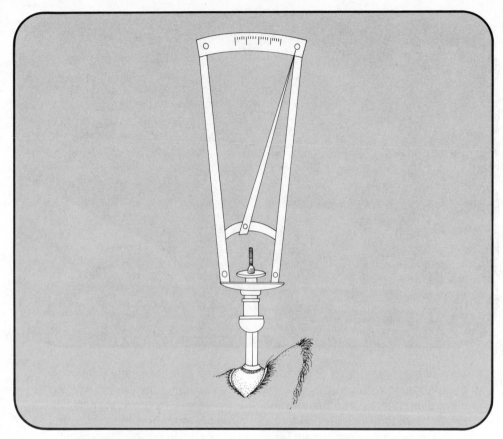

Figure 19-3. Measuring intraocular pressure by use of a tonometer.

tension within the eyeball, there is edema of the ciliary body and dilation of the pupil. Vision becomes blurred, and blindness will result if this problem is not corrected within a day. Diagnosis is confirmed by placing a tonometer on the anesthetized cornea to measure the intraocular pressure (Figure 19-3). The normal pressure is within 20 mmHg. A reading of from 20 to 25 mmHg is considered potential glaucoma. Another diagnostic test (gonioscopy) uses a contact lens and a binocular microscope to allow direct examination of the anterior chamber and differentiate angle-closure from open-angle glaucoma. In the past, if intraocular pressure did not decline within 24 hours, there would be surgical intervention. However, medications are now effective in treating the acute attack: carbonic anhydrase inhibitors, which reduce the formation of aqueous solution; and mannitol, urea, or glycerin, which reduce fluid due to their ability to increase osmotic tension in the circulating blood. An iridectomy may be performed after the acute attack to prevent future episodes of acute glaucoma.

Chronic glaucoma. Chronic glaucoma is the more common type. It often occurs so gradually that affected individuals are unaware that they have a visual problem. Peripheral vision becomes increasingly impaired so slowly that people may not realize for a long time why they bump or knock over items at their side. As the impairment progresses, central vision is affected. People may complain of a tired feeling in their eyes or of headaches or misty vision or of seeing halos around lights—symptoms which tend to be more pronounced in the morning. The cornea may have a cloudy appearance and the iris may be fixed and dilated. Although this condition usually involves one eye, both eyes can become affected if treatment is not sought. The same diagnostic procedures as mentioned with acute glaucoma are used to determine this problem. Treatment, aimed toward reducing the intraocular pressure, may consist of a combination of a miotic and a carbonic anhydrous inhibitor or of surgery to establish a channel to filter the aqueous fluid (e.g., iridectomy, iridencleisis, cyclodialysis, and corneoscleral trephining.)

Care and prevention. The vision lost due to glaucoma is not able to be restored. However, additional damage can be prevented by avoiding any situation or activity which increases intraocular pressure. Physical straining should be prevented, as should emotional stress. Mydriatics, stimulants, and agents which elevate the blood pressure must not be administered. It may benefit patients to carry a card or wear a bracelet indicating their problem to prevent administration of these medications in situations where they may be unconscious or otherwise unable to communicate. Abuse and overuse of the eyes must also be prevented. Periodic evaluation by an ophthalmologist is an essential part of the continued care of the patient with glaucoma.

Detached Retina
The aged may experience detachment of the retina, a forward displacement of the retina from its normal position against the choroid. The symptoms, which can be gradual or sudden, include the perception of spots moving across the eye, blurred vision, flashes of light, and the feeling that a coating is developing over the eye. There are blank areas of vision, progressing to complete loss of vision. The severity of the symptoms depends on the degree of retinal detachment. Prompt treatment is required to prevent continued damage and eventual blindness. Initial measures most likely to be prescribed are bedrest and the use of bilateral eye patches. The latter can be most frightening to the aged

265

patient, who may react with confusion and unusual behavior. The patient should be made to feel as secure as possible; frequent checks and communication, easy access to a call light or other means of assistance, and full, honest explanations will help provide a sense of well-being. After time has been allowed for the maximum amount of "reattachment" of the retina to occur, surgery may be planned.

Several surgical techniques are used in the treatment of detached retina. Electrodiathermy and cyrosurgery cause the retina to adhere to its original attachment; scleral buckling and photocoagulation decrease the size of the vitreous space. Eye patches remain on the patient for several days after surgery. Specific routines vary according to the type of surgery performed. The patient needs frequent verbal stimuli to minimize anxiety and enhance psychological comfort. Physical and emotional stress must be avoided. Approximately two weeks after surgery, the success of the operation can be evaluated. A minority of patients must undergo a second surgery. It is important for the patient to understand that periodic examination is important, especially since some patients later suffer a detached retina in the other eye.

Corneal Ulcers

Inflammation of the cornea, accompanied by a loss of substance, causes the development of a corneal ulcer. Febrile states, irritation, dietary deficiencies, lowered resistance, and cerebral vascular accident tend to predispose the individual to this problem. Corneal ulcers, which are extremely difficult to treat in the aged, may scar or perforate, leading to destruction of the cornea and blindness. This problem is responsible for 10 percent of all blindness. The affected eye may appear bloodshot on inspection and show increased lacrimation. Pain and photophobia are also present. Nurses should advise clients to seek assistance promptly for any irritation, suspected infection, or other difficulty with the cornea as soon as it is identified. Early care is often effective in preventing the development of a corneal ulcer and preserving visual capacity. Cycloplegics, sedatives, antibiotics, and heat may be prescribed to treat a corneal ulcer. Sunglasses will ease the discomfort associated with photophobia. It is important that the underlying cause be treated—be it an infection, abrasion, or presence of a foreign body. Corneal transplants are occasionally done for more advanced corneal ulcers.

HEARING DEFICITS

Hearing deficits can result from changes to the ear which occur with aging (Figure 19-4). The external ear does not undergo significant change, although cerumen secretion is somewhat altered. Cerumen,

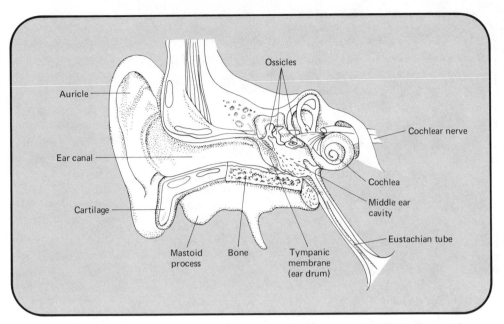

Figure 19-4. Anatomy of the ear. (Source: Barbara Bates, *A Guide to Physical Examination*, Lippincott, Philadelphia, 1974.)

secreted in lesser amounts, contains a greater amount of keratin in the aged which makes it harder and easily impacted. The middle ear may experience atrophy or sclerosis of the tympanic membrane. The inner ear and retrocochlear lose their efficiency, and there is a degeneration of the cells at the base of the cochlea. The changes affecting the inner ear are demonstrated first by a loss in the ability to hear high-frequency sounds; this is followed by a loss of middle and then low frequencies as well. *Presbycusis* is the commonly used term to describe this progressive hearing loss associated with aging.

Causes and Types of Deficits

Most aged have some degree of hearing loss, resulting from a variety of factors aside from aging. Exposure to noise, such as that of jets, traffic, and guns cause cell injury and loss. (The higher incidence of hearing loss in men may be associated with the fact that they are more often employed in occupations which subject them to loud noises, e.g., truck driving, construction, and heavy factory work.) Recurrent otitis media can damage hearing, as can trauma to the ear. Certain drugs may be ototoxic, including aspirin, streptomycin, neomycin, and karomycin; the delayed excretion of these drugs in many older persons may promote this effect. Diabetes, tumors of the nasopharynx, other disease pro-

267

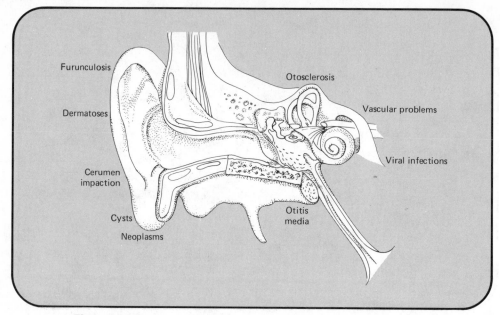

Figure 19-5. Problems affecting the ears of aged people.

cesses, and psychogenic factors can also contribute to hearing impairment.

There are particular problems which affect the aged ear (Figure 19-5). Vascular problems, viral infections and, as mentioned, presbycusis are often causes of inner ear damage. In otosclerosis an osseous growth causes fixation of the footplate of the stapes in the oval window of the cochlea. This may be a middle ear problem; it is a disorder, more common among women, that can progress to complete deafness. Middle ear infections are less common in older individuals; they usually accompany more serious disorders, such as tumors and diabetes. The external ear can be affected by dermatoses, furunculosis, cerumen impaction, cysts, and neoplasms.

The diagram below briefly outlines the normal transmission of sound through the ear. Interference with the transmission of the physical sound waves causes *conduction deafness*. Conduction deafness may be due to an easily correctable problem, such as infection or cerumen accumulation. *Perception deafness* is the term used to describe a problem with the nerve endings registering the electrical signals. Degeneration of the auditory nerve with age may be a factor in this form of deafness. The aged may have both conduction and perception deafness.

NORMAL TRANSMISSION OF SOUND

SOUND

↓

External Ear

↓

Middle Ear

↓

Inner Ear
(Here sound waves
are converted
from physical
waves to
electrical
signals.)

↓

Auditory Nerve

↓

BRAIN RECEIVES
NERVE IMPULSE

Methods of Care

The first measure to employ in caring for someone with a hearing deficit is to encourage audiometric examination. Hearing impairment should not be assumed a normal consequence of aging and ignored. It would be most sad and negligent if the cause of the hearing problem was easily correctable (e.g., removal of cerumen or a cyst) but was allowed to unnecessarily limit the life of the affected individual. The aged should be advised not to purchase a hearing aid without a complete audiometric evaluation. Many older persons invest money for a hearing aid from their limited budget just to discover that their particular hearing deficit can't be improved by this means.

Sometimes the underlying cause of the hearing problem can be

269

corrected. Frequently, however, the aged must learn to live with varying degrees of hearing deficits. Assisting the aged to live with these deficits is a challenge in gerontological care. It is not unusual for the impaired to demonstrate emotional reactions to their hearing deficits. Unable to hear conversation, patients may become suspicious of those around them and accuse people of talking about them. Anger, impatience, and frustration can result from repeatedly unsuccessful attempts to understand conversation. Patients may feel confused or react inappropriately upon receiving distorted verbal communications. Being limited in the ability to hear danger and protect themselves, they may feel insecure. Being self-conscious of their limitation, they may avoid social contact to escape embarrassment and frustration.

Social isolation can be a serious threat because people sometimes avoid the aged person with a hearing deficit due to the difficulty in communication. Even telephone contact may be threatened. (Approximately 10 percent of the aged have difficulty hearing telephone conversations.) Physical, emotional and social health can be seriously affected by this deficit.

Someone nearby should be alerted to the individual's hearing problem so that he or she can be protected in an emergency. In an institutional setting, such patients should be located near the nurse's station. People with hearing loss should be advised to request explanations and instructions in writing so that the full content is received. Those working with the aged can minimize the limitations caused by hearing deficits. To individuals with high-frequency hearing loss the speaker should talk slowly, distinctly, and in a low-frequency voice. Raising the voice or shouting will only serve to raise the high-frequency sounds more and compound the deficit. Methods for promoting more accurate and complete communication include talking into the least impaired ear; facing the individual when talking; using visual speech—sign language, gestures, and facial expressions; allowing the person to lipread; using flash cards, word lists, and other similar aids and devices.

Hearing Aids.   The otologist can determine if a hearing aid would be valuable for the given individual and recommend the particular aid best suited for his or her needs. The nurse is in a key position to educate the aged individual on the importance of consulting an otologist before purchasing a hearing aid (Figure 19-6). Patients must understand that even with a hearing aid their problems will not be solved. Hearing will not return to "normal"; speech may sound distorted through the aid because when speech is amplified, so are all environmental noises, and this can be most uncomfortable and disturbing to the individual. Sounds may be particularly annoying in areas where reverberation can easily occur (such as a church or a large hall). Some persons never make the

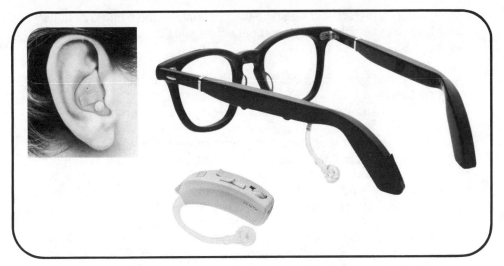

Figure 19-6. Types of hearing aids: (a) In-the-ear model. (b) Behind-the-ear model. (c) Eyeglass model. (Courtesy Zenetron, Manufacturer of Zenith Hearing Aids.)

adjustment to a hearing aid and choose not to wear the appliance rather than to tolerate these disturbances and distortions.

To facilitate adjustment to a hearing aid, an initial period should be provided for experimentation with the controls. This will help the wearer find the most beneficial setting. It may be useful for the person to wear the hearing aid for short periods of time at first, increasing the length of time as adjustment is made. To reduce the disturbances, the individual may find it useful to sit in the front rows of churches and meeting halls, where there is less reverberation. Lowering the amplification in a noisy environment—such as a train station, airplane terminal, or stadium—may also reduce annoyance and discomfort.

Like any fine instrument, the hearing aid must be well cared for. The ear mold can be separated from the receiver for daily washing with soap and water. The cannula should be checked for patency, since cerumen can accumulate in it and interfere with the function of the hearing aid. A pipe cleaner will effectively remove any particles from the cannula. The batteries should be periodically checked; it may not be a bad idea to install new batteries prior to the time the old ones are expected to wear out. The wearer may find it useful to carry extra batteries in a pocketbook or pocket. Prompt repair is advisable when damaged cords or faulty functioning are detected.

Prevention. Gerontological nurses have a responsibility to help

271

aging persons protect and preserve their hearing. Some hearing deficits in old age can be avoided by good care of the ears throughout life. Such care should include the following:

1. Prompt and complete treatment of ear infections should be obtained.
2. Trauma to the ear—from a severe blow, a foreign object in the ear, etc.—should be prevented.
3. Cerumen or particles should be removed by irrigating the external auditory canal rather than by using cotton tipped applicators, hairpins, and other similar devices. It should be remembered that a forceful stream of solution during this procedure can cause perforation of the eardrum.
4. People should be protected from exposure to loud noises, such as those associated with factory and construction work, vehicles, loud music, and explosions. Earplugs or other sound-reducing devices should be used when exposure is unavoidable.
5. Regular audiometric examinations should be scheduled.

Local chapters of hearing and speech associations and organizations serving the deaf can provide assistance and educational materials to those affected by and interested in hearing problems.

OTHER SENSORY DEFICITS AND RELATED CARE

Sight and hearing are not the only senses affected by the aging process; other sensations are also reduced with age. The number of functioning taste buds may be significantly decreased, most obviously by the reduced ability to taste sweet and salty flavors. Pain and pressure are not as easily sensed by the aged. Age-related effects on tactile sensation may also be noted by the difficulty some aged persons have in discriminating different temperatures. Some loss of olfactory function may be noted.

To compensate for the multiple sensory deficits the aged may be experiencing, special attention may be paid to stimulation of all the senses during part of daily living activities. The diet can be planned to include a variety of flavors and colors. Perfumes, fresh flowers and scented candles (safely used) can provide interesting fragrances to smell. In an institutional setting, having a pot brewing fresh coffee in the patients' area can provide a pleasant and familiar aroma during the early morning hours; likewise, a tabletop oven can allow for cookie baking and other cooking activities in the patients' area, providing a variety of stimuli. Different textures can be used in upholstery and clothing fabrics. Clocks that chime, music boxes, and windchimes can vary the environmental sounds which are heard. The design of facilities for the aged should take into consideration the use of different shapes and colors. Intellectual stimulation—through conversation, music, and books, for instance—is also vital.

Touch is not only a means of sensory stimulation, but also an expression of warmth and caring. Too frequently, the nurse may inadvertently only touch the patient during specified procedures, when doing *to* the patient. It is easy for this patient to begin to feel that others perceive him only in terms of tasks rather than as a total human being. How often are patients referred to as "a complete bath," "a foley irrigation," or "a feed"? How often are these labels nonverbally communicated to the patient when the nurse's only encounters with him are for the sake of these activities? To hold a hand, rub a cheek, and pat a shoulder, basic as they may seem, can convey a message to the patient that he is still perceived as a human being. Acceptance of the patient's efforts to touch is also important. The universal language of touch can often communicate a friendship, warmth, and caring which overcomes the most severe sensory deficit.

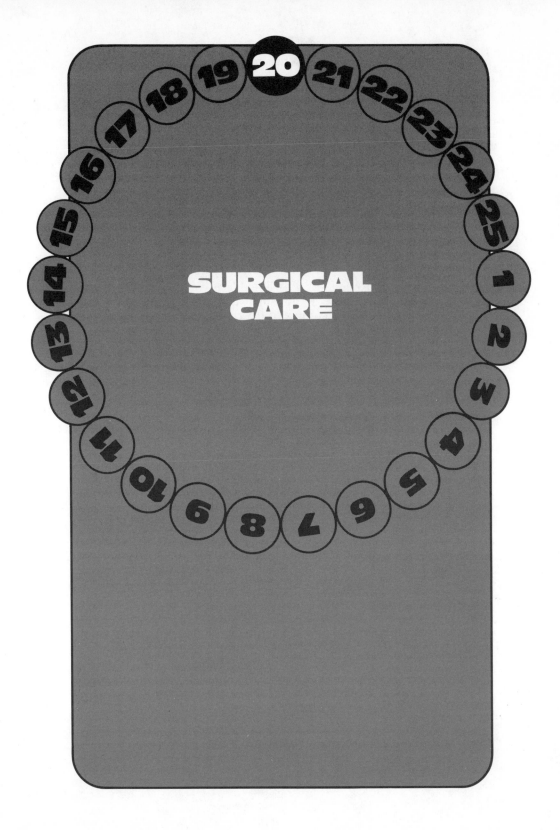

SURGICAL
CARE

The improvement of surgical procedures and the increased numbers of persons living to old age account for the fact that nurses are now confronted with many more aged surgical patients. People are no longer denied the benefit of surgery based on their age alone. Surgical intervention has provided many of our aged people not only with more years to their lives, but with more functional years. Successful surgical management of an older person's health problems is dependent on the nurse's understanding of the age-related factors that alter normal surgical procedures.

In general, the aged have a smaller margin of physiological reserve and are less able to compensate for and adapt to physiological changes. Infection, hemorrhage, anemia, blood pressure changes, and fluid and electrolyte imbalances are more problematic for the aged. Unfortunately, inelasticity of blood vessels, malnourishment, increased susceptibility to infection, and reduced cardiac, respiratory, and renal reserves cause complications to occur more frequently in the aged, especially during emergency or complicated surgical procedures. By strengthening their capacities preoperatively, maintaining these capacities postoperatively, and being alert to early signs of complications, the nurse can help reduce the risk of problems.

PREOPERATIVE PROCEDURES

The gerontological nurse must be sensitive to the fears many older patients have concerning surgery. Throughout their lifetimes, the aged may have witnessed severe disability or death in older persons having surgery, and they may be concerned about similar outcomes from their operation. Reassurance should emphasize the increased success of surgical procedures:

Better diagnostic tools facilitating earlier diagnosis and treatment
Improved therapeutic measures, including surgical techniques and antibiotics
Increased knowledge concerning the unique characteristics of the aged

In addition to reassurance, patients and their families should be taught what to expect before, during, and after the operative procedure:

Preoperative preparation—scrubs, medications, and nothing to eat by mouth
Types of reactions expected to anesthesia
Length of the surgery and a brief description
Routine recovery room procedures
Expected pain and its management

Turning, coughing, and deep-breathing exercises
Rationale for and frequency of dressing changes, suctioning, oxygen, catheters, and other anticipated procedures

Explanations given by the nurse should be communicated to others responsible for care through documentation in the patient's record. Concerns, questions, and fears should be identified by the nurse during assessment and preoperative preparation, and the physician should be made aware of these findings.

It is advisable for the nurse to review with the physician the medications the patient is receiving to determine those which must be continued throughout the hospitalization. Medications which the patient usually takes may need to be administered in spite of NPO restrictions. Sudden interruption of steroid therapy, for instance, can cause cardiovascular collapse and must be prevented. The nurse may learn that the patient has been taking antihypertensive, tranquilizing, or other medications prior to hospitalization. Occasionally, patients forget or are reluctant to tell the physician about these drugs. Since cardiac and pulmonary functions can be altered by certain drugs, it is important to make sure this information is communicated to the physician.

Due to the direct nature of the care she gives, the nurse may be the only person to recognize certain problems. She may discover loose teeth in an aged patient, and they can become dislodged and aspirated during the surgical procedure, causing unnecessary complications. This problem should be brought to the physician's attention in an effort to ensure preoperative dental correction. Another precaution during preparation for surgery is to pad the bony prominences of aged patients to protect them from the pressure of lying on a hard operating room table and subsequent skin breakdown.

OPERATIVE AND POSTOPERATIVE PROCEDURES

Since anesthesia produces depression of the already compromised functions of the cardiovascular and respiratory systems of the aged patient, it must be carefully selected. Close monitoring by the anesthesiologist during the surgery can detect and prevent difficulties in the patient's vital functions. Prolonged surgery for the aged patient is discouraged. Rough, frequent handling of the tissue during surgery is usually avoided since this stimulates reflex activity, increasing the demand for anesthesia. If inhaled agents are used for anesthesia, the nurse should be aware that the patient may remain anesthesized for a longer period of time due to the slower elimination of these agents; turning and deep breathing will facilitate a faster elimination of inhaled agents.

Frequent, close observation and monitoring is extremely important postoperatively. The decreased ability of the aged to manage stress reinforces the need to detect and treat symptoms of shock and hemorrhage promptly. While not being fully conscious from surgery, the aged patient may demonstrate restlessness as the primary symptom of hypoxia. It is important that this restlessness not be mistaken for pain; administration of a narcotic could deplete the body's oxygen supply even more. Prophylactic administration of oxygen may be a beneficial component of the postoperative therapy. Blood loss should be accurately measured, and if excessive, promptly corrected. Frequent checking of urinary output can help reveal the onset of serious complications. Fluid and electrolyte imbalances can be avoided and detected through strict recording of intake and output. (Output should include drainage, bleeding, vomitus, and all other sources of fluid loss.)

Routine care in the recovery phase of older patients is similar to that for all other adults. Activity is vital postoperatively; the benefits of surgery will be diminished if the patient becomes debilitated from the complications arising from immobility. Since the aged patient has a greater risk of developing infections, strict attention must be paid to caring for wounds and changing dressings. A good nutritional status is beneficial to tissue healing and should be encouraged. To conserve the patient's energy and provide comfort, relief of pain is essential. Maintaining regular bowel and bladder elimination, keeping joints mobile and assisting the patient in achieving a comfortable position can assist in pain control. If medications are employed for pain relief, attention should be paid to the reduced activity that may result and to the prevention of the ill effects of such immobilization. It is vital to observe the patient for respiratory depression if narcotic analgesics are administered.

There are several postoperative complications to which aged patients are particularly subject (Glenn, 1974; Mason, Gau, and Byrne, 1976). Respiratory complications include atelectasis, pulmonary emboli, and pneumonia. If pneumonia develops in an aged patient, it is more problematic than it would be for a younger adult and it requires a longer period for recovery. Cardiovascular complications include embolus, thrombus, myocardial infarction, and arrhythmias. Cerebrovascular accident and coronary occlusion occur, but less commonly. Reduced activity and lowered resistance can cause decubiti to develop easily. Paralytic ileus, accompanied by fever, dehydration, abdominal tenderness, and distention, is also a postoperative complication which the aged may experience.

It is not unusual for the positioning on the operating room table and the pulling and moving while unconscious to cause soreness of the aged patient's muscles and bones for several days postoperatively. The nurse should be aware that this is a normal consequence and should take steps to provide comfort. The nurse is in a key position to assist the geriatric patient in achieving maximum benefit from surgery. The most sophisticated surgical procedure in the world performed by the most skillful surgeon is of little value if poor rehabilitative care causes disability or death from avoidable complications. To combine the principles and practices of surgical nursing with the unique characteristics of the aged patient is an immense challenge to the gerontological nurse. To see the increased capacity and more meaningful life many aged persons derive from the benefits of surgery is an immense satisfaction.

REFERENCES

Mason, J. H., Gau, F. C., and Byrne, M. P. "General Surgery." In Steinberg, F. U. (ed.), Cowdry's, The Care of the Geriatric Patient, 5th ed. Mosby, St. Louis, 1976, pp. 236–244.

Glenn, F. "Surgical Principles for the Aged Patient." In Chinn, A. B. (ed.), Working with Older People, Vol. IV. U.S. Dept. of Health, Education, and Welfare, 1974, pp. 259–262.

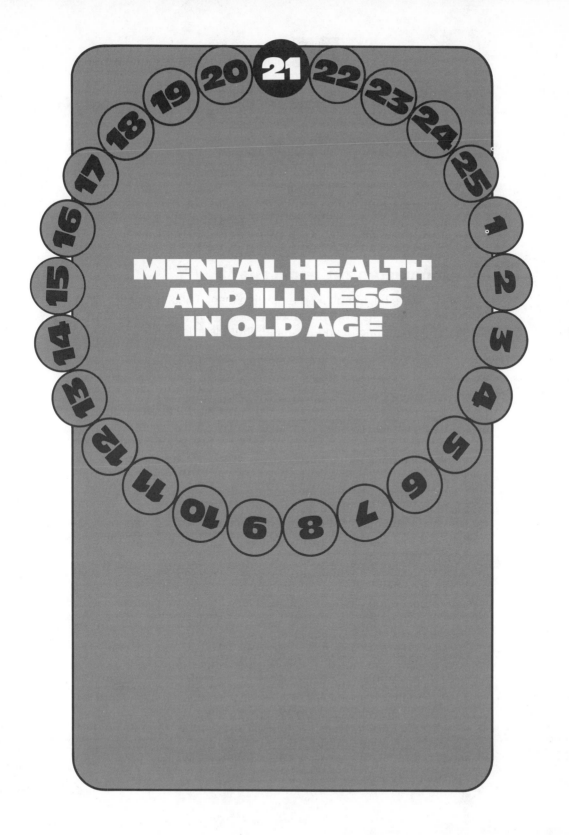

MENTAL HEALTH AND ILLNESS IN OLD AGE

Mental health in old age indicates a capacity to cope with and manage life's stresses in an effort to achieve a state of emotional homeostasis. The aged have an advantage over other age groups in that they have probably had more experience with coping, problem solving, and stress management by virtue of the years they have lived. Most older persons have no delusion regarding what they are or what they are going to be. They have integrity—knowing where they've been, what they've accomplished, and who they really are. Immigrating to a new country, fighting in a world war, and surviving the Great Depression may be among the multitudinous stresses that today's aged have managed to overcome. Such experiences have provided them with a unique emotional strength which should not be underestimated.

RECOGNIZING THE PROBLEMS

Many myths have prevailed regarding mental health and the aged. For instance, there has been a popular belief that with age there is a decline of mental functioning. Granted, there is a loss of neurons with age, but there actually is little correlation between the number of neurons lost and impaired mental function. Another myth propagated has had to do with personality changes with age. Statements have been made that as one grows old, one becomes "more rigid," "childlike," or "senile." These descriptions have been so widely accepted that when an aged person demonstrates these characteristics, it is often considered normal and no attempt is made to explore or treat the underlying cause; some reversible conditions are ignored for this reason. The aged experience the same organic and functional forms of mental illness that younger individuals experience, and they require the same prompt, thorough diagnostic and therapeutic actions employed for the young. At no time should the signs of mental illness be interpreted or accepted as "normal" for the aged. Aging alone does not necessitate a significant change in personality, and several studies have demonstrated personality to be stable over a lifetime (Birren, 1964; Neugarten, 1968). Nurses can promote a better understanding of the aging process by clarifying these misconceptions to the public and to professional persons.

Stresses

There are added stresses in old age, however, that challenge the elderly's coping capacities. Physiological changes may reduce energy reserves, impose physical limitations, and cause the onset of many new symptoms. Bodily changes may result in an alteration in body image and self-concept. Retirement and the independence of children are among the situations in old age which can alter roles and positions. Independence may be threatened by a loss of health or reduced income. The deaths of spouse and friends, as well as the realization of one's own mortality must be faced. Health problems may also produce emotional wear and tear. These stresses are above and beyond the usual stresses of daily living, such as managing a household, marketing, and meeting self-care demands.

Most aged persons cope with these stresses remarkably well; more are interested in working through their problems than surrendering to them. There are situations, however, when the aged individual is more vulnerable to these stresses and mental health can be threatened: illness and hospitalization; death of family, friends, or pets; loss of family or friends for reasons other than death; the illness of a spouse and other added burdens; a reduction in income or an increase in expenses; a change of environment.

The various types of therapeutic assistance that can benefit the aged individual in these situations include crisis intervention, counseling, diversional therapy, health care, psychotherapy, medications, and supplemental income. The most appropriate solution to the problem presented should always be sought. For example, let us say that an elderly man is depressed, and that in exploring the situation it is learned that he is depressed because he lost his part-time job and can't meet his expenses. Antidepressant medications may assist him, but the most appropriate solution would be to obtain financial assistance for him. This action may reestablish his emotional homeostasis and preserve his mental health. It must be remembered that no one approach or technique can be effective for all problems.

Grief.   Grief as a result of a loss can occur at any age. Sighing, choking, tightness of the throat, weakness, and gastrointestinal symptoms may occur in the grieving process. Although grief is most often associated with death, individuals can grieve at virtually any significant loss. Such losses may involve bodily function, appearance, a house, or a pet. It is important for the nurse to appreciate the impact of all losses to the aged and to understand the natural grieving process. (Grief is discussed further in Chapter 24.)

Signs of Mental Illness
Since nurses have close contact with the elderly and are often in a key position to detect changes in mental function, they need to be aware of the general signs of mental illness which the aged may demonstrate.

Disinterested in self-care activities
   Inattention to hygienic practices
   Not changing clothing
   Poor eating habits
Inappropriate behavior or speech

Deterioration of intellect
Poor judgment
Suspiciousness
Withdrawal

Careful, accurate documentation of specific changes observed by the nurse can facilitate diagnosis and treatment. It is essential, however, to assess the behaviors the individual demonstrates that are suggestive of mental illness. Is an elderly man suspicious because he can't hear what those around him are saying? Is the older woman withdrawn because the high-crime district in which she lives makes it unsafe for her to leave her apartment at night? If a person wears a coat on a warm July afternoon, is it because of poor judgment or because lower body temperature actually necessitates the added warmth? Is the individual's disinterest in self-care activities and inattention to hygienic practices due to the fact that the bathroom is unheated and it is too cold to shower or bathe? Quite frequently, the peculiar behaviors observed in aged persons make a great deal of sense if their origin is explored.

Diagnosis and Treatment

Increased interest is being shown in the relationship of physiological problems to mental illness. Among the factors that can cause an alteration in mental function or a manifestation of emotional disorders are hypotensive states, which decrease cerebral circulation; respiratory diseases, which interfere with full oxygenation of the blood; infections; fluid and electrolyte imbalances; uremia; compromised liver function; sensory deficits; arteriosclerosis; metabolic disorders; and certain medications. This emphasizes the necessity of a thorough physical examination whenever mental dysfunction is detected. Unfortunately, acceptance of mental dysfunction as "normal" for aged individuals often causes delayed or missed diagnosis and treatment of the correctable physiological problems that are at the root of the emotional problem—a profound disservice to the aged and a discredit to the helping professions!

Once detected, the mental illness should be specifically diagnosed in the aged. *Senility is not a diagnosis.* The term senility has served as a catch-all for any sign the aged display reflecting a decline in mental function. It has been used so indiscriminately that it is meaningless in communicating an exact, accurate description of the given individual. It has also been used carelessly at times, implying a decline in mental function as an anticipated outcome of the normal aging process. Senility is not unique to the aged, nor is it a normal state. Those working with other persons must be careful not to accept as normal levels of mental dysfunction which would prompt aggressive therapeutic action if noted in other age groups. The aged can be found to have any of the mental illnesses occurring in other age groups. Some people have been affected by an illness for a major portion of their life span; some have problems that first become apparent in old age. Only through an accurate differential diagnosis can effective therapeutic actions be determined.

Just as the aged have a right to the full diagnostic measures utilized for younger adults, they also have a right to the full range of treatment measures. In the past, medications and institutionalization have been the major approaches employed for the mentally ill aged. Psychotherapy has been used with the aged to a significantly lesser degree than with younger adults. The aged comprised a small minority of the private practice of psychiatrists (Butler, 1975). Community-based mental health programs concern themselves with only a small number of the aged in need of their services. Although approximately 30 percent of the persons in psychiatric hospitals are aged, only slightly more than 2 percent are in community-based programs. The aged can and do benefit from many different approaches. Creativity and variety should be used in the treatment of the mentally ill aged.

COMMON MENTAL HEALTH PROBLEMS OF OLD AGE AND RELATED NURSING ACTIONS

Depression

Depression is the most frequent problem psychiatrists treat in the elderly, and it increases in incidence with age (Butler, 1971a). Although depressive episodes may have been a problem for certain individuals throughout their lifespan, it is not uncommon for depression to be a new problem in old age. When one considers the adjustments and losses the aged face, often concurrently, it is not surprising that depression may occur, e.g., the independence of one's children; the reality of retirement; significant changes or losses of roles; reduced income restricting the pursuit of satisfying leisure activities and limiting the ability to meet basic needs; decreasing efficiency of the body; a changing self-image; the deaths of family members and friends, reinforcing the reality of one's own shrinking lifespan; and overt and covert messages from society that one's worth is inversely proportional to one's age. Under these circumstances, it is understandable that many persons slump into an emotional valley in old age.

Depression can be demonstrated in a variety of ways in older persons. "Vegetative symptoms" are the most common manifestations of this problem, including insomnia, weight loss, anorexia, and constipation. Apathy, self-depreciation, inertia, and remorse, often attributed to "growing old," can also indicate depression. Mental confusion resulting

TABLE 21-1: SUICIDE
RATES PER 100,000 POPULATION

Age	Males	Females
15–24	17.0	4.3
25–44	21.9	9.5
45–64	28.5	12.0
65 and over	38.1	7.8

Source: National Center for Health Statistics, *Vital Statistics of the United States, 1973.*

from malnutrition may have depression as its root. The nurse must remember that depressions do not assume a typical picture in the aged, although they do tend to last longer in aged persons. Therapy can help improve this condition quickly, and treatment includes any of the approaches utilized for other age groups. Psychotherapy and medications are successful in almost half of all depressions in aged persons. Treatment should not be withheld because the depression is assumed to be associated with a physical illness; alleviating the depression may help the individual better cope with and manage any other existing problem. It is essential to realize that physical health can be significantly threatened by untreated depression.

Suicidal impulses are sometimes associated with depression. The suicide rate increases with age and is particularly high in aged Caucasian males (Table 21-1). All suicidal threats in the aged should be taken seriously. In addition to recognizing obvious suicidal attempts, the gerontological nurse must learn to recognize those that are more subtle but equally destructive. Medication misuse, either in the form of overdosages or omission of dosages, may be a suicidal gesture. Starvation may be another sign. Engaging in activities that oppose a therapeutic need or threaten a medical problem—such as ignoring dietary restrictions or refusing a particular therapy—may indicate a desire to die. Walking through a dangerous area, driving while intoxicated, and subjecting oneself to other risks can also be signals of suicidal desires.

The suicidal aged need close observation, careful protection, and prompt therapy. The nurse can compliment other therapeutic measures by providing opportunities to increase the individual's self-worth and by offering activities from which satisfaction can be derived. It is important to recognize and comment favorably on a person's clothing, jewelry, hairstyle, or smile; and even the simplest arts and crafts creation should be complimented. The nurse can demonstrate sensitivity and reflect interest in the individual by remembering past and future satisfactions and events. Although aged individuals may feel that their life is meaning-

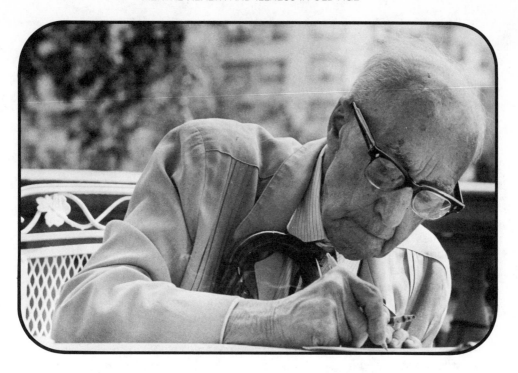

less at a given moment, commenting on how much they helped others at some previous time or on how much everyone is looking forward to some future action can balance the current negative feelings with the more positive feelings associated with other times. Gerontological nurses need to identify even the most minor positive behaviors which can be reinforced. While helping the aged face and manage the many problems which can cause stress and depression, the nurse can instill and help the aged maintain a faith and hope in the future.

Organic Brain Syndrome

Organic brain syndromes are among the most common form of mental illness in the aged. Associated with some impairment of brain tissue function, this disorder affects intellect, memory, judgment, orientation, comprehension, and general emotional stability. *Acute brain syndrome* usually has a rapid onset. Restlessness, night confusion, and a fluctuating level of awareness are demonstrated. There can be a misidentification of people. For instance, affected individuals may believe that their nurse is their sister, or they may not be able to recognize their children. If hallucinations are present, they tend to be visual rather than auditory. The causes of acute syndrome are multiple and include the following:

287

Fluid and electrolyte imbalances	Decreased respiratory function
Malnutrition	Decreased renal function
Anemias	Ingestion of toxic substances
Congestive heart failure	Hyper- and hypo-glycemia
Hormonal imbalances	Hyper- and hypo-thyroidism
Hypotension	Medications (e.g.
Infection	barbiturates, diuretics,
Trauma	L-Dopa, and steroids)
Decreased cardiac function	

Fortunately, acute brain syndrome is reversible. Treatment of the underlying cause frequently results in rapid and marked improvement. Families of aged persons who demonstrate signs of organic brain syndrome should be urged to take the affected individual for a thorough physical examination and not merely accept these signs as a natural consequence of the aging process.

Chronic brain syndrome, a disorder more commonly diagnosed in elderly women, involves a loss or malfunction of neurons in the brain cortex. The individual may demonstrate disorientation, memory deficits, misidentification, delusions, confabulation, and both visual and auditory hallucinations. There is a progressive change in behavior, although social behavior may not be affected. This degenerative brain disease usually has many causes. If cerebral arteriosclerosis is the underlying cause, there may be occasional improvements in the individual's mental function due to periodic improvements in cerebral circulation. Along with a history of symptoms, electroencephalography, echoencephalography, and brain scanning are among the diagnostic procedures employed to confirm this problem.

Unlike acute brain syndrome, chronic brain syndrome is irreversible. Medications and other therapeutic measures may be used to promote a limited degree of improvement. Affected individuals will need continued reevaluation of their changing capacity to meet self-care demands. As this disorder progresses and increased limitations develop, the nurse can plan interventions which promote health and safety and prevent threats to well-being. The difficulty family members and friends may have observing the progressive mental deterioration of this individual should be recognized, and appropriate support should be offered. It can be terribly painful for a husband to hear his wife tell a jumbled tale of how imaginary people appear in her room at night, or for a child not be recognized by his parent. Realistic explanations coupled with sensitive reassurance can help to ease the agonizing feelings of those involved with the impaired individual.

Anxiety

New problems and the adjustments to physical, emotional, and socioeconomic limitations in old age add to the variety of causes for anxiety. Anxiety reactions, not uncommon in aged persons, can be manifested in various ways, including somatic complaints, rigidity in thinking and behavior, insomnia, fatigue, hostility, restlessness, chain smoking, pacing, fantasizing, confusion, and increased dependency. There may be an increase in pulse, blood pressure, and the frequency of urination. Anxious individuals may excessively handle their clothing, jewelry, or utensils. They may become intensely involved with a minor task, such as folding a piece of linen, and may attempt to focus on an activity outside the one with which they are involved, such as watching the activity in another area while they are being interviewed.

Nurses can assist the anxious person by simplifying the environment through measures such as the following:

Allowing adequate time for conversations, procedures, and other activities
Preparing the individual for anticipated activities
Providing thorough, honest, and basic explanations
Controlling the number and variety of persons with whom the individual must interact
Preventing overstimulation of the senses by reducing noise, using soft lights, maintaining stable temperature, etc.
Keeping and using familiar objects

Paranoia

Paranoid states frequently occur in aged persons, especially in aged women (Butler, 1971b). Considering the realities of old age, it is not surprising that sensory losses, so common among the aged, can easily cause the environment to be misperceived; that illness, disability, living alone, a limited budget, and the regular encounters with ageism do not contribute feelings of security. Old people's mistrust of the environment may actually be quite a sensible and normal reaction to the fact that they are common victims of crime. It is difficult to say whether paranoia is a sign of a mental illness or a safe defense against the realities one faces in old age.

The initial consideration in working with paranoid aged individuals is to explore mechanisms which could reduce insecurity and misperception. Corrective lenses, hearing aides, supplemental income, new housing, and a stable environment are valuable improvements. Psychotherapy and medications can be employed when improvement is not achieved through other techniques. The nurse should be aware that

289

these states can threaten individuals with self-imposed isolation and that appropriate measures are needed to prevent and manage such a situation.

Hypochondriasis

Hypochondriasis, a problem frequently found among aged persons, is commonly associated with depression. However, it may be demonstrated for certain purposes. For some persons, it may be an attention getting mechanism. Often, health professionals reinforce this behavior by reacting to physical complaints but not recognizing or rewarding periods of health and good function. Some people may find hypochondriasis an effective means to control a spouse or children. Older people may use it as a means of socialization; if they do not have travels, professions, or interests they can share with others they can count on most of their peers appreciating or experiencing one ailment or another. Providing alternative interests and not reinforcing the associated behavior may assist individuals with hypochondriasis more than efforts to convince them that there is no physical cause for their symptoms.

NURSING CONSIDERATIONS

Mental health in old age implies a satisfaction and interest in life. This can be displayed in a variety of ways, ranging from quiet reflection to zealous activity. The quiet individual who stays at home does not necessarily have less mental health than the gregarious person who is actively involved in every senior citizen program. It is important to realize that there is no singular mold for the mentally healthy aged and that attempts to assess an older individual's mental status based on any given stereotype are to be avoided.

Good mental health practices throughout an individual's lifetime promote good mental health in old age. To preserve mental health, individuals need to maintain the activities and interests which they find satisfying. They need opportunities to prove their value as a member of society and to have their self-worth reinforced. Security through the provision of adequate income, safe housing, the means to meet basic human needs, and support and assistance through stressful situations will promote mental health. A basic ingredient in the preservation and promotion of mental health which must not be underestimated is optimum physical health.

The nurse must recognize that there are times in everyone's life when disturbances occur, altering the capacity to manage stress. The same techniques that would be employed in the presence of a physical problem should be employed by the nurse in an effort to restore emotional homeostasis:

1. Strengthen the individual's capacity to manage the problem.
2. Minimize or eliminate the limitations imposed by the problem.
3. Act for or do for the individual when necessary.

Efforts which strengthen the individual's capacity to manage an emotional problem include improvement of physical health, a good diet, thorough explanations, meaningful activity, income supplements, and socialization. Efforts which minimize or eliminate the limitations imposed by an emotional problem include providing consistency in care, not fostering hallucinations, reality orientation, and correction of physical problems. Efforts involving acting for or doing for the individual include choosing an adequate diet, bathing, managing finances, directing activities, and keeping the individual in a protective environment. These examples are by no means all inclusive and do not imply that an action which involves "acting for" can't also be used to "strengthen capacity" or "minimize a limitation."

Drugs may be used in the treatment of mental illness. As has been discussed in other chapters, drug therapy in the aged requires close monitoring and extreme caution. The nurse should observe for the effectiveness of the drug and the changes it may cause in the patient. Toxic effects must be observed for, and frequent evaluation to determine the patient's continued need for the drug is essential. Although drugs can be a beneficial compliment to other forms of therapy, they are not to be utilized as a singular means of treatment. The aged can benefit from psychiatric help. They, like any other age group, should be provided a fair opportunity to solve problems and work through their crises. As advocates for the aged, nurses can encourage the establishment of available, accessible, and affordable mental health services—in nursing homes, communities, and all geriatric care settings.

REFERENCES

Birren, J. E. *The Psychology of Aging.* Prentice-Hall, Englewood Cliffs, N.J., 1964.

Butler, R. N. "Clinical Psychiatry in Late Life." In Rossman, I. (ed.), *Clinical Geriatrics.* Lippincott, Philadelphia, 1971. (a) p. 442; (b) p. 446.

———— *Why Survive? Being Old in America.* Harper & Row, New York, 1975, pp. 233–234.

Neugarten, B. L. (ed.). *Middle Age and Aging.* Univ. of Chicago Press, 1968.

291

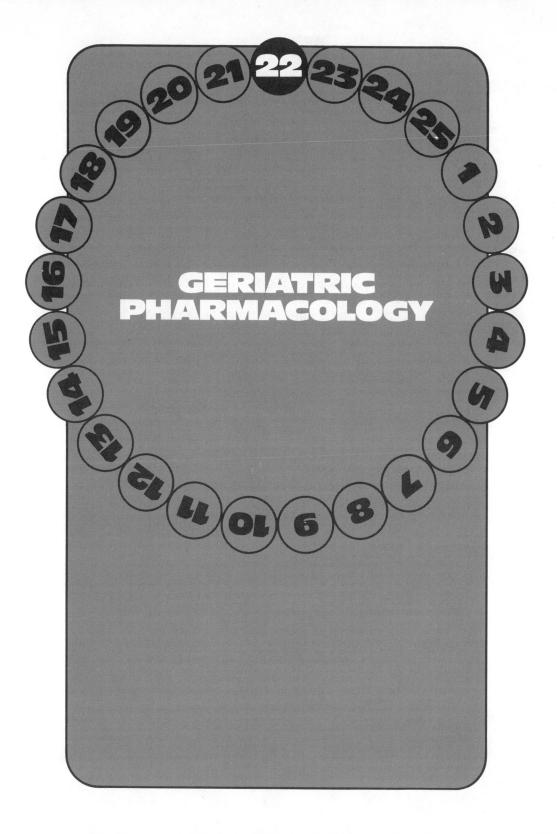

GERIATRIC
PHARMACOLOGY

Because of their many health problems, the elderly are likely to receive a greater quantity and variety of medications. Although they account for only 10 percent of the total population, 25 percent of all prescription medications ordered are for the elderly. In addition, they may self-medicate with over-the-counter drugs such as analgesics, antacids, antihistamines, and laxative preparations, in an attempt to manage the health problems they face. The risk of adverse reactions to medications always increases as the quantity increases, and since alterations during the aging process decrease the efficiency of the body, drug therapy is further complicated for the aged.

Investigators claim that adverse drug reactions are responsible for from 3 to 5 percent of all hospital admissions (Caranasos, Stewart, and Cluff, 1974; Hurwitz, 1969) and that there is a higher proportion among the aged. Studies report incidences of drug reactions in hospitalized individuals ranging anywhere from 10 to 30 percent (Hoddinott, 1967; Seidl et al., 1966). One study, involving 1160 patients in Belfast hospitals, reported an incidence of 10.2 percent (Hurwitz and Wade, 1969)—interestingly, only 6.3 percent were patients under age 60 while 15.4 percent were over 60, more than double (Hurwitz, 1969). It has been estimated that on one-seventh of all hospital days some type of drug reaction occurs, costing approximately three million dollars annually (Task Force on Prescription Drugs, 1969). This is in addition, of course, to the disability and discomfort that may result.

DRUG THERAPY AND RELATED NURSING CONSIDERATIONS

Complications associated with drug therapy emphasize the need for nurses to be familiar with the principles of geriatric pharmacology and with the relationship between these principles and the administration of drugs and their absorption, distribution, metabolism, detoxification, and excretion by the body.

Administering Drugs

The most common way to administer drugs is orally. Oral medications in the form of tablets, capsules, liquids, powders, elixers, spirits, emulsions, mixtures, and magmas are used either for their direct action on the mucous membrane of the digestive tract, as in the case of antacids, or for their systemic effects, as with antibiotics and tranquilizers. Although administration is simple, certain problems can interfere with the process. Dry mucous membrane of the oral cavity, not uncommon in older individuals, can prevent capsules and tablets from being swallowed. If they are then expelled from the mouth, there is no

294

therapeutic value; if they dissolve in the mouth, they can irritate the mucous membrane. Proper oral hygiene, ample fluids for assistance with swallowing and mobility, proper positioning, and an examination of the oral cavity after administration will ensure the medication of the full benefit of travel through the gastrointestinal system. Some elderly may not even be aware that a tablet is stuck to the roof of their dentures or under their tongue.

Large tablets, generally difficult for an older person to swallow, should be crushed and mixed with a small amount of soft food, such as applesauce or gelatin. As a rule, capsules should not be broken open and mixed. Medications are put into capsule form so that unpleasant tastes will be masked or so that the coating will dissolve when it comes into contact with specific gastrointestinal secretions. Breaking the capsule defies the purposes of using it, and perhaps another form of the drug should be prescribed if there is a swallowing problem. Some vitamin, mineral, and electrolyte preparations are bitter in taste, and even more so for older persons, whose taste buds for sweetness are lost long before those for sourness and bitterness. Combining the medication with foods and drinks such as applesauce and juices can make them more palatable and also prevent gastric irritation. Individuals should always be made aware that the food or drink they are ingesting contains a medication. Oral hygiene after the administration of oral drugs will prevent an unpleasant aftertaste.

Drugs prescribed in suppository form for local or systemic action are administered by insertion into various body cavities. They act either by melting from body heat or dissolving in body fluids. Because circulation to the lower bowel and vagina is decreased and the general body temperature reduced in older individuals, a prolonged period may be required for the suppository to melt. If there is no alternative route which can be utilized and the suppository form must be given, the nurse should try to remain with the individual until the suppository is thoroughly melted in order to prevent drug loss through expulsion.

Intramuscular and subcutaneous administration of drugs are necessary when immediate results are sought or when other routes aren't possible, either due to the nature of the drug or the status of the individual. The upper, outer quadrant of the buttocks is the best site for intramuscular injections, and the outer portion of the upper arm for subcutaneous injections. Frequently, the older person will bleed or ooze after the injection because of the decreased tissue elasticity; a small bandage with pressure may be helpful. Alternating the injection site will help reduce discomfort. Special attention should be paid to injecting a medication in an immobile limb because inactivity of the limb will reduce the rate of absorption. A person receiving frequent injections should be checked for signs of infection at the injection site; reduced cutaneous sensation in the aged or lack of sensation, as in a stroke patient, may prevent the individual from being aware of a complication.

Occasionally, intravenous administration of drugs is essential. In addition to observing the effects of this medication, the nurse needs to be alert to the amount of fluid in which the drug is administered. Declining cardiac and renal function make the aged not only more susceptible to dehydration, but also to overhydration. Signs of circulatory overload must be closely observed for, including elevated blood pressure, increased respirations, coughing, shortness of breath, and symptoms associated with pulmonary edema. Intake and output balance, body weight, and specific gravity should be monitored by the nurse. Of course, the complications associated with intravenous therapy in any age group—infiltration, air embolism, thrombophlebitis, pyrogenic reactions, etc.—are also observed for in the aged. Decreased sensation may mask any of these potential complications, emphasizing the necessity for close nursing observation.

Assessment. When administering medications to older individuals, the nurse should assess certain factors:

1. Ascertain whether the correct dosage has been prescribed—not only the normal dosage range but the *lowest dose* required for effectiveness. Generally, lower dosages are required for the elderly.
2. Ascertain whether the most effective route of administration is being utilized.
3. Determine whether the drug continues to be required.
4. Determine whether the drug continues to have a therapeutic effect.
5. Make sure adverse reactions to the drug aren't present. These sometimes develop suddenly from medications taken over a long period. Since they sometimes do not appear when expected they must be watched for. Side effects may not be similar in all individuals; what may cause a rash in one individual could cause mental confusion in another.

The nurse should reflect her continued assessment of these items in written documentation. If problems are detected or if there is any question as to the appropriateness of the drug's administration, the drug should be withheld until the physician can be consulted.

Safeguards. Special nursing action is warranted when older individuals are expected to administer medications themselves. A detailed description—verbal and written—should be given to the per-

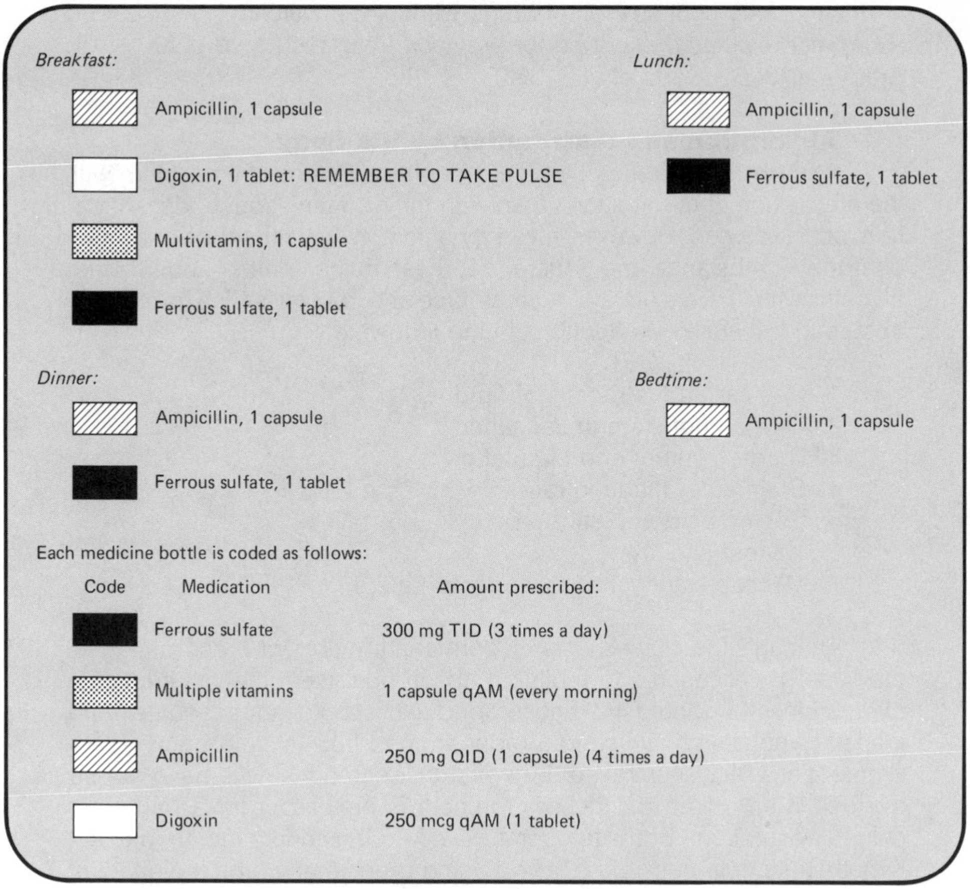

Breakfast:

▨ Ampicillin, 1 capsule

☐ Digoxin, 1 tablet: REMEMBER TO TAKE PULSE

▨ Multivitamins, 1 capsule

■ Ferrous sulfate, 1 tablet

Lunch:

▨ Ampicillin, 1 capsule

■ Ferrous sulfate, 1 tablet

Dinner:

▨ Ampicillin, 1 capsule

■ Ferrous sulfate, 1 tablet

Bedtime:

▨ Ampicillin, 1 capsule

Each medicine bottle is coded as follows:

Code	Medication	Amount prescribed:
■	Ferrous sulfate	300 mg TID (3 times a day)
▨	Multiple vitamins	1 capsule qAM (every morning)
▨	Ampicillin	250 mg QID (1 capsule) (4 times a day)
☐	Digoxin	250 mcg qAM (1 tablet)

Figure 22-1. Color-coded schedule of medication dosage for aged patients who are visually impaired or illiterate.

son, outlining the drug name, dosage schedule, route of administration, action, special precautions, and adverse reactions. Other drugs or foods incompatible with a given prescribed drug should be mentioned. A color-coded dosage schedule can be developed to assist persons who have visual deficits or who are illiterate (Figure 22-1). Medication labels with large print and caps that can be easily removed by weak or arthritic hands should be provided. The nurse should review the medication schedule and explore any new symptoms at every patient-nurse encounter. A variety of potential medication errors can be prevented or corrected by close monitoring. Several studies have revealed some common self-medication errors to guard against—errors in dosage administered, noncompliance due to misunderstanding, discontinuation

297

or unnecessary continuation of drugs without a physician's advice, and using medications prescribed for previous illnesses (Boyd et al., 1974; Brady, 1973, Schwartz et al., 1962).

Absorption and Distribution by the Body

Absorption. Generally older people have less of a problem with the absorption of medications than with their administration, detoxification, and excretion. However, a variety of factors will alter the absorption of drugs. For instance, the general decrease in the number and function of cells with increased age can reduce the rate at which drugs are absorbed because of reductions in the following:

1. Cellular and intracellular fluid
2. Oxygen uptake and utilization
3. Cardiac output and circulation
4. Glomerular filtration rate
5. Gastric acid secretion
6. Thyroid activity
7. Mechanisms that regulate temperature

Although the nurses cannot permanently correct these changes, they can use measures to facilitate absorption. Exercise will stimulate circulation and should be encouraged, as should an adequate fluid intake. Hypotension, which can reduce blood flow, should be avoided. Preparations that neutralize the gastric secretions will have to be avoided if an acidic gastric environment is necessary for a particular drug's absorption. Body temperature could be monitored to prevent hypothermia. It is possible to avoid using drugs that inhibit the effect of each other, such as tetracycline preparations and magnesium antacids, and foods that interfere with drug action, as with processed cheeses and monamine oxidase (MAO) inhibitors. When urinary tract antibiotics that require an acidic urine pH are prescribed, the nurse can offer juices and foods rich in vitamin C. One form of administration may prove to have greater absorption potential than another, and the nurse should bring this suggestion to the physician's attention. There is some thought that there is less efficient absorption of drugs through the gastrointestinal tract with advanced age, including substances such as fat, thiamine, glucose, iron, and 3-methylglucose (Bender, 1968).

Distribution. Although it is difficult to predict how drug distribution will differ among aged individuals, it is known that changes in circulation, membrane permeability, body temperature, and tissue structure can modify this process. As mentioned in earlier chapters, adipose tissue does replace other tissues with age; medications which accumulate in adipose tissue, such as certain barbiturates, can be of longer duration due to the slower distribution throughout the body.

Metabolism, Detoxification, and Excretion

The renal system is primarily responsible for the body's excretory functions, and among its activities is the excretion of drugs. Drugs filtered through the kidneys follow a process similar to that for most of the constituents of urine. After systemic circulation, the drug filters through the walls of glomerular capillaries into Bowman's capsule. It continues down the tubule, where substances beneficial to the body will be reabsorbed into the bloodstream through proximal convoluted tubules, and where waste substances that are excreted through urine will flow into the pelvis of the kidney. Capillaries surrounding the tubules reabsorb the filtered blood and join to form the renal vein. It is estimated that almost ten times more blood circulates through the kidneys, as compared with similar sized body organs, to promote this filtration process.

The reduced efficiency of body organs with advanced age affects the kidneys as well, complicating drug excretion in the elderly. The number of nephron units are decreased in number (Rossman, 1971) and as much as 64 percent of the nephrons can be nonfunctional in very old individuals (Hoffman, 1970). The glomerular filtration rate is reduced 46 percent between the ages of 20 and 90 (Davies and Shock, 1950), along with a reduction in tubular reabsorption (Miller, McDonald, and Shock, 1952). Decreasing cardiac function contributes to the almost 50 percent reduction in blood flow to the kidneys (Hoffman, 1970). The implications of the reduced kidney efficiency are important. Drugs are not as quickly filtered out of the blood stream and are present in the body longer. The biological half-life, or the time for one half of the drug to be excreted, can increase up to 40 percent. These factors can lead to an increased risk of adverse reactions.

The liver also has many important functions that influence drug detoxification and excretion. Carbohydrate metabolism in the liver converts glucose into glycogen and releases it into the bloodstream when needed. Protein metabolism in the parenchymal cells of the liver are responsible for the loss of the amine groups from amino acids, which aid in the formation of new plasma proteins, such as prothrombin and fibrinogen as well as in the conversion of some poisonous nitrogenous by-products into nontoxic substances, such as the conversion of ammonia into urea. Fatty acids and ketone bodies are metabolized in the liver to prepare essential substances such as vitamin B-12. Also important is the liver's formation of bile, which serves to break down fats through enzymatic action and to remove substances such as bilirubin from the blood. Although no significant effects have been reported, the liver's decrease in size and function with age might interfere with the formation of certain necessary body substances, such as prothrombin, albumin, and vitamins A, D, and B-12.

Certain enzymes may not be secreted, interfering with the metabolism of drugs requiring enzymatic activity. Most importantly, the detoxification and conjugation of drugs can be significantly reduced, so that the drug stays longer in the bloodstream. There is some evidence indicating larger drug concentrations at administration sites in aged individuals (Wade, 1972).

Adverse Reactions

The higher risk of adverse reactions to drugs in the elderly has already been discussed. Certain general factors related to adverse reactions should be kept in mind by the nurse:

1. The signs and symptoms of an adverse reaction to a given drug may differ in older individuals.
2. A prolonged period of time may be required for an adverse reaction to become apparent in older individuals.
3. An adverse reaction to a drug may be demonstrated even after a drug has been discontinued.
4. Adverse reactions to a drug that has been administered over a long period without problems can develop suddenly.

Varying degrees of mental dysfunction are often early symptoms of an adverse reaction to such commonly prescribed medications for the elderly as codeine, digitalis, lidocaine, methyldopa, phenobarbital, L-Dopa, valium, librium, and various diuretics. Any medication that can promote hypoglycemia, acidosis, fluid and electrolyte imbalances, temperature elevations, increased intracranial pressure, and reduced cerebral circulation can also produce mental disturbances. The nurse should be alert to changes in mental status and should consult with the physician regarding medications that could be responsible. The aged may easily be victims of drug-induced senility. Unfortunately, mental dysfunction in the aged is sometimes treated symptomatically; that is, with medications but without full exploration of the etiology. This will not correct an original drug-related problem, and it will predispose the individual to additional complications from the new drug.

COMMONLY USED DRUGS, REACTIONS, AND RELATED PROCEDURES

The nurse should be thoroughly knowledgeable about the drugs commonly prescribed for the elderly, including the actions of such drugs, the necessary precautions, and the adverse reactions. To sup-

300

plement the material presented in the following pages, it is advisable for the nurse to obtain more complete information from the pharmacology literature.

Analgesics

For the relief of rheumatic pain and similar discomforts that are common with aged people, various analgesics can be employed. Aspirin remains a major drug used by the aged, having antipyretic and anti-inflammatory actions in addition to its analgesic effects. When used for arthritic conditions, aspirin reduces pain and swelling, which promotes joint mobility. Aspirin's effectiveness and relatively low cost make it quite popular. Of the various side effects of this drug, gastrointestinal bleeding is one of the most serious. Iron deficiency anemia in an older individual should suggest an assessment of aspirin consumption to explore the existence of gastrointestinal hemorrhage. Using buffered or enteric-coated aspirin preparations and avoiding aspirin ingestion on an empty stomach are helpful measures in preventing gastrointestinal irritation and bleeding. Since older persons are very likely to prescribe and take aspirin on their own nurses should caution them on several points.

Aspirin should not be used for persons on anticoagulants unless it is closely monitored by a physician.

Probenecid has an antagonistic action with salicylates and should not be administered concurrently.

Sodium bicarbonate increases the rate of urinary excretion of salicylates, diminishing their action; therefore, older patients taking salicylates should be discouraged from using baking soda to relieve indigestion.

Since people can develop a tolerance for aspirin, the patient should discuss the need for a dosage increase with a physician and not increase the dosage independently.

Occasionally, disturbances of the central nervous system develop when individuals with decreased renal function use salicylates. Since renal function may be reduced in some older persons, symptoms of central nervous system problems should be observed for, including changes in mental status (most commonly, confusion), dizziness, tinnitus, and deafness. Acetaminophen may bring older persons relief. This drug is a nonsalicylate antipyretic and analgesic, with rare incidents of adverse reactions.

Codeine is sometimes prescribed as a mild analgesic. Two effects of this drug are of significance to the aged. First, codeine therapy may result in drowsiness, predisposing an elderly person to accidents. The

301

nurse should caution the person about this effect and advise against driving, climbing a ladder, or any other activity which could pose a risk. Second, constipation sometimes occurs when a person is taking codeine. Due to reduced peristalsis and an often limited intake of bulk foods, constipation is already a not uncommon problem for the aged; thus the probability of constipation while on codeine therapy is fairly high. The nurse should encourage the ingestion of fruit juices and bulk foods as a prevention and closely observe and record bowel elimination patterns to detect constipation early.

Narcotic analgesics are prescribed for the aged to relieve severe pain of short duration, such as occurs postoperatively or with a myocardial infarction, and to provide relief from pain during the terminal phase of an illness when analgesics of lesser potency aren't effective. These drugs must be used with extreme caution in the aged. Morphine sulfate, an opium derivative, is used for the relief of severe pain. In addition to its analgesic effect, it acts to produce euphoria and mild disorientation, reduce peristalsis, slow respirations, increase sphincter muscle tone, and reduce the heartbeat slightly while increasing the force of the beat. Since morphine sulfate can dull sensations and depress respirations, it should be used with extreme caution in older individuals. There is some belief that a lower dose of this drug should be prescribed for the aged, who tend to react more to its depressant effects; it is recommended that aged individuals should receive one-half the usual adult dosage and that morphine be avoided in persons 70 years of age or older.

Meperidine is a narcotic analgesic for mild to severe pain with actions similar to morphine but without the severe problems associated with morphine. Unlike morphine, meperidine does not produce deep sedation or respiratory depression; however,these effects will be seen if the drug is administered with other central nervous system depressants. In the aged especially, meperidine is known to cause hypotension, dizziness, nausea, and impaired mental and physical functioning. Precautions must be taken if the patient is receiving phenothiazines because these drugs will potentiate the action of meperidine. This drug should not be administered if the individual is receiving MAO inhibitors or has received them within the previous two weeks.

Nurses should employ alternative measures to relieve pain before resorting to analgesics. Sometimes, position changes, warm baths, back rubs, conversations, or diversional activity can make the intensity of pain less severe. Only after other measures are no longer able to relieve discomfort should drugs be used. Narcotic analgesics must always be used cautiously and selectively in the aged. The continued requirement for an analgesic should be frequently assessed. No patient should be denied the benefit of an analgesic on the basis of age alone. Instead, the goal of analgesic therapy in the aged is to provide the greatest possible comfort with the least possible number of adverse reactions.

Antianginal Drugs

Nitroglycerin and the long-acting organic nitrates are prescribed for acute angina pectoris episodes in patients with coronary insufficiency, coronary heart disease, coronary occlusion, and subacute myocardial infarction. Since it is not uncommon for many elderly individuals to use nitroglycerin outside of a health care facility, the nurse should include these points when educating the patient about this drug:

1. Nitroglycerin is administered and absorbed sublingually; its purpose is to provide relief in several minutes.
2. Persons should sit or lie down for a short period following administration of nitroglycerin as dizziness, flushing, and cranial throbbing are common reactions.
3. Nitroglycerin tablets should be stored in a closed dark container, away from heat, and not used if over six months old since potency is reduced over time.
4. Nitroglycerin should be used only when necessary since tolerance can develop.
5. If several nitroglycerin tablets do not relieve the attack, the nurse or physician should be promptly contacted.

Some of the adverse reactions to antianginal drugs of particular significance to the aged are irregular and rapid pulse, dizziness, hypotension, decreased respirations, rise in intraocular pressure, blurred vision, muscular weakness, and mental confusion.

Antiarrhythmic Drugs

Procainamide may be used to treat arrhythmias from a variety of conditions. It is known to produce a rapid hypotensive action, and close monitoring is warranted when it is administered to older persons. A reduced dose is recommended for the aged. *Lidocaine,* which does not produce the degree of hypotension that procainamide does, is used to treat multiple ectopic beats associated with acute infarction. This drug is administered parenterally. Particular adverse reactions demonstrated in the aged include mild hypotension, drowsiness, dizziness, and blurred vision. *Propranolol,* a beta-receptor blocking agent, is used to control atrial tachycardia. It is also used in the management of digitalis intoxication and postanesthesia arrhythmias. For hypertensive elderly individuals who have had difficulty with methyldopa, guanethidine, or bethanidine therapy, propranolol is often an effective hypotensive agent.

303

Bradycardia, depression, fatigue, gastrointestinal disturbances, and dizziness are some of the adverse reactions to this drug. *Quinidine* may be used for controlling ventricular ectopic beats and, prophylactically, for paroxysmal arrhythmias. It is recommended that a lower dose be administered to older persons. Adverse reactions include ringing in ears, headache, dizziness, and gastric upset.

Antibiotics

Similar principles guiding the use of antibiotics in other age groups apply to their use in the aged. Liquid forms of certain antibiotics may prove beneficial to older persons who frequently have difficulty swallowing large capsules. The intramuscular dosages for antibiotic drugs may have to be lowered since the aged obtain higher blood levels of these drugs. Altered tissue structure in aged persons warrants care in the intramuscular injection of these drugs to make sure accidental subcutaneous or intravenous injection doesn't occur. Adverse reactions should be closely observed for because reduced kidney efficiency may promote the accumulation of toxic levels of these drugs.

There are some special considerations for the nurse to remember when an aged person is receiving antibiotic therapy. The oral form of ampicillin remains stable in the presence of gastric acid; the nurse should advise older patients that the use of antacids may change the acidity of the gastric contents, thus threatening the potency of this drug. The excretion of ampicillin can be slowed if the patient is receiving probenecid, and if penicillin is being administered, ampicillin will be totally inactivated. Klebsiella infections may develop following ampicillin therapy and symptoms of this problem should be closely observed for. Gentamicin has a high potential for toxicity and should be used with caution in the elderly, especially in those with impaired renal function. As vestibular and auditory ototoxicity may be caused by gentamicin, it should be avoided for use in patients receiving potent diuretics because many of these agents contribute to ototoxicity as well. The aged are also especially subject to the ototoxic effects of streptomycin. The incidence of adverse reactions is significant in elderly persons receiving the long-acting sulfonamide drugs which are commonly prescribed for the treatment of urinary tract infections.

Tetracycline can depress plasma prothrombin activity, necessitating adjustment if the patient is also receiving anticoagulant therapy. Excessive accumulation and possible liver toxicity can occur in patients with impaired renal function. Signs of hepatic and renal damage—potential complications of tetracycline therapy—should be closely observed for, especially during intravenous administration of this drug. Antacids containing aluminum, calcium, or magnesium will impair the absorption of tetracycline, as will certain foods and dairy products; the

304

nurse should caution patients about this problem and recommend that the drug be administered from one to two hours before or after meals.

Oral forms of penicillin must be administered at regular intervals to maintain a constant blood level of the drug. This may be of particular problem to the aged who must self-administer the drug and remember how and when to do so. A medication calendar or assistance from a family member can compensate for poor memory and increase the likelihood of accurate and regular administration of the drug. If penicillin is to be administered intramuscularly, it is essential that the site of injection be rotated each time; reduced muscle tissue in the aged contributes to poor absorption and pain from injection of this drug. Accidental subcutaneous injection of penicillin may cause a "sterile abscess," and accidental intravenous injection can be extremely dangerous. It should be remembered that although an elderly person might not have experienced a problem with penicillin in the past, an allergic reaction can develop suddenly; close nursing observation is essential.

Anticoagulants

Anticoagulants are used with caution in the aged due to the higher risk of anticoagulant bleeding. There is a greater possibility of a lowered prothrombin time being produced in atherosclerotic individuals, many of whom are in the geriatric population. Some physicians discourage anticoagulant therapy in persons over age 70, while others believe the cautious utilization of these agents may be of great benefit to the aged.

Heparin is usually prescribed for rapid anticoagulation, followed by a coumarin drug for prolonged results. Heparin does not dissolve existing clots but rather inhibits the formation of clots by preventing the conversion of fibrinogen to fibrin. The same general principles applied to heparin therapy in the general population are also applied with the aged. Aspirin should be avoided or given with extreme caution because acetylsalicylic acid can interfere with platelet aggregation and cause bleeding. Digitalis, antihistamines, nicotine, and tetracyclines will partially counteract the effects of heparin. Higher dosages of this drug are required when the patient is febrile, emphasizing the importance of nursing observation and communication regarding vital signs. Heparin will also block the eosinophilic response to ACTH (adrenocorticotropic hormone) adrenocorticosteroids, and insulin. Osteoporosis and spontaneous fractures are known to occur when heparin has been used over a long period of time. Older females should be carefully observed during heparin therapy as they tend to have a higher incidence of bleeding.

Warfarin may also be prescribed for anticoagulant therapy. It inhibits fibrin clotting but has no effect on established thrombus, nor does it reverse ischemic tissue damage. Caution is necessary when this

305

drug is administered in the presence of infectious disease, trauma, an indwelling catheter, hypertension, and moderate to severe hepatic or renal insufficiency. Alcohol, antibiotics, MAO inhibitors, phenothiazines, salicylates, sulfonamides, and thyroxine are some of the drugs that increase warfarin's sensitivity; barbiturates, corticosteroids, diuretics, and multivitamins can decrease its sensitivity. As several of these drugs are regularly used by older individuals, it is essential that a complete assessment of all medications the individual is taking be performed to prevent interference with anticoagulant therapy. For outpatients, the capacity of the individual to use an anticoagulant accurately and to detect side effects readily should be carefully assessed in order to avoid serious errors and consequent threats to health status.

Anticonvulsants

Seizure disorders in the aged are sometimes a reflection of a lifelong history of epilepsy and sometimes a result of cerebral arteriosclerosis, hemiplegia, or other disease processes. Anticonvulsant drugs are used, singularly or in combination, to sustain a blood level that is able to control seizures with the least amount of adverse reactions. Phenobarbital is not as popular in treating the aged as it is with younger adults because it can cause emotional disturbance, delirium, disorientation, ataxia, and coma. Mysoline, of lesser toxicity, is the drug of choice for long-term anticonvulsant therapy in the aged. Dilantin is widely used to control seizure disorders; a common side effect of this drug is gingival hyperplasia, which can be minimized and controlled by regular, thorough oral hygiene.

Other drugs, such as sulthiame and carbamazepine, may also be prescribed for anticonvulsant therapy in the aged. Most oral anticonvulsants are known to cause some degree of gastric irritation. Administering these drugs with food or immediately after a meal may reduce this problem. Blurred vision and diplopia should be noted because these visual disturbances may indicate the need for a dosage adjustment. Fatigue, easy bruising, sore throat, pallor, and unusual bleeding may indicate the development of blood dyscrasias, frequently associated with this drug group; routine urinalyses and blood sample evaluation should be performed.

Antihistamines

Since the aged more frequently experience side effects such as dizziness, disturbed coordination, sedation, and hypotension from antihistamines, these drugs are used with care. Patients should be advised to monitor activities and not subject themselves to situations which could threaten their safety, such as working with a power tool or driving an automobile. These drugs are available without prescription, and self-medication may be a problem. Older persons especially should consult with their nurse or physician before using them. Misuse of antihistamines can produce a tolerance which lessens the effectiveness necessary of other drugs the patient may be taking and can mask symptoms of disease, which delays diagnosis.

Antihypertensive Drugs

As mentioned in earlier chapters, a rise in blood pressure normally occurs with advanced age and that which may be a hypertensive level for a younger adult may be normal for an elderly person. Higher blood pressure levels are often necessary to compensate for the blood flow resistance resulting from arteriosclerosis. Thus, a high blood pressure alone does not warrant the use of antihypertensive drugs. When antihypertensive drugs are indicated, aggressive therapy is discouraged. Thiazide diuretics are commonly used for the management of hypertension in the aged. These drugs work by interfering with the renal tubular mechanism of electrolyte reabsorption. There is an increase in the excretion of sodium and chloride and, to a lesser extent, of potassium, magnesium, and bicarbonate. The excretion of calcium and ammonia, on the other hand, is reduced. The increased excretion of ammonia may increase the concentration of blood ammonia. Other antihypertensive drugs may be potentiated by the thiazides.

Elderly people are at a greater risk of developing a fluid and electrolyte imbalance, and diuretics increase this risk considerably. The nurse should attempt to prevent this by recognizing the signs of an imbalance early and by employing prompt measures to correct it. Signs include dryness of the mouth, mental confusion, thirst, weakness, lethargy, drowsiness, restlessness, muscle cramps, muscular fatigue, hypotension, oliguria, nausea, vomiting, slow pulse rate, and gastrointestinal disturbances. Potassium depletion can be prevented by potassium supplements and citrus juices. Hypokalemia could sensitize the heart to the toxic effects of digitalis, which is a significant consideration for the patient being given both digitalis and diuretics. Thiazides may increase blood glucose levels, and the nurse should be aware that insulin requirements for the diabetic patient may need adjusting if the patient is receiving these drugs. Symptoms of diabetic complications should be closely observed for. Latent diabetes mellitus could be manifested during thiazide therapy.

As the onset of action is rapid and frequent voiding is expected, these drugs should be given in the morning. Bedtime administration may predispose the older person to falls while attempting to reach the bathroom or embarrassing bed-wetting incidents. It is helpful for the nurse to offer the bedpan at least every two hours and to plan activities so that easy access and availability of a toilet is provided. Fear of

307

incontinence or absence of a bathroom facility can discourage the older person from engaging in social activities. The nurse should note whether patients are decreasing their fluid intake to avoid the annoying need for frequent voiding and should help them understand the importance of maintaining a good fluid intake.

Reserpine can either be combined with a thiazide diuretic or used alone in the management of mild hypertension. This drug produces tranquilizing effects, in addition to lowering the blood pressure, and frequently causes mental depression. Since the risk is greater with advanced age, close monitoring of aged patients receiving this drug is important. The nurse should be alert to the most subtle indications of depression, closely noting any withdrawal, agitation, lack of interest in activities or self-care, new questions or conversations about death, and suicidal behaviors.

Methyldopa may be prescribed for moderate to severe hypertension in the aged. Frequent evaluation of hematocrit and hemoglobin should be done, since hemolytic anemia may develop in patients receiving this drug. The breakdown of methyldopa or its metabolites may cause the urine to darken when exposed to air; it is helpful for the nurse to prepare the patient, the family and those providing care for the patient to expect this condition. Close observation of individuals with angina pectoris is required because methyldopa may aggravate this problem. Tolerance to methyldopa may develop when used for several months, emphasizing the necessity of continued nursing evaluation of this drug's effectiveness.

Occasionally, monoamine oxidase (MAO) inhibitors are prescribed for moderate to severe hypertension in the aged; they are also employed as antidepressants. MAO inhibitors must be used with extreme caution in the aged. The nursing staff and patient should be taught that certain foods must be avoided during therapy with these drugs, including chocolate, yeast extract, avocado, pickled herring, pods of broad beans, chicken livers, and processed or aged cheeses. No food or drink requiring the action of bacteria or molds for preparation or preservation, such as alcoholic beverages, can be ingested. Cream cheese, ricotta, and cottage cheese are acceptable. MAO inhibitors are not administered to patients who are receiving methyldopa, dopamine, meperidine, centrally acting sympathomimetic amines (such as the amphetamines), or peripherally acting sympathomimetics (such as ephedrine, frequently contained in cold remedies), or to patients who have received L-Dopa within a one-month period prior to initiating MAO inhibitors. Antihistamines, hypnotics, caffeine, sedatives, tranquilizers, and narcotics must be used carefully in combination with MAO inhibitors and in lower dosages. Febrile illness can potentiate the actions of these drugs. MAO inhibitors can also cause orthostatic hypotension, and induce hypo-glycemia and increase symptoms of parkinsonism.

Close monitoring of older patients on antihypertensive therapy is essential. A severe reduction in blood pressure may decrease cerebral circulation, threatening mental functioning; frequent evaluation of blood pressure—preferably in lying, sitting, and standing positions—is necessary. Patients should be advised against rising from a sitting or lying position rapidly, so as to prevent falls resulting from orthostatic hypotension. The nurse should be familiar with the side effects of drugs in this group and facilitate their prompt correction if they occur.

Anti-inflammatory Drugs

Of the musculoskeletal problems in the aged for which anti-inflammatory drugs are used, arthritic conditions are the most common. The salicylates (discussed above under analgesics) are the most popularly chosen anti-inflammatory drugs. For more severe problems, steroids and other potent drugs may be used, but with extreme caution due to the many serious effects they produce. The steroids have profound metabolic effects, modifying the body's immune response. Resistance to infection may be reduced and symptoms of infection masked. Sodium and fluid retention tends to occur, and nursing attention should be given to daily weights, limited sodium intake, monitoring of fluid intake and output, evaluation of blood pressure, and observation for edema. A demineralization of the bones may occur during steroid therapy, predisposing the older person to pathologic fractures. Patients with ocular herpes simplex who receive prednisone may experience corneal perforation; prolonged use of prednisone can cause glaucoma, with possible damage to the optic nerve, and posterior subcapsular cataracts.

Phenylbutazone and indomethacin are potent nonsteroids that are effective for relief in arthritic conditions. Phenylbutazone commonly produces side effects, the incidence of which increases with age. These include nausea, epigastric pain, stomatitis, gastrointestinal bleeding (especially when the patient has had a peptic ulcer in the past), sodium and fluid retention, agranulocytosis, and a variety of other blood dys-crasias. Administration of this drug with meals or with milk reduces the amount of gastric irritation. Nursing observations for the patient receiv-ing phenylbutazone should focus on the development of a sore throat, temperature elevation, mouth lesions, weight gain, change in blood pressure, and the passage of black and tarry stools. Frequent blood evaluations are essential, and it is recommended that phenylbutazone be used selectively, and for short periods of time. Although indometha-cin is of lesser toxicity than phenylbutazone, it is not without serious side

309

effects, and it should also be used cautiously in the aged. Adverse reactions to this drug include headache, nausea, gastric irritation, abdominal pain, diarrhea, and gastrointestinal bleeding in patients who have a history of peptic ulcers. The suppository form of this drug is beneficial in alleviating gastric intolerance. The nursing observations and considerations necessary in the use of phenylbutazone are applicable with indomethacin.

Antiparkinsonism Drugs

No drugs are presently available to alter the course of Parkinson's disease. Those that will diminish the symptoms and limitations of the disease include: trihexyphenidyl (Artane), methylphenidate hydrochloride (Ritalin), and amantadine hydrochloride (Symmetrel). Most of these drugs reduce muscular rigidity to improve coordination, posture, and balance; tremor is less effectively helped by drug therapy. While they may be valuable, these drugs are likely to produce side effects in older individuals. Common side effects are dryness of the mouth, nausea, vomiting, epigastric distress, and blurred vision. Administering these drugs during or after meals may reduce gastric discomfort; and providing fluids, hard candy, and frequent oral hygiene may reduce dryness of the mouth. Urinary retention and altered mental function, including confusion, dizziness, excitement, and drowsiness, are symptoms which should be particularly observed for in the aged. These drugs should not be administered to patients with glaucoma, mental confusion, tachycardia, or urinary retention. (The aged are more subject to the atropinelike effect that many of these drugs have on the eye and bladder.) In antiparkinsonism drug therapy, the beginning dosage should be low and increases should be gradual; the dosage should be gradually tapered when the drugs are discontinued in order to prevent a Parkinsonian crisis.

Larodopa (L-Dopa) is increasingly successful for relief of the symptoms of Parkinson's disease. It is used selectively in patients with severe cardiovascular or respiratory disease, bronchial asthma, glaucoma, and renal, hepatic, and endocrine disease; it is contraindicated in patients with a history of organic brain disease or psychosis. MAO inhibitors must be discontinued at least two weeks prior to initiating larodopa—these two drugs cannot be administered concurrently. Patients having a peptic ulcer are in greater risk of upper gastrointestinal hemorrhage when given larodopa. Symptoms of depression and suicidal tendencies should be closely observed for by the nurse when this drug is used.

Debriding Agents

Enzymes are sometimes applied to decubiti to assist in debridement efforts. Elase is a fibrinolytic enzyme which acts on the denatured proteins in necrotic decubiti. Santyl is a collagenase ointment which dissolves the collagen matter attaching the necrotic tissue to the wound. The objective of these agents is to remove the necrotic tissue which allows granulation and epithelization to occur, facilitating wound healing. Neither of these agents affects living cells. The nurse should closely observe the patient who has wounds being debrided for signs of infection. Specific directions, precautions, and adverse reactions accompany these agents.

Digitalis

Digitalis preparations are used in the treatment of congestive heart failure, atrial flutter and fibrillation, supraventricular tachycardia, and extrasystoles, to increase the force of myocardial contraction through direct action on the heart muscle. The resulting improvement in circulation helps to reduce edema as well. These drugs are absorbed from the intestinal tract within 2 hours after administration, reaching their peak in from 1 to 12 hours. The most popularly used drug from this group is digoxin. The biological half-life of digoxin is normally 34 hours but may be as long as 45 hours in the elderly. This implies the need for a lower dose of this drug in the aged and indicates that the risk of adverse reactions may be greater. Continued administration of digoxin can cause a heart block because of the slowing effect this drug has on the heart. Anorexia may develop, followed by nausea and vomiting several days later. Excessive and copious salivation may occur, as may diarrhea.

Other signs of toxicity include headache, fatigue, malaise, drowsiness, neuralgic pain, blurred vision, aphasia, and hallucination. Confusion, vision problems, and disorientation are the most common adverse reactions in the aged; and it is here that keen nursing assessment and communication with the physician can correct drug-induced senility. When potassium is lost, which sensitizes the heart to the toxic effects of digoxin, digitalis toxicity is promoted. Offering potassium-rich foods or supplements may prevent this problem. In order to reduce gastric discomfort, digoxin can be administered with meals. Digitalis preparations are quite irritating to the tissues and should not be given subcutaneously. Intramuscular forms should be given deep into the gluteal muscles and used only when absolutely necessary, due to the discomfort, the possible development of sterile abscesses, and the uncertainty regarding absorption.

In addition to observing for adverse reactions, an important nursing measure is checking the pulse rate prior to the administration of digoxin. Apical pulse is recommended, and when the apical pulse rate is lower than 60, the drug should be withheld until the physician is consulted and makes a decision. If patients are being prescribed digoxin on an outpatient basis, careful instruction is required. Older persons must be able to find and take their radial pulse and must have the visual capacity to see the second hand on a clock in order to count a minute. Confusion or memory problems can interfere with the accurate counting of the pulse rate, and it is wise to obtain a periodic return demonstration from other individuals to evaluate their capacity for this skill. Families can assist with this procedure and they should receive instruction and be made aware of the signs of toxicity.

General Anesthetics, Hypnotics, and Sedatives

The aged respond differently to general anesthesia. Absorption, distribution, and elimination are delayed, and older persons frequently remain anesthetized longer than desired. Since the risk of respiratory and cardiovascular depression is high, a significantly reduced dose of the anesthetic has to be used. The nurse should evaluate vital signs frequently and promote activity in all body systems.

The aged are often prescribed hypnotics and sedatives for the treatment of insomnia, nocturnal restlessness, anxiety, acute confused states, and related disorders. The drug serves as either a hypnotic or sedative, depending on the dose prescribed. Unlike sedatives, hypnotics do not suppress mental activity, limit attention span, or diminish the ability to concentrate. Since a tolerance to sedatives can develop after several weeks of use, continued evaluation of their effectiveness is required. Nurses should be aware that restlessness, insomnia, and nightmares may occur after sedatives are discontinued. Some aged persons, especially those with some degree of mental impairment, demonstrate residual effects of these drugs for days after they are administered. The nurse should observe for limitations in cognitive functioning on the day following the administration of a sleeping medication; it is unwise to forfeit daytime awareness or independent functioning solely for a full night's sleep, especially since the lack of daytime activity and stimulation may be the cause of insomnia in the first place. As the aged are more vulnerable to the many hazards of immobility, the nurse should note reductions in body movements when these drugs are used. Many of these drugs produce hypotension, drowsiness, and impaired coordination, and nurses should provide assistive measures and educate patients regarding safety considerations.

Chloral hydrate is an effective sedative and hypnotic used in the aged. This drug tends to produce less toxicity and fewer residual effects than many other similar drugs. Usually, chloral hydrate is not prescribed for patients with cardiac disease because it has a depressant action on the heart. The nurse should monitor vital signs and carefully observe for signs of decreased cardiac function. Chloral hydrate is avoided or cautiously used with patients receiving anticoagulant therapy.

Barbiturates. Since an older person reacts more sensitively to barbiturates, they are used carefully. Barbiturates are stored in adipose tissue, and the increased proportion of adipose tissue in an aged person's body can result in an accumulation of these drugs. Since barbiturates are detoxified in the liver, they should be used cautiously if a patient's liver functioning is impaired. Their depressant action warrants caution if a patient has respiratory difficulties. Barbiturates should not be given if other depressants to the central nervous system are being used. Nurses should be aware that barbiturates lower the basal metabolic rate, blood pressure, and mental activity, and that care has to be adjusted accordingly, allowing ample time for activities. Since barbiturates will reduce peristalsis, predisposing the patient to constipation, the nurse should also observe bowel patterns.

A dependence on these drugs can cause symptoms of barbiturate poisoning, including decreased physical and mental function, anxiety, insomnia, amnesia, and cardiac and gastrointestinal disorders. Acute barbiturate poisoning can cause respiratory depression, apnea, severe central nervous system depression, and circulatory collapse. Less severe but important adverse reactions include lethargy, nausea, vomiting, bronchospasm, residual sedation, and general allergic reactions. Barbiturates may decrease the potency of anticoagulant therapy, which could subject the individual to other health threats as well. If a tolerance to these drugs develops with prolonged use, there may be a tendency for the individual to increase the dosage; this can produce adverse reactions and should be discouraged.

Barbiturates are serious drugs and must be used selectively and cautiously, especially with the elderly, whose functioning is already declined and who may be more susceptible to adverse reactions. Nurses should attempt to find alternative means to relax the older individual, with back rubs, warm milk, a quiet environment, etc., using barbiturates only when absolutely necessary and not as a routine measure. Glutethimide is sometimes employed as a barbiturate substitute, producing beneficial and less toxic effects. Paraldehyde and bromides are rarely used as hynotics or sedatives in the aged.

Insulin and Oral Hypoglycemic Agents

Hypoglycemia is a more probable and serious problem than ketosis in older diabetics. Unfortunately, the classic signs and symptoms of hypoglycemia are sometimes replaced by other ones in the

313

aged. Instead of restlessness, tachycardia, and profuse perspiration, symptoms may include speech disorders, confusion, and disorientation; these may be easily mistaken for "senility" in the aged. Keen nursing observation and thorough education for patient and family are essential. Some medications—such as antibacterial sulfonamides, phenyl-butazone, salicylates, propranolol, probenecid, dicoumarol, and MAO inhibitors—are capable of potentiating a hypoglycemic reaction. The action of barbiturates and alcohol may be prolonged by some oral hypoglycemics.

For a more thorough discussion of these drugs, see Chapter 12.

Laxatives

A reduction of peristalsis, activity, and bulk and fluids in the diet are among the causes of constipation in the aged. Add to these factors the belief of many aged persons that a daily bowel movement is essential, and it is easy to understand why laxatives are so widely used, and abused, in the older population. Measures to promote bowel elimination without the use of laxatives (discussed in Chapter 7) should be implemented before resorting to medications. When laxatives are necessary, they should be selectively chosen and used. Diocytyl sodium sulfosuccinate (Colace) is a stool softener often prescribed for older persons. It is not irritating to the intestinal tract and usually promotes a bowel movement in from one to three days after administration of the initial dose. Peri-Colace has the stool softening action of Colace but adds a mild stimulant which provides gentle peristalsis. A bowel movement usually results in from 8 to 12 hours following the administration of Peri-Colace.

Bisacodyl (Dulcolax) stimulates peristalsis and is available in tablet or suppository form; the oral form is effective in approximately 6 hours, and the suppository form in from 15 to 60 minutes. Supportive measures, such as exercise, drinking plenty of fluids, and ingesting bulk foods, are beneficial. The nurse should observe for the effectiveness of these agents and consult with the physician if results are not obtained within a reasonable time. Mineral oil should be discouraged as a laxative for the aged because it interferes with the absorption of fat-soluble vitamins. Bulk laxatives are also not advised because many of them require chewing of a pellet form, a difficult activity for most older individuals. Magnesium preparations should be used carefully; they may reduce the already reduced acidity of the gastric environment and interfere with the digestive process or the effectiveness of medications requiring gastric acidity for action.

General Principles

There are many risks associated with drug therapy in the aged. On the other hand, there are many benefits derived by the aged from the use of medications. The benefits must be weighed with the problems in assessing whether or not a given drug is advantageous. If an older individual is able to maintain an active life style as a result of the relief aspirin provides his arthritic joints, he may be willing to tolerate the slight gastric discomfort from the drug. However, he may not be willing to tolerate dulled mental activity throughout the day to benefit from a sedative which provides a full night's sleep.

At no time should a valuable drug be withheld due to an individual's age. The aged should have the same opportunity as the young to benefit from drug therapy and achieve their optimum level of well-being. Rather than fearing or completely discouraging drug use in the aged, those providing care should use drugs discreetly, selectively, and intelligently.

REFERENCES

Bender, A. D. "Effect of Age on Intestinal Absorption: Implications for Drug Absorption in the Elderly." *Journal of the American Geriatrics Society,* 16:1331, 1968.

Boyd, J. R., Covington, T. R., Stanaszek, W. F., and Coussons, R. T. "Drug Defaulting, II: Analysis of Noncompliance Patterns." *American Journal of Hospital Pharmacy,* 31:485–491, 1974.

Brady, E. S. "Drugs and the Elderly." In Davis, R. S. (ed.), *Drugs and the Elderly.* Andrus Gerontology Center, Univ. of Southern Calif. Los Angeles, 1973, pp. 2–3.

Caranasos, G. J., Stewart, R. B., and Cluff, L. E. "Drug Induced Illness Leading to Hospitalization." *Journal of the American Medical Assoc.,* 228:713–717, 1974.

Davies, D. E., and Shock, N. W. "Age Changes in Glomerular Filtration Rate. Effective Renal Plasma Flow and Tubular Excretory Capacity in Adult Males." *Journal of Clinical Investigation,* 29:496, 1950.

Hoddinott, B. C., Gowdey, C. W., Coulter, W. K., and Parker, J. M. "Drug Reactions and Errors in Administration on a Medical Ward." *Canadian Medical Assoc. Journal,* 97:1001–1006, 1967.

Hoffman, A. M. (ed.). *The Daily Needs and Interests of Older People.* Thomas, Springfield, Ill., 1970, pp. 200–201.

Hurwitz, N. "Admissions to Hospital Due to Drugs." *British Medical Journal,* 1:539–540, 1969.

———— and Wade, O. L. "Intensive Hospital Monitoring of Adverse Reactions to Drugs." *British Medical Journal,* 1:531–536, 1969.

Miller, J. H., McDonald, R. K., and Shock, N. W. "Age Changes in the Maximal Rate of Renal Tubule Reabsorption of Glucose." *Journal of Gerontology,* 7:196, 1952.

Rossman, Isadore (ed.). *Clinical Geriatrics.* Lippincott, Philadelphia, 1971, p. 24.

Schwartz, D., Wang, M., Zeitz, L., and Goss, M. E. W. "Medication Errors Made by Elderly, Chronically Ill Patients." *American Journal of Public Health,* 52:2018–2029, 1962.

315

Seidl, L. G., Thornton, G. F., Smith, J. W., and Cluff, L. E. "Studies on the Epidemiology of Adverse Drug Reactions, III. Reactions in Patients on a General Medical Service." *Johns Hopkins Hospital Bulletin*, 119:229–315, 1966.

Task Force on Prescription Drugs. *Final Report.* U.S. Dept. of Health, Education, and Welfare, 1969.

Wade, O. L. "Drug Therapy in the Elderly." *Age and Ageing*, 1:65, 1972.

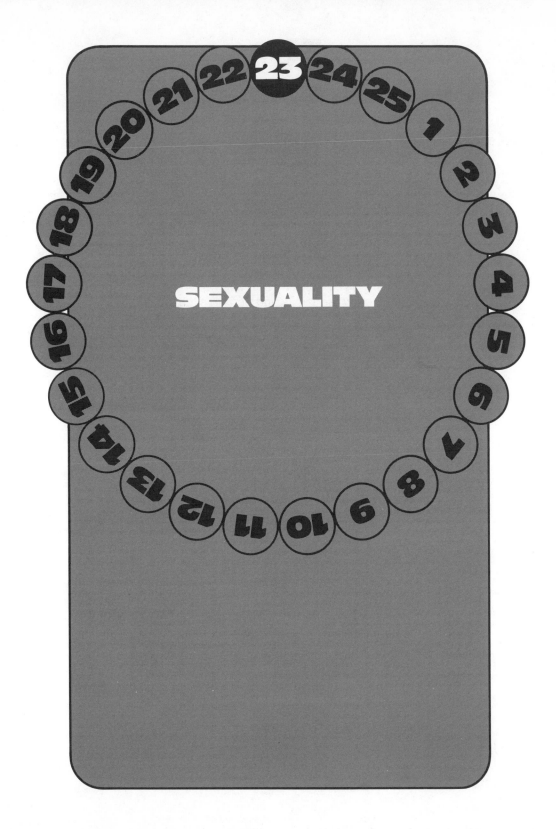

SEXUALITY

For many years, sex was a major conversational taboo in our country. Discussion and education concerning this natural, normal process was discouraged and avoided in most circles. Literature on the subject was minimal and usually secured under lock and key. An interest in sex was considered sinful and highly improper. There was an awareness that sexual intercourse had more than a procreative function, but the other benefits of this activity were seldom openly shared and sexual expression outside of wedlock was viewed as disgraceful and indecent. The reluctance to accept and intelligently confront human sexuality led to the propagation of numerous myths, the persistence of ignorance and prejudice, and the relegation of sex to a vulgar status.

Fortunately, attitudes have changed over the years, and sexuality has come to be increasingly understood, and accepted as natural and pleasurable. Education has helped erase the mysteries of sex for both adults and children, and magazines and books on the topic flourish. Sex courses, workshops, and counselors throughout the country are helping people gain greater insight and enjoyment of sex. Not only has the stigma attached to premarital sex been greatly reduced, but increasing numbers of unmarried couples are living together with society's acceptance. Sex is now viewed as a natural, good, and beautiful shared experience.

Natural, good, and *beautiful* for the varied individuals in society—seldom are these terms used to describe the sexual experiences of *aged individuals.* When the topic of sex and the aged is confronted, many old ignorances and prejudices concerning sex reappear. Education about the sexuality of old age is minimal; literature abounds on the sexuality of all individuals in the society *except the elderly.* Any signs of interest in sex or open discussions of sex by older persons are discouraged, and often labeled as lecherous. The same criteria which would make a man a "playboy" at age 30 makes him a "dirty old man" at age 70. Unmarried young and middle-aged adults who engage in pleasurable sexual experiences are accepted—but widowed grandparents seeking the same enjoyment are often viewed with disbelief and disgust. Myths run rampant. How many times do we hear that women lose all desire for sex after menopause, that older men can't achieve an erection, that older people aren't interested in sex anyhow? Somehow the aged are neutered—by the lack of privacy afforded them, by the lack of credence given to their sexuality, and by the lack of acceptance, respect, and dignity granted to their continued sexual expression. The myths, ignorance, and vulgar status previously associated with sex in general have been conferred on the sexuality of the aged.

Such misconceptions and prejudices are an injustice to persons of all ages. They reinforce any fears and aversion the young have to growing old, and they impose conformity on the aged which require that

318

they either forfeit warm and meaningful sexual experiences or suffer feelings of guilt and abnormality. Nurses can play a significant role in educating and counseling about sexuality and the aged; they can encourage attitudinal changes by their own example. A good perspective regarding sexuality is required because sexuality encompasses much more than a physical sexual act. It includes the love, warmth, caring, and sharing between people; a seeing beyond the gray hair, wrinkles, and other manifestations of aging; an exchange of words and touches by sexual human beings. Feeling important to someone else and wanted by him or her promotes security, comfort, and emotional well-being. With the multiple losses of roles and functions that the aged experience, the comfort and satisfaction derived from a meaningful relationship are especially significant.

Sexuality also includes expressing oneself and being perceived as man or woman, although many persons are currently attempting to eliminate masculine and feminine stereotypes. Today's aged were socialized into masculine and feminine roles—the aged have had a lifetime of experience with the understanding that men are to be aggressive, independent, and strong and that women are to be pretty, dainty, and dependent on their male counterparts. It is difficult and just as unfair to try to alter the roles of aged persons as it is to try to convince today's liberated woman that she is limited to the roles of wife and mother. The socialization of today's older population and their role expectations must be recognized and respected. Yet nurses may witness subtle or blatant violations of respect to the aged's sexual identity. Examples of such a lack of respect are not hard to find:

> Belittling the aged's interest in clothing, cosmetics, and hairstyles
> Dressing men and women residents of an institution in similar and asexual clothing
> Denying a woman's request for a female aide to bathe her
> Forgetting to button, zip, or fasten clothing when dressing the elderly
> Unnecessarily exposing aged individuals during examination or care activities
> Discussing incontinent episodes when the involved individual's peers are present
> Ignoring a man's desire to be cleaned and shaved before his female friend visits
> Not recognizing attempts by the aged to look attractive
> Joking about two aged persons' interest in and flirtation with each other

Why is it so difficult to understand that a recognition of sexual identity is

319

important to the aged? It is not unusual for a 30-year-old to be interested in the latest fashions, for two 35-year-old's to be dating, or for a 20-year-old female to prefer a gynecologist who is a woman. Most any younger woman would panic if a new date saw her before she had time to adjust her cosmetics, hair, and clothing. Chances are that no care provider would walk into the room of a 25-year-old in traction and precede to undress and bathe him in full view of other patients in the room. The aged require the same dignity and respect and appreciate the same recognition as sexual human beings that is afforded to persons of other ages. The aging process does not negate one's sex or alter the significance of sexual identity.

SEXUAL INTERCOURSE

With the exception of the outstanding work done by Pearl in 1925, Kinsey in 1934, and Masters and Johnson in 1966, there has been minimal exploration into the realities of sex in old age. Research has primarily involved small numbers of persons, and valid data are scarce. Possibly contributing to the lack of research and information are the following factors:

1. The acceptance and expansion of sexology has been relatively recent.
2. Impropriety was formerly associated with open discussions of sex.
3. There is a misconception on the part of professionals, the aged, and the general public that the aged are neither interested in nor capable of sex.
4. Practitioners lack experience in, and do not have an inclination for, discussing sex with any age group. Even today, medical and nursing assessments frequently do not reflect inquiry into sexual history and activity.

Nurses should be aware of recent interest and research in the area of sex in old age and communicate these research findings to colleagues and clients in an effort to promote a more realistic understanding of the aged's sexuality. Research has disproven the belief that aged persons are not interested in, or capable of, engaging in sex; older individuals can enjoy the pleasures of sexual foreplay and intercourse. Since the general pattern of sexual behavior is found to be basically consistent throughout life, individuals who were disinterested in sex and had infrequent intercourse throughout their lifetime will not usually develop a sudden insatiable desire for sex in old age. On the other hand, a couple who has maintained an interest in sex and continued regular coitus throughout their adult life will most likely not forfeit this activity at any particular age. Homosexuality, masturbation, a desire for a variety of sexual partners, and other sexual patterns also continue into old age. Sexual styles, interests and expression must be placed in the perspective of a total life experience.

Although clinical data is minimal and additional research is necessary, some general statements can be made about sex in the later years. According to Masters and Johnson (1966a), there tends to be a decrease in sexual responsiveness and a reduction in the frequency of orgasm. Older males are slower to erect, mount, and ejaculate, and older females may experience dyspareunia as a result of less lubrication and a decreased distensibility and thinning of the vaginal walls. Many older females gain a new interest in sex, possibly because they no longer have to fear an unwanted pregnancy or because they have more time and privacy with their children grown and gone. While there are individual differences in the intensity and duration of sexual response in older people, for both sexes, regular sexual expression is important in promoting sexual capacity and maintaining sexual function. With good health and the availability of a partner, sexual activity can continue well into the seventh and eighth decades.

The findings from Masters and Johnson's clinical investigations into the sexual responses of older persons are presented in their fine book *Human Sexual Response.* Since only a brief summary is be presented in this text, the nurse is encouraged to review their work for more specific information. The sexual response cycle was divided arbitrarily into four phases to provide a means of description:

1. ***Excitement phase***   The initial excitement phase results from stimulation from any source.
2. ***Plateau phase***   Sexual tensions are intensified during the plateau phase, and if they reach an extreme, orgasm will be well achieved; if the tension level drops, the individual will enter the resolution phase.
3. ***Orgasmic phase***   In the orgasmic phase, which lasts a few seconds, sexual stimuli are released. Although the entire body is involved to varying degrees, the orgasm is primarily concentrated in the clitoris, vagina, and uterus of the female and in the penis, prostate, and seminal vesicles of the male.
4. ***Resolution phase***   Sexual tensions are lost during the resolution phase; the female is capable of additional orgasms if stimulated during this period.

Using these phases as a framework, some of the changes in the sexual cycle of the aged can be discussed.

321

The Aged Female

During the excitement phase, older women experience clitoral response and nipple erection similar to that of younger women. Sex flush, caused by superficial vasocongestive skin response, does not occur as frequently, and there is less muscle tension elevation in response to sexual stimuli. Whereas the labia majoris separates, flattens, and elevates in response to sexual tensions in younger women, these responses do not occur in older women. The reactions of the labia minoris are also reduced. The secretory activity of the Bartholin's gland is reduced, and to a greater degree, so is vaginal lubrication. The vaginal wall expansion of the excitement phase occurs to a lesser degree.

As with all phases of the sexual cycle, the intensity of the plateau phase is also reduced. The older female does not demonstrate the intensity of areolae engorgement that a younger female does. During the orgasmic phase, the older woman has vaginal contractions in the same fashion as the young woman; these contractions are of lesser duration in the aged female. As in the younger woman, there is a small degree of involuntary distension of the external urinary meatus. In the resolution phase, nipple erection continues to exist, possibly for hours after the orgasm. The older female may experience urinary frequency, urgency, and burning for several hours after intercourse.

The Aged Male

The aged male may require more direct stimulation to achieve an erection than the younger male. During the excitment phase, it may take two to three times longer to achieve full penile erection, although once achieved, it can be maintained for a longer period of time before ejaculation. There is a significant reduction in the scrotal vasocongestive response to sexual tension. Like the older female, the older male experiences a sex flush less frequently. The plateau phase tends to be slower in the older male, and it is possible that a full erection will not occur until just before ejaculation. Although the physiologic response during orgasm is similar to that of the younger male, the older male does have a slower orgasmic phase. During ejaculation there may be more of a seepage of semen rather than a forceful emission; the entire ejaculatory process may be less forceful. Orgasm may not occur during every intercourse, especially if there is frequent intercourse. The most significant difference in the resolution phase of the older male is that it is of longer duration.

In general, it can be stated that "if elevated levels of sexual activity are maintained from earlier years and neither acute nor chronic physical incapacity intervenes, aging males usually are able to continue some form of active sexual expression into the 70- and even 80-year age

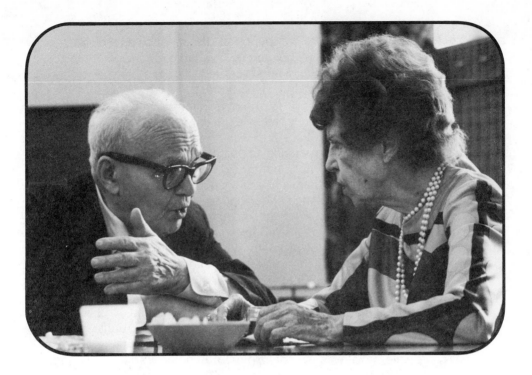

groups" (Masters and Johnson, 1966b). When there is a problem in the aged male's sexual functioning, the causes generally fall into one of six categories (Masters and Johnson, 1966c):

1. Monotony of a repetitious sexual relationship
2. Preoccupation with career or economic pursuits
3. Mental or physical fatigue
4. Overindulgence in food or drink
5. Physical or mental infirmities of either partner
6. Fear of performance associated with or resulting from any of the above

SEXUAL PROBLEMS

Impotence

The greatest sexual problem for males at any age is impotency. Although older males more frequently have organic causes for their impotency, psychological factors are most commonly responsible for this problem in males of all ages. Slower sexual response, less frequent and less forceful ejaculations, and irregular patterns of orgasms with

323

intercourse are among the factors that may contribute to performance anxiety in the older male. A long period of disuse, such as which may occur when there has been no partner available, can contribute to impotency when an opportunity for sexual activity does arise. A single impotent experience may alarm or embarrass the aged male to the degree that he is discouraged from further attempts; this experience may also erroneously be interpreted as a signal of ceasing sexual function due to "old age."

The older male experiencing impotency needs reassurance that this does not necessarily imply that sexual function is lost forever. This male and his partner need realistic explanations regarding the possible causes of impotency and encouragement to continue their efforts. The partner should be made aware of the importance of patience and sensitivity in helping the male with this problem. The value of sexual counselors must not be overlooked in helping the aged male with impotency. Coupled with the need for reassurance, the aged male who is impotent can benefit from a thorough physical examination. Neurological disorders, undiagnosed diabetes, obesity, alcoholism, medications, and other organic causes for impotency can be treated, and sexual functioning can be improved in some situations. If the organic cause results in impotency which cannot be improved, the possible implantation of a penile prosthesis may be explored. At no time should an aged male's impotency be written off to "old age" or regarded as something which isn't really important to an older person.

Prostate problems are discussed in Chapter 16 and will not be repeated here. However, it is important to emphasize that a prostatectomy does not have to result in impotency. Some change in the pattern of ejaculation may be noted, but in most cases satisfying intercourse is possible. The male undergoing a prostatectomy needs reassurance and a realistic understanding regarding the effects of this surgery on his sexual performance. While understanding that his sexual capacity will not necessarily be destroyed, he must also be aware that he will not have a sudden or drastic improvement of sexual functioning following this surgery.

Physical and Mental Barriers

There are some factors which can interfere with sexual performance in both sexes. Drugs, such as many of the antihypertensives and tranquilizers, and alcohol can depress sexual capacity. Malnutrition, anemia, diabetes, and other physical disorders can interfere with sexual function, as can physical and emotional stress. Misconceptions, such as beliefs that intercourse is not possible after a hysterectomy or prostatectomy or that sexual activity is harmful to a cardiac disorder, may discourage sexual enjoyment. A practical problem, particularly common among women who traditionally marry older men and consequently are left widowed, is lack of a partner. Another barrier to sexual expression is the lack of privacy. In addition, the impact of concerns over how others will perceive one's interest in sex may significantly interfere with sexual performance.

Whenever possible, health problems should be identified and corrected; poor health can interfere with sexual interest and capacity at any age. Older persons may benefit from counseling regarding the effects of poor diet and alcohol on sexual capacity—factors they may not have considered as related to sex at all. Specific information concerning capacities and limitations of sexual activity in the light of any existing health problem is an important component of patient education. The nurse can help aged individuals by demonstrating an understanding, acceptance, and respect for them as sexually active human beings.

NURSING CONSIDERATIONS

There are a variety of ways in which the nurse can foster sexuality in the aged, some of which have already been discussed. Basic education can help the aged understand the effects of the aging process on sexuality by providing a realistic framework of sexual functioning. A willingness on the nurse's part to discuss sex openly with the aged demonstrates acceptance and respect for their sexuality. Physical, emotional, and social threats to the aged's sexuality should be recognized, and solutions should be sought for problems—whether caused by the disfigurement of surgery, obesity, depression, poor self-concepts, fatigue, or having no lock on a bedroom door to guarantee privacy.

Consideration must be given to the sexual needs of older persons in institutional settings. Too often, couples admitted to the same facility are not able to share a double bed, and frequently they aren't even able to share the same room if they are evaluated as requiring different levels of care. How unnatural, unreal, inhumane, and unfair to be forced to travel to another wing of a building to visit a person who has intimately shared 40, 50, or 60 years of one's lifetime. Where in most institutional settings can two such individuals find a place where they will not be interrupted or in full view of others? The aged in institutional settings have a right to privacy. They should be able to close and lock a door, feeling secure that this action will be honored. They should not be made to feel guilty or foolish by their expressions of love and sexuality. They should not have to have their sexuality sanctioned, screened, or severed by any other person.

There have been recommendations for "petting rooms" in institutional settings to provide an area for couples to have privacy. Although the value of such rooms in providing privacy is positive, their artificiality must be examined. How many young couples could relax and thoroughly enjoy sex in a room specifically labeled for such a purpose? Is privacy really provided when curious minds realize a couple is in this room and fantasize about the activities behind the closed doors? Perhaps it would be more natural and beneficial to respect the aged's privacy in their bedrooms and to designate periods of the day when residents know that they will not be disturbed unless an emergency develops. Nursing staff in such facilities should not overlook the basic courtesy of knocking on a person's door before entering a room.

Masturbation is often beneficial in releasing sexual tensions and maintaining continued function of the genitalia. The nurse can convey her acceptance and understanding of the value of this activity. The nurse's approving attitude and open view can help eliminate feelings of guilt or abnormality related to masturbation activities.

As mentioned throughout this chapter, it is vital for the nurse to be aware of, respect, and encourage the aged's sexuality. The nurse, as a role model, can foster a positive attitude regarding sex and the aged. Improved understanding, increased sensitivity, and humane attitudes can help today's and tomorrow's aged population realize the full potential of sexuality in the later years.

REFERENCES

Masters, W. H., and Johnson, V. E. *Human Sexual Response.* Little, Brown, Boston, 1966. (a) pp. 223–270; (b) p. 264; (c) p. 261.

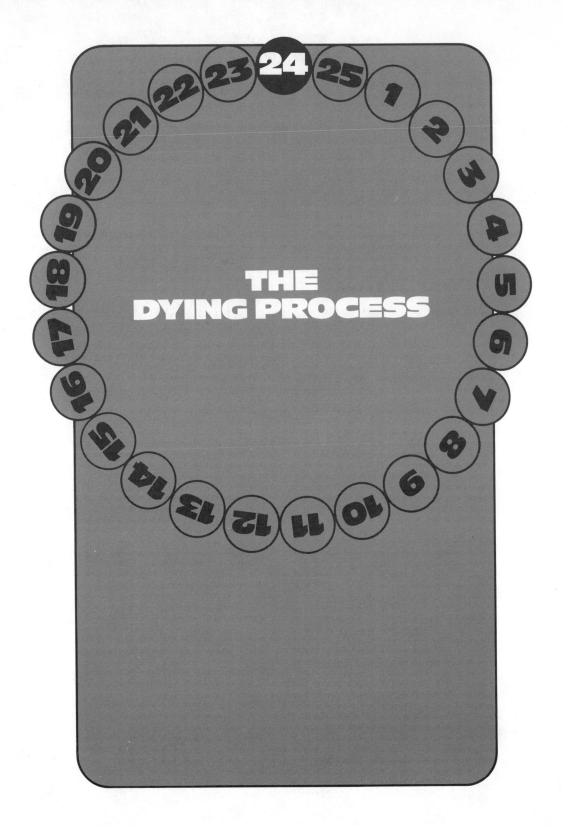

$\mathbf{D}$eath is an inevitable, unequivocal, and universal experience, common to all humanity. It is difficult for human beings to face, perhaps the most difficult and painful reality of all. Although a certainty, the cessation of life is often dealt with in terms of fury, fear, and flight. So reluctant are mortals to accept their mortality. . . .

It is difficult for the gerontological nurse to avoid facing the reality of death since over 80 percent of all who die are aged (Schultz, 1976). But it is not only the final event of death the gerontological nurse must learn to deal with; it is the entire dying process—the complex of experiences which dying individuals, their family, their friends, and all others involved with them must go through. It is far from easy to work with this complicated process, and it requires a fine blend of sensitivity, insight, and knowledge of the vast topic of death.

WHAT IS DEATH?

The final termination of life . . . the cessation of all vital functions . . . the act or fact of dying—these are definitions the dictionary offers concerning death, attempts at succinct explanations of this complex experience (McKechnie, 1974). But we humans are often reluctant to accept such simple descriptions of this inescapable thief of life. For example, the world of literature reflects many eloquent words on the topic:

> Now I am about to take my last voyage,
> a great leap in the dark.
>> THOMAS HOBBS

> Do not go gentle into that
> good night,
> Old age should burn and
> rave at close of day;
> Rage, rage against the dying
> of the light.
>> DYLAN THOMAS

> Down, down, down into the
> darkness of the grave,
> Gently they go, the beautiful,
> the tender, the kind;
> Quietly they go, the intelligent,
> the witty, the brave.
> I know. But I do not approve.
> And I am not resigned.
>> EDNA ST. VINCENT MILLAY

Death hath this also, that it
openeth the gate to good fame,
and extinguisheth envy.
    FRANCIS BACON

Each person is born to one
possession which outvalues
all the others—his last breath.
    MARK TWAIN

The night comes on that
knows not morn,
When I shall cease to be
all alone,
To live forgotten, and love forlorn.
    TENNYSON

For so the game is ended
That should not have begun.
    A. E. HOUSMAN

For as we well wot, that
a young man may dye
soon: so be we very sure
that an olde man cannot
live long.
    SIR THOMAS MORE

Thou shalt come to thy grave
in a full age, like as a shock
of corn cometh in his season
    JOB 5:26

The silence of that dreamless sleep
I now envy too much to weep.
    BYRON

Death is fortunate for the
child, bitter to the youth,
too late to the old.
    PUBLILIUS SYRUS

Death is the mother of beauty.
    WALLACE STEVENS

329

Throughout Shakespeare's voluminous works there is a recurrent mention of death:

> ... *death—*
> *The undiscover'd country, from*
> *whose bourne*
> *No traveller returns.*
> HAMLET

> *The stroke of death is as*
> *a lover's pinch,*
> *Which hurts, and is desir'd.*
> ANTONY AND CLEOPATRA

> *A man can die but once:*
> *We owe God a death.*
> HENRY IV

Dramatic, or amusing, the descriptions of death offered in popular literature have done little to enhance our knowledge of its true meaning. Current scientific literature does not provide much more in the way of specific, definite definitions of death. There is the United Nations Vital Statistics definition that death is the permanent disappearance of every vital sign. But then there are terms such as *brain death,* death of brain cells determined by a flat electroencephalograph reading; *somatic death* determined by the absence of cardiac and pulmonary functions; and *molecular death,* determined by the cessation of cellular function. The controversy lies in deciding at which level of death a person is considered dead. There are situations in which an individual with a flat EEG still has cardiac and respiratory functions; could this individual be said to be dead? There are also situations in which individuals with flat EEGs and no cardiopulmonary functions still have living cells that permit their organs to be transplanted; are individuals really dead if they possess living cells? The answers to these questions are not easy or simple. Much current thought and investigation is focused on the need for a single criterion in the determination of death.

THE REALIZATION OF MORTALITY

There was a time when most births and deaths occurred in the home. In extended family living, more older persons were part of the household and could be naturally observed as they grew old and died. Direct contact with births and the dying process was not uncommon. Viewed as natural processes, these events were managed by familiar

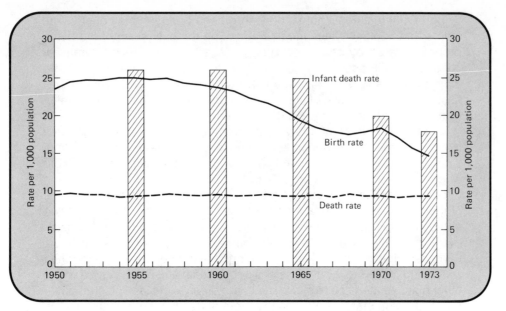

Figure 24-1. Changes in birth and death rates from 1950 to 1973. (Source: U.S. Bureau of the Census, *Statistical Abstract of the United States, 1975*, p. 52.)

faces in familiar surroundings. Intimate encounters with the beginning and end of life were rich experiences that provided insights and helped foster understanding of these realities. Perhaps the family felt a certain comfort and closeness by being with and doing for the life about to begin or end. And who can determine the benefit to the infant or the dying individual of being comforted and cared for by close loved ones? A high mortality rate also made experiences with the dying process more common in days past (Figure 24-1). Not only were living conditions poor, health care facilities inadequate, disease control techniques limited, and technologies to fight and control nature's elements unheard of, but there were fewer numbers of hospitals and other institutions in which people could die.

As Figure 24-1 indicates, the mortality rate has decreased over the years. Health and medical care are now more available and accessible, and new medications and therapeutic interventions increase the possibility of surviving an illness. Sophisticated and widespread life-saving technologies and improved standards of living have also lowered the number of deaths in the population. The declining mortality rate is one of several factors that have limited our experience with the dying process. Another factor is that our more mobile nuclear families are frequently comprised of young members, with older parents and grandparents living in different households, often in different parts of the country. The funeral of the older family members may be the only event of the dying process shared by other age groups. Aged persons in the family or community will most likely not die in their familiar environment. With a majority of deaths occurring in an institutional setting, and over half in a hospital setting, rarely do family and friends remain with the individual or witness the dying process (Butler, 1975a).

The separation of individuals from their loved ones and their familiar surroundings during the dying process seems discomforting, stressful, and unjust. "The final indignity in hospitals is to isolate the old when they are dying" (Butler, 1975b). How inhumane to remove dying persons from intimate involvement with their support systems at the time of their greatest need for support. As our direct experiences with dying and death are lessened, death becomes a more impersonal and unusual event. Its reality is difficult to internalize; it is held at arm's distance. Perhaps this explains why many persons have difficulty accepting their own mortality. Avoiding discussions about death and not making a will or other plans related to one's own death are clues to the lack of internalization of one's mortality. Although the topic of death can be confronted on an intellectual level, it is often this internalization of life's finiteness that remains difficult.

In order to assist the dying and their families effectively, nurses should analyze their own attitudes toward death. Denying their own mortality or feeling angry about it, nurses may tend to avoid dying persons or discourage their efforts to deal realistically with their death or instill false hopes in them and their families. The difficult process of confronting and realizing one's own mortality need not be viewed as depressing by the nurse; it can provide a fuller appreciation of life and the impetus for making the most of every living day. Nurses who understand their own mortality are more comfortable helping individuals through their dying process. A very special book that may be helpful to nurses is *Gramps,* which depicts an aged man's dying experience narratively and photographically (Jury and Jury, 1976). With honesty and sensitivity, the family supports this dying man in his familiar surroundings as his life is declining. The children, grandchildren, and great-grandchildren who share Gramp's dying experience do so with extraordinary warmth, love, and naturalness. One cannot help but marvel at how these individuals learn to accept their own mortality by sharing this process.

SUPPORTING THE DYING INDIVIDUAL

For a long time nurses were more prepared to deal with the care of a dead body than with the dynamics involved with the dying process. Not only was open discussion of an individual's impending death rare, but it was not unusual for the dying person to be moved to a separate and often isolated location during the last few hours of life. If the family was present, they were frequently left alone with the dying person, without benefit of a professional person. Rather than planning for additional staff support for the dying person and his family, nurses were concerned with whether a patient would live until their next shift and require postmortem care. When death did occur, the body was removed from the unit in secrecy so that other patients wouldn't be aware of the event. Nurses were discouraged from "showing emotion" when a patient died. A detached objectivity was promoted as part of nursing the dying patient.

Nursing has now moved toward a more humanistic approach to caring for the dying patient. Emphasis on meeting the total needs of the patient has stimulated greater concern for the psychosocial care of the dying. There is now recognition that family and "significant others" play a vital role in the dying process, and must be considered by the nurse. Knowledge has increased in the field of thanatology (the study of death and dying), and more nurses are exposed to this body of knowledge. The nursing profession has come to realize that professionalism does not negate human emotions in the nurse-patient relationship. These factors have contributed to increased nursing involvement with the dying individual. Since the dying process is unique for every human being, individualized nursing intervention is required. Previous experiences with death, religious beliefs, philosophy of life, age, and health status are among the multitude of complex ingredients affecting the dying process. The nurse must carefully assess the particular experiences, attitudes, beliefs, and values that all individuals bring to their dying process. Only through this assessment can the most therapeutic and individualized support be given to the dying person.

Coping Mechanisms and Related Nursing Intervention
Although the dying process varies in each individual, common reactions that have been observed to occur provide a basis for generalizations. Elizabeth Kubler-Ross, after several years of experiences with dying patients, developed a conceptual framework outlining the coping mechanisms of dying in terms of five stages (1969). It behooves the nurse to be familiar with these stages and to understand the most therapeutic nursing interventions during each stage. Not all dying persons will progress through these stages in an orderly sequence. Neither will every dying person experience all of these stages. However, an awareness of Kubler-Ross' conceptual framework can assist the nurse in supporting dying individuals as their many complex reactions to death are demonstrated. A brief description of these stages is provided below, along with pertinent nursing considerations.

333

Denial and isolation. Upon becoming aware of their impending death, most individuals initially react by denying the reality of the situation. "It isn't true" and "there must be some mistake" and "they're wrong, not me" are among the comments reflective of this denial. Patients sometimes "shop" for a physician who will suggest a different diagnosis or invest in healers and fads that promise a more favorable outcome. Denial serves several useful purposes for the dying person: it is a shock absorber after learning the difficult and shocking news that one has a terminal condition; it provides an opportunity for people to test the certainty of this information; it allows people time to internalize this information and mobilize their defenses.

Although the need is strongest during the early stages, dying persons may use denial at various times throughout their illness. They may fluctuate between wanting to discuss their impending death and denying its reality. The nurse must be sensitive to the person's need for defenses while also being ready to participate in dialogues on death when the person needs to do so. Contradictions may occur, and although these can be confusing, the nurse should try to accept the dying person's use of defenses rather than focus on the conflicting messages. People's individual life philosophy, their unique coping mechanisms, and the knowledge of their condition will determine when denial will be replaced for less radical defense mechanisms. Perhaps the most important nursing action during this stage is to accept the dying individual's reactions and provide an open door for honest dialogue.

Anger. The stage of denial is gradually replaced, and the "No, not me" reaction is substituted for one of "Why me?" The second stage, anger, is often extremely difficult for individuals surrounding the dying person since they are frequently the victims of displaced anger. In this stage, the dying person expresses the feeling that nothing is right. Nurses don't answer the call lights soon enough; the food tastes awful; the doctors don't know what they're doing; and visitors either stay too long or not long enough. Seen through the eyes of the dying person, this anger is understandable. Why wouldn't people resent not having what they want when they want it when they won't be wanting it very much longer? Why wouldn't they be envious of those who will enjoy a future they will never see? Their unfulfilled desires and the unfinished business of their life may cause outrage. Perhaps their complaints and demands are used to remind those around them that they are still living beings.

During this time, the family may feel guilt, embarrassment, grief, and anger as a result of the dying person's anger. They may not understand why their intentions are misunderstood or their actions unappreciated. It is not unusual for them to question whether they are doing things correctly. The nurse can help the family gain insight into

334

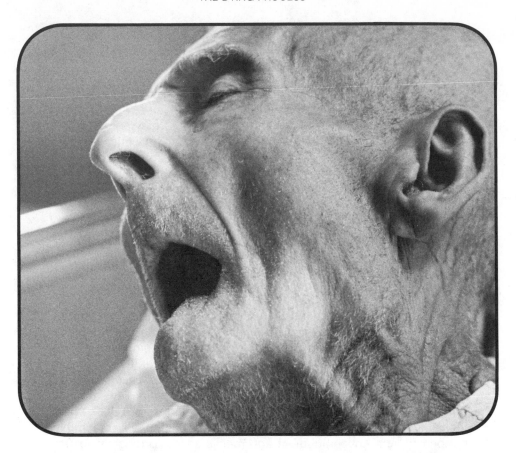

the individual's behavior which will relieve their discomfort and, thereby, create a more beneficial environment for the dying person. If the family can be brought to a realization that the person is reacting to impending death and not to them personally, it may facilitate a supportive relationship and prevent guilt feelings.

The nurse should also guard against responding to the dying person's anger as a personal affront. The best nursing efforts may receive criticism for not being good enough; cheerful overtures may be received with scorn; the call light goes on the minute the nurse leaves the room. It is important that the nurse assess such behavior and understand that it may reflect the anger of the second stage of the dying process. Instead of responding to the anger, the nurse should be accepting, implying to the dying person that it is all right to vent these feelings. Anticipating needs, remembering favorite things, and maintaining a pleasant attitude can counterbalance the anticipated losses that are becoming more apparent to the dying individual. It may be useful for the

335

nurse to discuss her feelings about the patient's anger with an objective colleague who can serve as a sounding board; and to validate that the relationship continues to be therapeutic.

Bargaining. After recognizing that denying and being angry don't change the reality of impending death, dying persons may attempt to negotiate a postponement of the inevitable. They may agree to be a better Christian if God lets them live through one more Christmas; they may promise to help themselves more if the physician initiates aggressive therapy to prolong life; they may promise anything in return for an extension of life. Most bargains are made with God and usually kept a secret. Sometimes such agreements are shared with clergymen. The nurse should be aware that dying persons may feel disappointed at not having their bargain honored or guilty over the fact that having gained time, they want an additional extension of life, even though they agreed that the request would be their last. It is important that these often covert feelings be explored with the dying person.

Depression. When a patient is hospitalized with increasing frequency and has a declining functional capacity and a greater prevalence of symptoms, the reality of the dying process is emphasized. The aged patient may already have had many losses and experienced depression. Not only may lifetime savings, pleasurable pastimes, and a normal lifestyle be gone, but bodily functions and even bodily parts may be lost. All this quite understandably leads to depression. Unlike other forms of depression, however, the depression of the dying person may not benefit from encouragement and reassurances. Urging dying persons to cheer up and look at the sunny side of things implies that they shouldn't contemplate their impending death. It is unrealistic to believe that since most of us normally grieve the loss of a significant person or object, dying people shouldn't be deeply saddened by the most significant loss of all—their life.

The depression of the dying person is usually a silent one. It is important for the nurse to understand that cheerful words may be far less meaningful to dying individuals than holding their hand or silently sitting with them. Being with this person as he openly or silently contemplates his future is a significant nursing action during this stage. The nurse may also have to help the family understand this depression, explaining that their efforts to cheer the dying person can hinder his or her emotional preparation rather than enhance it. The family may require reassurance for the helplessness they feel at this time. The nurse might emphasize that this type of depression is necessary in order for the individual to be able to approach death in a stage of acceptance and peace. An interest in prayer and a desire for visits from a clergyman are commonly seen

336

during this stage. The nurse should be particularly sensitive to the dying person's religious needs and facilitate the clergy-client relationship in every way possible.

Acceptance. For many dying persons, there comes a time when the struggling ends and relief ensues. It is as though a final rest is being taken to gain the strength for a long journey. This acceptance should not be mistaken for a happy state; it implies that the individual has come to terms with his or her death and found a special peace. During this stage, patients may benefit more from nonverbal than verbal communication. It is important that their silence and withdrawal not result in isolation from human contact. Touching, comforting, and being near the person are valuable nursing actions. An effort to simplify the environment may be required as the dying person's circle of interests gradually shrinks. It is not unusual for the family to need a great deal of assistance in learning to understand and support their loved one during this stage.

Hope during the five stages of dying. Significantly, hope commonly permeates all the stages of the dying process. Hope can be used as a temporary but necessary form of denial; as a rationalization for enduring unpleasant therapies; and as a source of motivation. It may provide a sense of having a special mission to comfort an individual through the last days. A realistic confrontation of impending death does not negate the presence of hope. In Cicero's succinct words, "While there's life, there's hope."

SUPPORTING FAMILY AND FRIENDS

Thomas Mann's comment that "a man's dying is more the survivors' affair than his own" is a reminder that the family and friends of the dying person should be considered in the nursing care of that person. They too may have needs requiring therapeutic intervention during the dying process of their loved one. Offering the appropriate support throughout this process may prevent unnecessary stress and provide immense comfort to those involved with the dying person. Just as dying persons experience different reactions as they cope with the reality of their impending death, so may the family and friends pass through the stages of denial, anger, bargaining, and depression before they are ready to accept the fact that a very special person in their lives is going to die. The reactions described below may be demonstrated by family and friends.

Denial and isolation This stage may involve discouraging patients from talking or thinking about death; visiting patients less

337

frequently; stating that patients will be better as soon as they return home, start eating, have their intravenous tube removed, etc.; and "shopping" for a doctor or hospital who will have a special "cure" for the terminal illness.

Anger Reactions may include criticizing staff for the care they are giving; reproaching a family member for not paying attention to the patient's problem earlier; and questioning why someone who has led such a good life should have this happen.

Bargaining People may tell the staff that if they could take patients home they know they could improve their condition. Through prayers or open expression they may agree to take better care of the patient if given another chance. They may consent to take some particular action (go to church regularly, volunteer for good causes, give up drinking) if only the patient could live to a particular time.

Depression Family and friends may become more dependent on the staff. They may begin crying and limiting contact with the patient.

Acceptance In this stage people may react by wanting to spend a great deal of time with the dying person; telling the staff of the good experiences they've had with the patient and how they're going to miss him or her. They may request the staff to do special things for the patient (arrange for favorite foods, eliminate certain procedures, provide additional comfort measures). They may frequently remind the staff to be sure to contact them when "the time comes." They may begin making specific arrangements for their own lives without the patient (change of housing, plans for property, strengthen other relationships for support).

Obviously the type of nursing support will vary depending on the stage a family member or friend is assessed to be in. While the nursing actions described for the dying individual during each stage may be applicable for family and friends, the stages experienced by those involved with the dying person may not coincide with the patient's own timetable for these stages. For instance, patients may have already worked through the different stages, come to accept the reality of death, and be ready to openly discuss the impact of their death and make plans for their survivors. However, family members and friends may be at very different stages and not be able to deal with the patient's acceptance. The nurse must be aware of these discrepancies in stages and provide individualized therapeutic interventions. While providing appropriate support to family and friends as they pass through the stages, the nurse can offer opportunities for dying persons to discuss their death openly with a receptive party.

Helping the Family After a Death

When patients die, the nurse should be available to provide any needed support to the family. Some people wish to have several minutes in private with deceased patients to view and touch them. Others want the nurse to accompany them as they visit the deceased. Still others may not want to enter the room at all. The personal desires of the family and friends must be respected; nurses should be careful not to make value judgments of the family's reaction based on their own attitudes and beliefs. It is beneficial to encourage the family and friends to express their grief openly. Crying and shouting may help people cope with and work through their feelings about the death more than suppressing their feelings to achieve a calm composure. (Unfortunately, public figures have often been presented as reacting in a composed and stoical manner to a death, thus providing poor role models.)

Funeral and burial arrangements may require guidance by a professional also. The survivors of the deceased may be experiencing grief, guilt, or other reactions which place them in a very vulnerable position. At this time they are especially susceptible to sales pitches equating their love for the deceased to the cost of the funeral. Funerals may be arranged costing thousands of dollars more than survivors can actually afford, either depleting any existing savings or leaving a debt which will take years to repay. The family may need to have the extravagant plans presented by a funeral director counterbalanced by realistic questions concerning the financial impact of such a funeral. Someone must take the role of reminding the family that life does go on, and that their future welfare must be considered. Whether it be the nurse, a clergyman, or a neighbor, it is valuable to identify some person who can be an advocate for the family at this difficult time, and prevent them from being taken advantage of. (Rather than waiting for a death to occur before thinking through reasonable funeral plans, people should be encouraged to learn about the funeral industry and plan in advance for funeral arrangements.) In addition to books on the topic (e.g., Morgan, 1973), there are a number of memorial societies which can assist individuals in their planning.*

In addition to assisting the family through the funeral, someone should be available to check on family members several weeks after the death. After the excitement of the funeral has diminished and fewer visitors are calling to pay their respects, the full impact of the death may first be realized. Gorer (1965) has described the three stages of mourning as (1) a period of shock during the first few days following the

---

* More information on memorial societies can be obtained by contacting the Continental Association of Funeral and Memorial Societies, 59 East Van Buren Street, Chicago 60605.

death; (2) a period of intense grief lasting six to eight weeks; and (3) a period of reawakening of interest in life. As can be noted, intense grief occurs during that letdown period when fewer resources may be available to provide support. Several studies have revealed higher mortality rates in widowers, especially during the first year following the death (Glick et al., 1974; Hobson, 1964; Maddison and Viola, 1968; Parkes, 1976; Parkes and Brown, 1972). Since there are potential threats to the mourning individual's well-being, planned interventions may prove valuable. The gerontological nurse can arrange for a visiting nurse, a church member, a social worker, or some other resource to contact the family members several weeks following the death to make sure they are not experiencing any crisis. Widow-to-widow and similar groups support individuals through their grieving process. It may also be beneficial to provide the phone number of a person who the family can contact if assistance is required.

Edwin Schneidman, who has done considerable "postventive" work with survivors, offers some concise guidance in working with the family and friends of the deceased (Shneidman, 1976):

1. Total care of a dying person needs to include contact and rapport with the survivors-to-be.
2. In working with survivor-victims of dire deaths, it is best to begin as soon as possible after the tragedy; within the first seventy-two hours if possible.
3. Remarkably little resistance is met from survivor-victims; most are willing to talk to a professional person, especially one who has no ax to grind and no pitch to make.
4. The role of negative emotions toward the deceased—irritation, anger, envy, guilt—needs to be explored, but not at the very beginning.
5. The professional plays the important role of reality tester. . . not so much the echo of conscience as the quiet voice of reason.
6. Medical evaluation of the survivors is crucial. One should be alert for possible decline in physical health and in overall mental well-being.

SUPPORTING THE NURSE

The staff working with the dying individual have their own set of feelings regarding this significant experience. It may be extremely difficult for nurses, not only to accept a particular patient's death, but to come to terms with the whole issue of death. As was discussed earlier in this chapter, some nurses share the difficulty many persons have realizing their own mortality. Nurses' experiences with death may be limited, as may their exposure to the subject through formal education. In a health profession where the emphasis is primarily on "curing," death may be viewed as a dissatisfying failure. Nurses may feel powerless as they realize that their best efforts can do little to overcome the reality of impending death.

It is not unusual for a nurse who is involved with a dying patient to also experience the stages of the dying process described by Elizabeth Kubler-Ross. Nurses are commonly observed to avoid contact with dying patients, tell a patient to "cheer up" and not think about death, continue to practice "heroic" measures although a patient is nearing death, and grieve at the death of a patient. Nurses may be limited in their ability to support patients and their families if they are at a different stage from them. For example, the nurse may be unable to accept that the patient is dying, and avoidance of the topic and unrealistic plans for the patient's future reflect this denial. The patient, however, may be at the point of accepting the reality of the dying process and may want to discuss personal feelings. Recognizing that the nurse is still denying, the patient may avoid an open discussion of death and be deprived of an important therapeutic activity.

The nurse working with a dying patient requires a great deal of support. Colleagues should help nurses explore their own reactions to dying patients and recognize when those reactions interfere with a therapeutic nurse-patient relationship. The attitude of colleagues and the climate of the environment should be such that nurses can retreat from a situation which is not therapeutic either for them or the patient. To encourage the nurse to cry or show emotions in other forms may be extremely beneficial. The utilization of thanatologists and other resource people may also be valuable in providing support to nurses as they assist an individual through the dying process.

REFERENCES

Butler, R. N. *Why Survive? Being Old in America.* Harper & Row, New York, 1975. (a) p. 218; (b) p. 191.

Glick, I. O., Weiss, R. S., and Parkes, C. M. *The First Years of Bereavement.* Wiley, New York, 1974.

Gorer, G. *Death, Grief and Mourning.* Doubleday (Anchor Books), New York, 1965.

Hobson, C. J. "Widows of Blackton." *New Society,* September 14, 1964.

Jury, Mark, and Jury, Dan. *Gramp.* Grossman, New York, 1976.

Kubler-Ross, E. *On Death and Dying.* Macmillan, New York, 1969.

Maddison, D., and Viola, A. "The Health of Widows in the Year Following Bereavement." *Journal of Psychosomatic Research,* 12:297, 1968.

Marris, P. *Widows and Their Families.* Routledge, London, 1958.

McKechnie, J. L. (ed.). *Webster's New Twentieth Century Dictionary of the*

English Language, Unabridged, 2nd ed. World Publishing Co., New York, 1974.

Morgan, E. *A Manual of Death Education and Simple Burial.* Celo Press, Chicago, 1973.

Parkes, C. M. "The Broken Heart." In Shneidman, E. S. (ed.), *Death: Current Perspectives.* Aronson Jason, New York, 1976, pp. 333–347.

——— and Brown, R. J. "Health After Bereavement: A Controlled Study of Young Boston Widows and Widowers." *Psychosomatic Medicine,* 34:449–461, 1972.

Schultz, R. "Meeting the Three Major Needs of the Dying Patient." *Geriatrics,* 31(6):132, June 1976.

Shneidman, E. S. "Postvention and the Survivor-Victim." In Shneidman, E. S. (ed.), *Death: Current Perspectives.* Aronson Jason, New York, 1976.

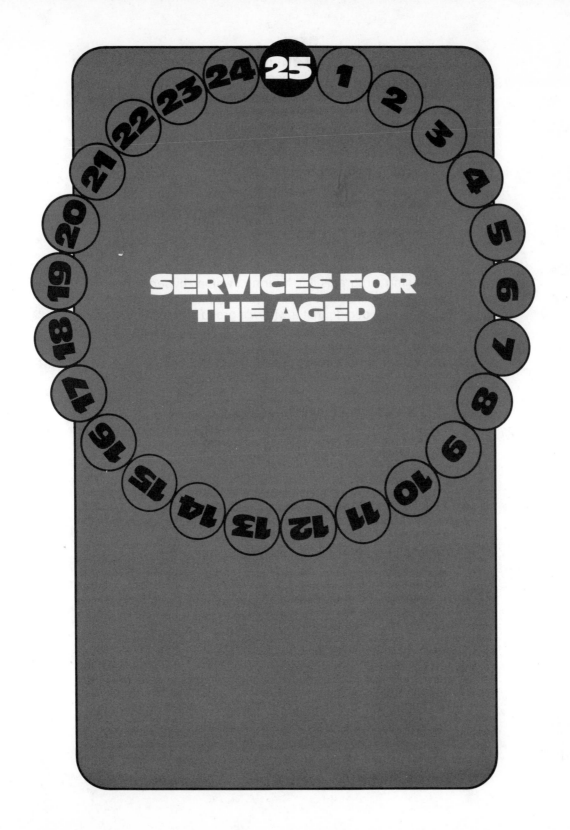

SERVICES FOR
THE AGED

The needs of the aged population are diverse and multitudinous, and the needs of any one aged individual are in a dynamic state, fluctuating in different periods of time as the individual's capacities and life demands change. A wide range of services is essential to meet the complex and changing needs of this group. The continuum of care for the aged takes several factors into consideration:

1. *Physical, emotional, and social factors* Services must be available to meet the unique physical, emotional, and social needs of the aged. They should be planned to deal with whatever problems the aged are most likely to develop and implemented in a manner that is relevant to the unique characteristics of the aged. For instance, a local health department interested in meeting the unique needs of the aged would add screening programs for hearing, vision, hypertension, and cancer to their existing services. Likewise, a social services agency may decide that a widow's group and retirement counseling services are more relevant for the aged than marriage counseling services.

2. *Individual differences* Flexibility is necessary to provide physical, emotional, and social care services according to the individual's needs at a given time, recognizing that priorities are not fixed. An aged individual may be attending a clinic for hypertension control. During a clinic visit, the individual may express concern regarding a recent increase in rent. Unless assistance is obtained to provide additional income or lower-cost housing, the potential effects of this social problem—such as stress and dietary sacrifices—may have deleterious effects on his hypertension problem. Ignoring this individual's need for particular social services can minimize the effectiveness of the health services provided.

3. *Timing* An opportunity must exist for the aged individual to move along the continuum of care, depending on capacities and limitations at different times. Perhaps an elderly woman lives with her children and attends a senior citizen recreational program during the day. If this woman should fracture her hip, she may move along the continuum to hosptialization for acute care, and then to nursing home care for convalescence. As her condition improves and she becomes more independent, she may then move along the continuum to home care and then possibly to a geriatric day care program.

4. *Matching needs to services* Individualization must be practiced to match the unique needs of the individual with specific services. Just as it is inappropriate to assume that at the age of 65 all people need nursing home placement, it is equally

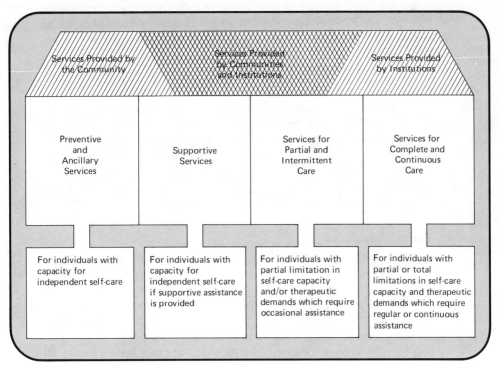

Figure 25-1. Continuum of care services for the aged.

inappropriate to assume that all aged persons would benefit from counseling, sheltered housing, home delivered meals, a geriatric day care program, or any other service. Aged individuals' unique capacities and limitations, and most importantly their preferences, are assessed to identify the most appropriate services for them.

The continuum of care provides for community care services, institutional care services, or a combination of both. Figure 25-1 depicts this continuum. The nurse working with the aged must have an understanding of the various forms of care available for this age group in order to plan effectively. Although services may vary from one area to another, some general forms of geriatric care delivery can be briefly described.

PREVENTIVE AND ANCILLARY SERVICES

The services in this category are those which provide assistance to individuals with independent self-care capacity in an effort to maintain their capacity and prevent physical, emotional, and social problems from developing. The services described below are planned to meet the unique interests and concerns of the aged, and may be free or of nominal cost.

Banking Services

By completing a direct-deposit form at their bank, the aged can have the Social Security Administration mail Social Security and Supplemental Security Income checks directly to the bank. This service can save the aged from traveling to the bank and serve as a protection from theft. Many banks offer free checking accounts and other special services to senior citizens. It is advisable for older persons to explore the details of such services with their individual banks.

Burial Services

Various agencies provide financial assistance for burial and funeral expenses. For instance, wartime veterans are eligible for some assistance from the Veterans Administration, and the Social Security Administration will provide some payment for burial expenses to those who have been insured by that program; local offices of these administrations should be contacted for information. Also, social service agencies and religious organizations often provide services for persons with insufficient funds to pay for burial expenses.

Consumer Services

The aged are frequent victims of unscrupulous persons who profit by making promises which are convincing but not valid. It is important for older persons to investigate cure-alls, retirement villages, and get rich quick schemes before investing their funds. Local offices of the Better Business Bureau can provide useful information to prevent fraud and deception and can offer counseling if these activities do occur. Various consumer counseling services also provide a variety of services to older persons, ranging from money management to assistance in filing suit for fraud.

Counseling Services

Financial problems, the need to find new housing, strained family relationships, death, adjusting to a chronic illness, and retirement are among the situations which may necessitate professional counseling. Local departments of social services, and religious organizations are among the resources that may offer assistance.

346

Educational Services

Some public schools offer literacy, high school equivalency, vocational, and personal interest courses for older adults. In addition, many colleges have free tuition for the elderly. Individual schools should be contacted for more details.

Employment Services

State employment services and the Over-60 Employment Counseling Service conduct programs which provide employment counseling and job placement. Various states also have foster grandparent programs, older businessmen associations, and senior aide projects. Local offices on aging can direct older persons to employment programs and opportunities in their vicinity.

Financial Aid Services

The Social Security Administration may be able to assist the aged in obtaining retirement income, disability benefits, supplemental security income, and Medicare or other health insurances. The district office of the Social Security Administration can provide direct assistance and information. The Veterans Administration can provide financial aid to aged veterans and their families; the aged should be directed to the local VA office. Various communities offer discounts to senior citizens at department stores, pharmacies, theaters, concerts, restaurants, and for bus and taxicab services. Lists of such discounts may be obtained from local offices on aging.

Food, Health, Housing, and Transportation Services

Departments of social services can supply information and applications for food stamps to help the elderly purchase an adequate diet within the constraints of their budget. These departments may also provide shopping services and nutrition classes. Many senior citizen clubs and religious organizations offer a lunch program which combines socialization with a nutritious meal. The local office on aging or health department may be able to direct persons to the sites of such programs.

The aged should be encouraged to engage in preventive health practices for the purposes of preventing illness and detecting health problems in an early stage. Health services for the aged is provided by health departments, hospital clinics, and private practitioners. In addition to health services, these providers may assist the elderly in obtaining transportation and financial assistance for their health care. Aged persons should inquire about such services at their nearest health care office.

347

Local departments of social services, and departments of housing and community development can assist aged persons in locating adequate housing at an affordable cost. These agencies may also be able to direct the aged homeowner to resources to assist in home repairs and may provide information regarding property tax discounts. A variety of planned communities, villages, mobile home parks, and apartment complexes, specifically designed for older persons, are available throughout the country. Some of these housing complexes include special security patrols, transportation services, health programs, recreational activities, and architectural aids, (e.g., low cabinets, grab bars in bathrooms, tinted windows, slopes instead of curbs or stairs, and a call bell for emergencies). There may be one initial purchase price or a monthly fee. The aged person exploring retirement housing should be advised that sound facts are more important to his decision making than exciting promises. Visits to the housing complex and a full investigation of benefits and costs prior to a contractual commitment are essential.

Information and Referral Services
Local offices on aging, commissions on retirement education, and health departments usually provide assistance to the aged in learning about available services. Older persons should be encouraged to utilize these resources for any questions and problems and for any form of help that is needed.

Legal and Tax Services
Local legal aid bureaus and lawyer referral services of the Bar Association may help older persons obtain competent legal assistance at a nominal cost. The Internal Revenue Bureau can help older persons prepare federal tax returns and the State Comptroller's Office can assist with state tax returns; local offices should be called for additional information. Various colleges and law schools should be investigated for free legal and tax services which they may offer for senior citizens.

Recreational Services
Bureaus of recreation, religious organizations, and other groups may sponsor clubs and activities expressly for senior citizens. Local commissions or offices on aging may be able to provide information related to the availability of such programs, their activities, meeting dates, and persons to contact for more details. Local chapters of the American Association of Retired Persons can provide valuable information on services that keep older persons active and independent—ranging from creative leisure endeavors at home to discount travel opportunities. (Information on leisure pursuits is just one of the many services provided by the AARP).

348

The Young Men's (or Women's) Christian Association offers recreational activities for persons of all ages; the aged should explore the opportunities available at their nearest association. Art museums, libraries, theaters, concert halls, restaurants, and travel agencies should be explored for special programs offered to senior citizens.

Services by Mail

Persons who are homebound or geographically isolated from services may find it useful to obtain services by mail. Shopping by mail services have a long tradition and may reduce the inconveniences and risks associated with traveling to a shopping district, maneuvering in stores, handling large sums of money in public, and carrying packages. The postage and handling charge for this service may be no greater than the transportation (not to mention the energy) costs expended for direct shopping. Many libraries have a service by which books can be borrowed by mail; the aged should be encouraged to inquire about such services at their local branch. The United States Postal Service provides a service by which stamps can be ordered by mail. There is a nominal fee for this service. Order blanks for stamps by mail can be obtained by contacting the local postal station.

Transportation Services

Older persons are often given discounts for bus, taxicab, subway, and train services; individual agencies should be contacted for more information. Commissions or offices on aging, health departments, departments of social services, and local chapters of the American Red Cross may be able to direct persons to services accommodating wheelchairs and other special needs. Various health and medical facilities provide transportation for persons utilizing their services; individual facilities should be explored for specific details.

Volunteer Services

The wealth of knowledge and experiences possessed by older persons makes them especially good at volunteer work. Not only do older volunteers provide valuable services to other persons, but they may achieve a sense of self-worth from their contributions to society. Communities offer numerous opportunities for senior volunteers in hospitals, nursing homes, organizations, schools, and other sites. The aged should be encouraged to inquire about volunteer opportunities at the agency in which they are interested in serving. Frequently agencies without a formal volunteer program are able to utilize a volunteer's services if contacted. National programs also provide meaningful volunteer services in which older persons can participate. The American National Red Cross, Service Corps of Retired Executives (SCORE), and

349

Retired Senior Volunteer Program (RSVP) are a few such programs. Local offices of these programs should be consulted for details.

SUPPORTIVE SERVICES

The services in this category offer assistance to individuals who if aided are capable of self-care, but who are at risk of physical, emotional, and social problems without some planned intervention.

Chore Services
Departments of social services, health departments, private homemaker agencies, and religious organizations have services for older persons which help them remain in their homes and maintain independence. These services include light housekeeping, minor repairs, errands, and shopping. Local agencies should be contacted for specific information.

Day-Care Programs
Geriatric day-care programs provide services to persons with moderate physical or mental handicaps who live alone or with families in the community. Individuals attend the program for a portion of their day and enjoy a safe, pleasant, therapeutic environment under the supervision of qualified personnel. The programs attempt to maximize the existing self-care capacity of aged individuals while preventing further limitations. Although the primary focus is social, there usually is some health component to these programs. Rest periods and meals accompany the planned therapeutic activities. Older persons attending day care programs are provided with transportation to the site, and usually the buses are equipped with lifts and adjusted for wheelchairs.

In addition to helping the aged person avoid further limitations and institutionalization, day-care programs are extremely beneficial to the families of the individual. Families interested in caring for their aged relative may be able to continue their routine life-style (e.g., maintaining a job), knowing that the older person is safe and cared for. They may also be comforted knowing that they and the aged person have some respite from each other. Since day care programs vary in their schedule, activities, costs, and sponsoring agency, individual programs should be contacted for specific information. Health departments, departments of social services, and commissions or offices on aging may be able to provide lists of geriatric day care programs.

Foster Care Services
Adult foster care programs offer services to individuals who are capable of self-care but who require supervision to protect them from

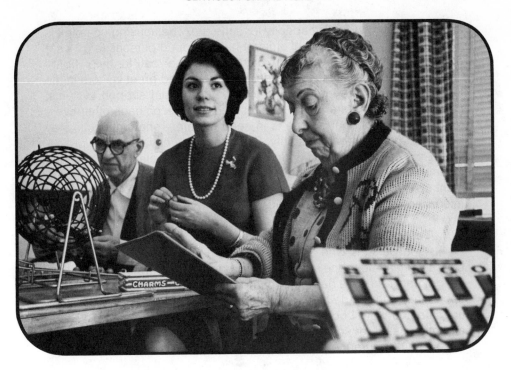

harm. Older persons placed in foster homes may need someone to direct their self-care activities (e.g., remind them to bathe and dress and encourage and provide good nutrition); they may also need someone to oversee their judgments (e.g., financial management). Foster care serves as a short- or long-term alternative to institutionalization for older persons unable to manage independently in the community. The local department of social services can supply details for adult foster care programs.

Home Delivered Meals Services

Persons unable to shop and prepare meals independently may benefit from having meals delivered to their homes. Such a service not only facilitates good nutrition, but also provides an opportunity for a social contact. Meals on Wheels is the most popularly known program for home delivery of meals, although various community groups provide a similar service. If a local Meals on Wheels is not available, departments of social services, health departments, and commissions or offices on aging should be consulted for alternative programs.

Sheltered Housing

Sheltered housing, frequently in the structure of an apartment complex, supplements independent living with special services which

351

maximize an individual's capacity for self-care. The housing complex is adjusted to meet the needs of older or handicapped persons (e.g., wide doors, low cabinets, grab bars in bathroom, and a "call for help" light). There is a guard, hostess, or resident to screen and greet visitors in the lobby. Residents are encouraged to develop mutual support systems; one example is a system by which residents check on each other every morning to ensure that no one is in need of help. Tenant councils may determine policies for the facility. Some facilities have a health professional on call or on duty during certain hours; social programs and communal meals may also be available. The local office of the Department of Housing and Urban Development (HUD) may be able to direct interested persons to such facilities.

Telephone Reassurance Programs

Aged persons who are homebound, handicapped, or lonely may benefit from a telephone reassurance program. Those who participate in the program receive a daily telephone call—usually at a mutually agreed upon time—to provide them with a social contact and ensure that they are safe and well. Local chapters of the American National Red Cross and other health or social service agencies should be consulted for the telephone reassurance programs they may conduct.

SERVICES FOR PARTIAL AND INTERMITTENT CARE

The services in this category are those which provide assistance to individuals with a partial limitation in self-care capacity and a therapeutic demand for which occasional assistance is required. Either due to the degree of the self-care limitation or the complexity of the therapeutic action required, the individual would be at risk of institutionalization if some assistance wasn't provided at periodic intervals. Such services can be for day treatment or home care.

Day treatment offers social and health programs, with a primary focus on the latter. Assistance is provided with self-care activities (e.g., bathing and feeding) and therapeutic needs (e.g., medication administration, dressing change, and vital signs monitoring). Physicians, nurses, occupational therapists, and physical therapists are among the care providers affiliated with programs for day treatment. Like geriatric day-care programs, geriatric day hospitals usually provide transportation services for the participants. Day hospitals can be used as alternatives to hospitalization and nursing homes. In addition, earlier discharge from an institution may be facilitated if an individual has an opportunity for continued therapeutic supervision in this type of program. These programs are sponsored by hospitals, nursing homes, or other agencies.

The local commission or office on aging can guide persons to programs of day treatment in their community.

Home care is for persons who are confined to their homes but in need of therapeutic assistance. The programs vary, and services can include bedside nursing, home health aides, physical therapy, health education, family counseling, and medical services. Visiting nurse associations have a long reputation of providing care in the home, and are able to assist many aged persons to remain in their homes rather than enter an institution. Offices or commissions on aging, health departments, and social work agencies may be able to answer inquiries about other available programs for home care.

SERVICES FOR COMPLETE AND CONTINUOUS CARE

The services in this category provide regular or continuous assistance to individuals with some limitation in self-care capacity whose therapeutic needs require 24-hour supervision by a health professional. These services provide hospital care or long-term institutional care.

Hospital care for older persons may be required when diagnostic procedures and therapeutic actions indicate a need for specialized technologies or frequent monitoring. Local medical societies and state hospital associations can answer inquiries about specific hospitals.

Long-term institutional care varies from one region to another, differing in the quality and quantity of medical, nursing, and other services provided. State health departments may be able to answer inquiries about specific long-term care facilities. Hospitals for chronic diseases and rehabilitation, nursing homes, and facilities for extended and intermediate care provide long-term institutional care. While this form of care for the aged with health problems is not the only kind, it is appropriate and quite beneficial for some aged persons. It is essential to match the unique needs of the aged individual with the particular services offered by a long-term care facility. Older persons and their families should be actively involved with the selection of the facility. It is important to examine the costs, services, and quality of the institution prior to admission. The guidelines below are helpful in choosing a nursing home.

Shopping Guide for Nursing Homes

Physical Considerations
    1. Location: pleasing to patient; near patient's doctor, family, friends; near cooperating hospital

353

2. Accident prevention: ample, nonglare lighting in all areas; nonslippery floors; no hazards underfoot; handrails, grab bars where appropriate
3. Fire-safety measures: meeting federal and/or state codes; clearly marked, unobstructed exits; emergency evacuation plan posted throughout facility; frequent fire drills; exterior doors unlocked on inside, with emergency opening devices; enclosed stairways, with doors kept closed; interior doors unlocked; sufficient staff always on hand to aid nonambulatory patients in an emergency; cigarette smoking by staff and patients regulated
4. Cleanliness—though with lived-in look; free of unpleasant odors or heavy disinfectant odor; incontinent patients given prompt attention
5. Lobby and lounge areas pleasant, welcoming; being used by residents; furniture attractive, comfortable, arranged to encourage conversation; seating easy to get into and out of; televisions, radios in working order; game boards, recent magazines, etc., available; quiet area for resting; plants, flowers, wall decoration
6. Hallways well lighted, wide enough for two wheelchairs to pass easily, with handgrip railings along walls
7. Bedrooms open onto hall; windows; no more than four beds per room; care used in selecting roommates; easy access to each bed, with room for wheelchair; drapery, nurse call bell, fresh drinking water by each bed; at least one comfortable chair per patient; reading lights; clothes closet, drawers for each resident; telephones; television and radio, with special attachments for patients with hearing loss
8. Toilet facilities convenient to bedrooms, preferably with separate facilities for each bedroom; easy for wheelchair patient to use; sink with hot and cold running water; nurse call bell; handgrips on or near toilets; nonslip surfaces, handgrips in bathtubs and showers
9. Dining room: attractive, inviting; comfortable chairs and tables; easy to move around in; tables convenient for those in wheelchairs; menus posted; those needing help receiving it; separated from food-preparation area
10. Kitchen: food preparation, dishwashing, garbage areas separated; food needing refrigeration not standing on counters; kitchen help observing sanitation rules
11. Activity rooms available and being used; equipment such as games, easels, yarn, kiln, etc., available

354

12. Special-purpose rooms available for physical examination or therapy, for private visits with family and friends, and being used for stated purpose
13. Isolation room: at least one bed and bathroom for patients with contagious illness
14. Grounds attractive, ramps to help handicapped; outdoor furniture in both sun and shade; hazardous objects away from areas where patients may walk; handrails where needed; residents using outdoor areas

Services

1. Medical: medical director on staff; physician available in emergency; private physicians allowed; regular visits from specialists; regular medical attention assured; thorough physical immediately before or soon after the patient's admission; medical records, plan of care kept up-to-date; patients involved in treatment plans; special equipment readily available; other medical services available regularly; freedom to buy prescribed drugs elsewhere
2. Hospitalization: arrangement with nearby hospital for transfer when necessary; emergency transportation readily available
3. Nursing services: registered nurse responsible for nursing staff in skilled nursing home; licensed practical nurse on duty day and night in skilled nursing home; preemployment and in-service training given nurses' aides and orderlies, with evaluation given regularly
4. Physical and rehabilitation therapy: full-time program of physical therapy under direction of qualified physical therapist; programs for special needs, such as speech therapy, bowel and bladder retraining, occupational therapy
5. Activities program: individual patient preferences observed; group and individual activities, with posted schedule; special observances on holidays; residents encouraged but not forced to participate; outside trips for those able to go; volunteer program; library service, including material in large print, talking books
6. Religious observances: arrangements for patients to worship as they please, either in the home or elsewhere; chaplain on staff
7. Social services: certified social worker available to aid residents and families; prospective resident counseling given; relatives notified of change in patient's condition
8. Food: tasty and attractively served; menus followed as posted;

355

personal likes, dislikes considered; dietitian-planned menus for those needing special diet; variety from meal to meal; meals served efficiently (hot foods hot, etc.) at normal times; plenty of time for each meal; nutritious snacks available; food delivered to those unable or unwilling to eat in dining room; help with eating given when needed

9. Grooming: assistance in bathing available; barbers, beauticians available; encouragement, and help if needed, given toward neat appearance

Attitudes and Atmosphere

1. General atmosphere warm, pleasant, cheerful
2. Staff respond quickly to patient calls for assistance; show interest in, affection for individual patients; are courteous, respectful; treat patients as adults; chat with patients; talk with families about their patient's progress, concerns
3. Administrator courteous and helpful; knows patients by name; available to answer questions, hear complaints, discuss problems
4. Residents appear alert, active, involved unless very sick; can decorate own bedrooms according to personal tastes and with personal belongings, can wear clothes of their choice; evidence self-expression; communicate freely with each other, the staff, and persons outside the home
5. Rules reasonable; visiting hours generous and convenient for residents and guests; precautions taken to prevent loss of clothing, other possessions; civil rights regulations observed

From Virginia E. Beverley, *Helping Your Patient Choose and Adjust to a Nursing Home.* Reprinted from *Geriatrics* © 1976 by Harcourt Brace Jovanovich, Inc.

Recognizing that services may vary from one area to another, gerontological nurses should become acquainted with the full range of services for the aged in their region. When necessary services are lacking, the nurse can serve as an advocate for the aged by stimulating the interests of consumers, professional colleagues, and policy makers in program development. A wide spectrum of services must exist to ensure that the appropriate level of assistance is available for the given level of need. The continuum of geriatric care services should reflect the varied and changing needs of this population. Opportunities exist along all points of the continuum for nursing to demonstrate competency and leadership in the care of the aged.

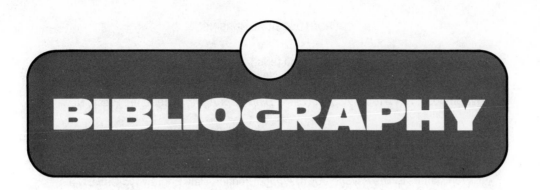
BIBLIOGRAPHY

CHAPTER 2:
Theories of Aging

Andrew, Warren. *The Anatomy of Aging in Man and Animals*. Grune & Stratton, New York, 1971.

Birren, James E. *The Psychology of Aging*. Prentice-Hall, Englewood Cliffs, N.J., 1964.

Birren, James E. (ed.). Handbook of Aging and the Individual. Univ. of Chicago Press, 1959.

Botwinick, Jack. *Aging and Behavior*. Springer, New York, 1973.

Clark, Margaret, and Anderson, Barbara G. *Culture and Aging*. Thomas, Springfield, Ill. 1967.

Comfort, A. *Aging: The Biology of Senescence*. Holt, Rinehart and Winston, New York, 1964.

Curtis, H. J. *Biological Mechanisms of Aging*. Thomas, Springfield, Ill., 1966.

Kastenbaum, Robert (ed.). *Contributions to the Psychology of Aging*. Springer, New York, 1965.

Kent, Donald P. "The Elderly in Minority Groups: Variant Patterns of Aging." *Gerontologist,* 11:(1) 26–29, 1971.

Krohn, Peter L. (ed.). *Symposium on Topics in the Biology of Aging*. Wiley, 1966.

Miller, Stephen J. "The Social Dilemma of the Aging Leisure Participant." In Rose, A. and Peterson, W. (eds.), *Older People and Their Social World,* Davis, Philadelphia, 1965, pp. 77–92.

Neugarten, Bernice L. *Middle Age and Aging,* Univ. of Chicago Press, 1968.

Shock, Nathan W. (ed.). *Aging: Some Social and Biological Aspects*. American Association for the Advancement of Science. Horn-Shafer, Baltimore, 1960.

Tibbitts, Clark (ed.). Handbook of Social Gerontology. Univ. of Chicago Press, 1960.

Tibbitts, Clark, and Donahue, Wilma (eds.). *Social and Psychological Aspects of Aging.* Columbia Univ. Press, New York, 1962.

Walford, R. L. "Immunologic Theory of Aging." *Gerontologist,* 4:195–197, 1964.

Woolhouse, H. W. (ed.). *Aspects of the Biology of Aging.* Academic Press, New York, 1967.

CHAPTER 3:
Adjustments in Aging

Barrett, J. *Gerontological Psychology.* Thomas, Springfield, Ill. 1972.

Birren, James E. *The Psychology of Aging.* Prentice-Hall, Englewood Cliffs, N.J., 1964.

Blau, Zena. *Old Age in a Changing Society.* New Viewpoints, New York, 1973.

Burnside, Irene M. "Accountrements of Aging." *Nursing Clinics of North America,* 7(2):291–301, June 1972.

Cameron, P., et al. "Consciousness of Death Across the Life Span." *Journal of Gerontology,* 28(1):92–95, January 1973.

Cavan, R. "Family Tensions Between the Old and Middle-Aged." In Vedder, C. (ed.), *Problems of the Middle Aged.* Thomas, Springfield, Ill., 1965.

Clark, M., and Anderson, B. *Culture and Aging: An Anthropological Study of Older Americans.* Thomas, Springfield, Ill., 1967.

Conti, Mary Louise. "The Loneliness of Old Age." *Nursing Outlook,* 18:28–30, August 1970.

Curtin, Sharon. *Nobody Ever Died of Old Age.* Little, Brown, Boston, 1972.

de Beauvoir, Simone. *The Coming of Age.* Warner Paperback Library, New York, 1973.

Erikson, Erik. *Childhood and Society,* 2nd ed. Norton, New York, 1950.

Geist, H. *The Psychological Aspects of the Aging Process.* Warren H. Green, St. Louis, 1968.

Golden, H. "The Dysfunctional Effects of Modern Technology on the Adaptability of the Aging." *Gerontologist,* 13:136, Summer 1973.

Havighurst, R., and Glasser, R. "An Exploratory Study of Reminiscence." *Journal of Gerontology,* 72(2):245–253, 1972.

Heilbrun, Alfred B., Jr., and Lais, Charles V. "Decreased Role Consistency in the Aged." *Journal of Gerontology,* 19:325–329, 1964.

Jury, Mark, and Jury, Don. *Gramp.* Grossman, New York, 1976.

Kopelke, Charlotte E. "Retirement As A Nursing Concern." *Journal of Gerontological Nursing,* 4:13–19, 1975.

"The Middle Years," *American Journal of Nursing.* 75:993–1024, June 1975.

Morrison, Esther. "Old, Aged, or Elderly . . . What's In A Name?" *Journal of Gerontological Nursing,* 2:25–27, 1975.

Neugarten, Bernice (ed.). *Middle Age and Aging.* Univ. of Chicago Press, 1968.

Neugarten, Bernice, et al. *Personality in Middle and Late Life.* Atherton Press, New York, 1964.

Reichard, S., et al. *Aging and Personality.* Wiley, New York, 1962.

Rosow, Irving. "Old Age: One Moral Dilemma of an Affluent Society." *Gerontologist,* 2:182–191, 1962.

Rosow, Irving. *Social Integration of the Aged.* Free Press, New York, 1967.

Schonfield, D. "Future Commitments and Successful Aging." *Journal of Gerontology,* 28(2):189–196, April 1973.

Soddy, K., and Kidson, M. *Men In Middle Life.* Lippincott, Philadelphia, 1967.

Stone, Virginia. "Give the Older Person Time." *American Journal of Nursing,* 69:2124–2127, October 1969.

Tibbitts, Clark (ed.). *Handbook of Social Gerontology.* Univ. of Chicago Press, 1960.

Walters, Dolores. "Life Is Beautiful at 87." *Journal of Gerontological Nursing,* 2:23–24, 1975.

CHAPTER 4:
Changes Associated with the Aging Process

Agate, J. N. *The Practice of Geriatric Medicine,* 2nd ed. Heinemann Medical, London, 1970.

Brocklehurst, J. C. (ed.). *Textbook of Geriatric Medicine and Gerontology.* Churchill Livingstone, Edinburgh and London, 1973.

Clark, M., and Anderson, B. G. *Culture and Aging.* Thomas, Springfield, Ill., 1967.

Eisdorfer, C. "Verbal Learning and Response Time in the Aged." *Journal of Genetic Psychology.* 107:15, 1965.

Kastenbaum, R. *Contributions to the Psychology of Aging.* Springer, New York, 1965.

Lansing, Albert (ed.). *Cowdry's Problems of Aging.* Williams & Wilkens, St. Louis, 1952.

Loether, H. J. *Problems of Aging.* Dickenson, Belmont, Calif., 1967.

Neugarten, B. L. (ed.). *Personality in Middle and Late Life.* Atherton Press, New York, 1964.

Shanas, E., Townsend, P., Wedderburn, D., Friis, H., Milhj, P., and Stehouwer, J. *Old People in Three Industrial Societies.* Atherton Press, New York, 1968.

Tibbitts, C., and Donahue, W. (eds.). *Social and Psychological Aspects of Aging.* Columbia Univ. Press, New York, 1962.

Williams, R. H., Tibbitts C., and Donahue, W. (eds.). *Processes of Aging,* Vols. I and II. Atherton Press, New York, 1963.

CHAPTER 6:
The Nursing Process

Birren, J. E. *The Psychology of Aging.* Prentice-Hall, Englewood Cliffs, N.J., 1964.

Blainey, Carol Gohrke. "Site Selection in Taking Body Temperature." *American Journal of Nursing,* 74(10):1859–1861, October 1974.

Burnside, Irene. "Interviewing the Aged." In Burnside, Irene (ed.), *Psychosocial Nursing Care of the Aged.* McGraw-Hill, New York, 1973.

Caird, F. I., and Judge, T. G. *Assessment of the Elderly Patient.* Pitman Medical Publishing Co., New York, 1974.

Carrieri, Virginia K., and Sitzman, Judith. "Components of the Nursing Process." *Nursing Clinics of North America,* 6(1):115–124, March, 1971.

Carter, J. H., et al. *Standards of Nursing Care: A Guide for Evaluation.* Springer, New York, 1972.

Cowdry, E. V., and Steinberg, Franz U. (eds.) *The Care of the Geriatric Patient.* Mosby, St. Louis, 1971.

Donabedian, Avedis. Part 1: "Some Issues in Evaluating the Quality of Nursing Care." *American Journal of Public Health,* 59:1833–1836, October 1969.

Evans, D. M. "Haematological Aspects of Iron Deficiency in the Elderly." *Gerontologia Clinica,* 13:12–20, 1971.

Gaitz, C. M., and Baer, P. E. "Diagnostic Assessment of the Elderly: A Multifunctional Model." *Gerontologist,* 10:47–52, 1970.

Knowles, Lois N. (ed). "Symposium on Putting Geriatric Nursing Standards Into Practice." *Nursing Clinics of North America,* 7(2):201–309, June 1972.

Little, Dolores E., and Carnevali, Doris. *Nursing Care Planning.* Lippincott, Philadelphia, 1969.

Mann, George V. "Relationship of Age to Nutrient Requirements." *American Journal of Clinical Nutrition,* 26:1096–1097, October 1973.

Moses, D. F. "Assessing Behavior in the Elderly." *Nursing Clinics of North America,* 7(2):225–233, June 1972.

Neugarten, Bernice. *Middle Age and Aging.* Univ. of Chicago Press, 1972.

Nichols, Glennodee A. "Taking Adult Temperatures—Rectal Measurements." *American Journal of Nursing,* 72(6):1092–1093, June 1972.

——— et al. "Oral, Axillary and Rectal Temperature Determinations and Relationships." *Nursing Research,* 15:307–310, Fall 1966.

——— and Kucha, Delores H. "Taking Adult Temperatures—Oral Measurements." *American Journal of Nursing,* 72(6):1091–1092, June 1972.

Orem, Dorothea E. *Nursing: Concepts of Practice.* McGraw-Hill, New York, 1971.

Phaneuf, M. C. *The Nursing Audit: Profile for Excellence.* Prentice-Hall (Appleton), Englewood Cliffs, N.J., 1972.

Rossman, Isadore (ed.). *Clinical Geriatrics.* Lippincott, Philadelphia, 1971.

Shock, N. W., and Yiengst, M. J. "Age Changes in the Acid-Base Equilibrium of the Blood of Males." *Journal of Gerontology,* 5:1–4, 1950.

Taylor, Joyce W. "Measuring the Outcomes of Nursing Care." *Nursing Clinics of North America,* 9(2):337–348, June 1974.

Yura, Helen, and Walsh, Mary B. *The Nursing Process: Assessing, Planning, Implementing and Evaluating,* 2nd ed. Prentice-Hall (Appleton), Englewood Cliffs, N.J., 1973.

Wandelt, M. S., and Phaneuf, M. C. "Three Instruments for Measuring the Quality of Nursing Care." *Hospital Topics,* 50:20–29, August 1972.

CHAPTER 7:
Assisting the Aged with Universal Self-Care Demands

Barrows, C. H. "Nutrition, Aging and Genetic Program." *American Journal of Clinical Nutrition,* pp. 829–833, August 1972.

Bates, J. F. et al. "Studies Relating Mastication and Nutrition in the Elderly." *Gerontologica Clinica,* 13:227–232, 1971.

Birren, J. E. *The Psychology of Aging.* Prentice-Hall, Englewood Cliffs, N.J., 1964.

DeWalt, Evelyn M. "Effect of Timed Hygienic Measures on Oral Mucosa in a Group of Elderly Subjects." *Nursing Research,* 24(2):104–108, 1975.

Exton-Smith, A. N. "Physiological Aspects of Aging: Relationship to Nutrition." *American Journal of Clinical Nutrition,* 25:853–859, August 1972.

Fisher, Seymour, and Cleveland, Sidney E. *Body Image and Personality.* Dover, New York, 1968.

Fuerst, Elinor V., and Wolff, Lu Verne. *Fundamentals of Nursing,* 3rd ed. Lippincott, Philadelphia, 1964.

Greenberg, Barbara. "Reaction Time in the Elderly." *American Journal of Nursing,* 73:2056–2058, December 1973.

Jaeger, Dorothea, and Simmons, Leo W. *The Aged Ill.* Prentice-Hall (Appleton), Englewood Cliffs, N.J., 1970.

Jennings, Muriel, Nordstrom, Margene J., and Shumake, Norine. "Physiological Functioning in the Elderly." *Nursing Clinics of North America,* 7(2):237–251, June 1972.

Kornzweig, Abraham L. "The Eye in Old Age." In Rossman, Isadore (ed.), *Clinical Geriatrics,* Lippincott, 1971.

Leonard, B. J. "Body Image Changes in Chronic Illness." *Nursing Clinics of North America,* 7(4):687–695, December 1972.

Lofholm, Paul. "Self-Medication by the Elderly." In Davis, Richard H. (ed.), *Drugs and the Elderly.* Andries Gerontology Center, Univ. of Southern California, Los Angeles, 1973.

Masters, W. H., and Johnson, V. *Human Sexual Response.* Little, Brown, Boston, 1966.

Orem, Dorothea E. *Nursing: Concepts of Practice.* McGraw-Hill, New York, 1971.

Rao, Dodda. "Problems of Nutrition in the Aged." *Journal of the American Geriatrics Society,* 21:362, August 1973.

Rossman, Isadore (ed.). *Clinical Geriatrics.* Lippincott, Philadelphia, 1971.

"Symposium on Nutrition." *Geriatrics,* 29, May 1974.

Wylie, Ruth C. *The Self Concept.* Univ. of Nebraska Press, 1961.

CHAPTER 8:
Cardiovascular Problems

Adatto, I. J., Poske, R. M., Pouget, J. M., Pilz, C. G. and Montgomery, M. M. "Rheumatic Fever in the Adult." *Journal of the American Medical Assoc.,* 194:1043, 1965.

Agate, J. A. (ed.). *Medicine in Old Age.* Lippincott, Philadelphia, 1966.

Anderson, W. F. *Practical Management of the Elderly.* Davis, Philadelphia, 1967.

Bedford, P. D., and Caird, F. I. *Valvular Disease of the Heart in Old Age.* Little, Brown, Boston, 1960.

Beland, Irene L. *Clinical Nursing: Pathophysiological and Psychosocial Approaches,* 3rd ed. Macmillan, New York, 1975.

Bell, William R. "Reaching the Correct Diagnosis of Pulmonary Thromboembolism." *Geriatrics,* 30:49–53, September 1975.

Brunner, Lillian S., and Suddarth, Doris S. *Textbook of Medical-Surgical Nursing,* 3rd ed. Lippincott, Philadelphia, 1975.

———*The Lippincott Manual of Nursing Practice.* Lippincott, Philadelphia, 1974.

Chobanian, Aram V. "Hypertension: Major Risk Factor for Cardiovascular Complications." *Geriatrics,* 31:87–95, January 1976.

Dall, J. L. C. "Digitalis Toxicity in Elderly Patients." *Lancet,* 1:194, 1965.

Dock, W. "How Some Hearts Age." *Journal of the American Medical Assoc.,* 195:442, 1966.

Fisch, C., Genovese, P. D., Dyke, R. W., Laramore, W., and Marvel, R. J. "The Electrocardiogram in Persons Over 70." *Geriatrics,* 12:616, 1957.

Fowler, N. O. "Chronic Cor Pulmonale." *Geriatrics,* 22:156, 1967.

Freeman, J. T. (ed.). *Clinical Features of the Older Patient.* Thomas, Springfield, Ill., 1965.

Harris, R. "Special Features of Heart Disease in the Elderly Patient." In Chinn, A. B. (ed.), *Working with Older People,* Vol. IV. U.S. Dept. of Health, Education, and Welfare, 1974, pp. 81–102.

———*The Management of Geriatric Cardiovascular Diseases.* Lippincott, Philadelphia, 1970.

Henry, James P. "Understanding the Early Pathophysiology of Essential Hypertension." *Geriatrics,* 31:59–72, January 1976.

Landowne, M., Brandfonbrener, M. and Shock, V. W. "Relation of Age to

361

Certain Measures of the Performance of the Heart and Circulation." *Circulation,* 12:567, 1955.

Librach, G., Schadel, M., Seltzer, M., and Hart, A. "Assessing Incidence and Risk Factors in Myocardial Infarction." *Geriatrics,* 30:79–93, September 1975.

McMillan, J., and Leo, H. "The Aging Heart, II: The Valves." *Journal of Gerontology,* 19:1, 1964.

Moidel, Harriet C., Giblin, Elizabeth C., and Wagner, Berniece M. (eds.). *Nursing Care of the Patient with Medical-Surgical Disorders,* 2nd ed. McGraw-Hill, New York, 1976.

Pathy, M. S. "Clinical Presentation of Myocardial Infarction in the Elderly." *British Heart Journal,* 29:190, 1967.

Perloff, Dorothee. "Diagnostic Assessment of the Patient with Hypertension." *Geriatrics,* 31:77–83, January 1976.

Remington, Richard D. "Blood Pressure: The Population Burden." *Geriatrics,* 31:48–54, January 1976.

Rodstein, Manuel. "Heart Disease in the Aged." In Rossman, Isadore (ed.), *Clinical Geriatrics,* Lippincott, Philadelphia, 1971.

Shafer, Kathleen N., et al. *Medical-Surgical Nursing,* 5th ed. Mosby, St. Louis, 1971.

Syzek, Barbara J. "Cardiovascular Changes in Aging: Implications for Nursing." *Journal of Gerontological Nursing,* 2(1):28, 1976.

White, Paul D. "Cardiovascular Disorders." In Cowdry, E. V., and Steinberg, F. U. (eds.), *The Care of the Geriatric Patient.* Mosby, St. Louis, 1971.

CHAPTER 9:
Peripheral Vascular Disease

Beland, Irene L. *Clinical Nursing: Pathophysiological and Psychosocial Approaches,* 3rd ed. Macmillan, New York, 1975.

Blumenthal, Herman T. "Aging and Peripheral Vascular Disease." In Chinn, Austin B., *Working with Older People. A Guide to Practice,* Vol. IV. U.S. Dept. of Health, Education, and Welfare, Rockville, Md., 1974 pp. 103–112.

Brunner, Lillian S., and Suddarth, Doris S. *Textbook of Medical-Surgical Nursing,* 3rd ed. Lippincott, Philadelphia, 1975.

——— *The Lippincott Manual of Nursing Practice.* Lippincott, Philadelphia, 1974.

Cobey, James C., and Cobey, Janet H. "Chronic Leg Ulcers." *American Journal of Nursing,* 74:258–259, February 1974.

Compere, C. L. "Early Fitting of Prosthesis Following Amputation." *Surgical Clinic of North America,* 48:215, 1968.

Haimovici, Henry. "The Peripheral Vascular System." In Rossman, Isadore, *Clinical Geriatrics.* Lippincott, Philadelphia, 1971, pp. 165–181.

Harris, P., et al. "The Fate of Elderly Amputees." *British Journal of Surgery,* 61:665–668, 1974.

Kerstein, M. D., Zimmer H., Dugdale, F. E., and Lerner, E. "What Influence Does Age Have on Rehabilitation of Amputees?" *Geriatrics,* 30:67–71, December 1975.

Lofgren, Eric P., and Lofgren, Karl A. "Alternatives in the Management of Varices." *Geriatrics* 30:111–113, September 1975.

Moidel, Harriet C., Giblin, Elizabeth C., and Wagner, Berniece M. (eds.). *Nursing Care of the Patient with Medical-Surgical Disorders,* 2nd ed. McGraw-Hill, New York, 1976.

Rose, Mary Ann. "Home Care After Peripheral Vascular Surgery." *American Journal of Nursing,* 74:260–262, February 1974.

Shafer, Kathleen N., et al. *Medical-Surgical Nursing,* 5th ed. Mosby, St. Louis, 1971.

CHAPTER 10:
Cancer

Beland, Irene L. *Clinical Nursing: Pathophysiological and Psychosocial Approaches,* 3rd ed. Macmillan, New York, 1975.

Bouchard, Rosemary, et al. *Nursing Care of the Cancer Patient.* Mosby, St. Louis, 1972.

Browning, Mary, and Lewis, Edith P. (eds.). "The Nurse and the Cancer Patient." *American Journal of Nursing,* New York, 1973.

Brunner, Lillian S., and Suddarth, Doris S. *Textbook of Medical-Surgical Nursing,* 3rd ed. Lippincott, Philadelphia, 1975.

——— *The Lippincott Manual of Nursing Practice.* Lippincott, Philadelphia, 1974.

Clifford, G. O. "Hematologic Problems in the Elderly." In Rossman, Isadore (ed.), *Clinical Geriatrics.* Lippincott, Philadelphia, 1971, pp. 261–264.

Donovan, C. "What's New in Cancer Control." *American Journal of Nursing,* 76(6):962, June 1976.

Exton-Smith, A. N., and Windsor, A. C. M. "Principles of Drug Treatment in the Aged." In Rossman, Isadore (ed.), *Clinical Geriatrics.* Lippincott, Philadelphia, 1971, pp. 383–384.

Jarvik, L. "Genetic Aspects of Aging." In Rossman, Isadore (ed.), *Clinical Geriatrics.* Lippincott, Philadelphia, 1971, pp. 99–100.

Moidel, Harriet C., Giblin, Elizabeth C., and Wagner, Berniece M. (eds.). *Nursing Care of the Patient with Medical-Surgical Disorders,* 2nd ed. McGraw-Hill, New York, 1976.

Ostfield, A. M., and Gibson, D. C. (eds.). *Epidemiology of Aging.* U.S. Dept. of Health, Education, and Welfare, Publication (NIH) 75–711, Bethesda, Md., 1972.

Pelner, L. "Specific Aspects of Malignancy in the Older Body." In Freeman, Joseph (ed.), *Clinical Features of the Older Patient.* Thomas, Springfield, Ill., 1965, pp. 345–352.

Rinear, Eileen. "Helping the Survivors of Expected Death." *Nursing,* 75, 3:60–65, March 1975.

Shafer, Kathleen N., et al. *Medical-Surgical Nursing,* 5th ed. Mosby, St. Louis, 1971.

Zippin, Calvin, et al. "Identification of High Risk Groups in Breast Cancer." *Cancer,* 1381–1387, December 1971.

CHAPTER 11:
Respiratory Problems

Beland, Irene L. *Clinical Nursing: Pathophysiological and Psychosocial Approaches,* 3rd ed. Macmillan, New York, 1975.

Brunner, Lillian S., and Suddarth, Doris S. *Textbook of Medical-Surgical Nursing,* 3rd ed. Lippincott, Philadelphia, 1975.

——— *The Lippincott Manual of Nursing Practice.* Lippincott, Philadelphia, 1974.

Henshaw, H. C. *Diseases of the Chest.* Saunders, Philadelphia, 1969.

Moidel, Harriet C., Giblin, Elizabeth C., and **Wagner, Berniece M.** (eds.). *Nursing Care of the Patient with Medical-Surgical Disorders,* 2nd ed. McGraw-Hill, New York, 1976.

Report of the Surgeon General. The Health Consequences of Smoking. U.S. Government Printing Office, Washington, D.C., 1972.

Rodman, T., and **Sterling, F. H.** *Pulmonary Emphysema and Related Lung Diseases.* Mosby, St. Louis, 1969.

Schwaid, M. C. "The Impact of Emphysema." *American Journal of Nursing,* 70:1247–1250, June 1971.

Sedlock, Stephanie A. "Detection of Chronic Pulmonary Disease." *American Journal of Nursing,* 72(8):1407–1411, August 1972.

Shafer, Kathleen N. et al. *Medical-Surgical Nursing,* 5th ed. Mosby, St. Louis, 1971.

Stolley, Paul D. "Asthma Mortality." *American Review of Respiratory Disease,* 105:883–890, 1972.

Ungvarski, P. "Mechanical Stimulation of Coughing." *American Journal of Nursing,* 71:2358–2361, December 1971.

CHAPTER 12:
Diabetes

American Diabetes Association. *Diabetes Mellitus: Diagnosis and Treatment,* Vol. 3. New York, 1971.

Davies, D. "Advances Toward Understanding Diabetes Mellitus." *Geriatrics,* 30(11):79–83, November 1975.

Ellenberg, M. "Diabetes in the Older Age Group." *Geriatrics,* 19:47, 1964.

Gitman, Leo. "Diabetes Mellitus in the Aged." In Chinn, A. B., *Working with Older People: A Guide to Practice,* Vol. IV. U.S. Dept. of Health Education, and Welfare, Rockville, Md. 1974, p. 219.

Marble, A., et al. (eds.). *Joslin's Diabetes Mellitus,* 11th ed. Lea and Febiger, Philadelphia, 1971.

Rafkin, H., and **Ross, H.** "Diabetes in the Elderly." In Rossman, I. (ed.), *Clinical Geriatrics.* Lippincott, Philadelphia, 1971, pp. 391–403.

CHAPTER 13:
Musculoskeletal Problems

Avioli, L. V. "Aging, Bone, and Osteoporosis." In Steinberg, F. U. (ed.), *Cowdry's, The Care of the Geriatric Patient,* 5th ed. Mosby, St. Louis, 1976, pp. 119–132.

Ball, B. "Helping Patients Adjust to Rheumatoid Arthritis." *Nursing,* 72(2)11–17, October 1972.

Beckenbaugh, R. D. "Reconstructing the Crippled Arthritic Hand." *Geriatrics,* 31(3):89–93, March 1976.

Beland, Irene L. *Clinical Nursing: Pathophysiological and Psychosocial Approaches,* 3rd ed. Macmillan, New York, 1975.

Bennage, B. A., and **Cummings, M. E.** "Nursing the Patient Undergoing Total Hip Arthroplasty." *Nursing Clinics of North America,* 8:107–116, March 1973.

Brewerton, D. A. "Rheumatic Disorders." In Rossman, I. (ed.), *Clinical Geriatrics.* Lippincott, Philadelphia, 1971, pp. 301–307.

Brunner, Lillian S., and **Suddarth, Doris S.** *Textbook of Medical-Surgical Nursing,* 3rd ed. Lippincott, Philadelphia, 1975.

——— *The Lippincott Manual of Nursing Practice.* Lippincott, Philadelphia, 1974.

Cabanela, M. E. "Superiority of Total Hip Replacement Arthroplasty." *Geriatrics,* 31(3):61–66, March 1976.

Chamberlin, G. W. "Bone: Radiological and Clinical Aspects." In Freeman, J. T. (ed.), *Clinical Features of the Older Patient.* Thomas, Springfield, Ill., 1965, pp. 359–376.

Chao, E. Y. S. "The Biomechanics of Total Joint Replacement Surgery." *Geriatrics,* 31(3):48–57, March 1976.

Devas, M. "Orthopedics." In Steinberg, F. U. (ed.), *Cowdry's, Care of the Geriatric Patient,* 5th ed. Mosby, St. Louis, 1976, pp. 258–274.

Ford, L. T. "Orthopedic Surgery." In Cowdry, E. V., and Steinberg, F. U. (eds.), *The Care of the Geriatric Patient.* Mosby, St. Louis, 1971.

Freehafer, A. A. "Injuries to the Skeletal System of Older Persons." In Chinn, A. B. (ed.), *Working with Older People,* Vol. IV. U.S. Dept. of Health, Education, and Welfare, Rockville, Md., 1974, pp. 180–193.

Grob, D. "Common Disorders of Muscles in the Aged." In Chinn, A. B. (ed.), *Working with Older People,* Vol. IV. U.S. Dept. of Health, Education, and Welfare, Rockville, Md., 1974, pp. 156–162.

———"Prevalent Joint Diseases in Older Persons." In Chinn, A. B. (ed.), *Working with Older People,* Vol. IV. U.S. Dept. of Health, Education, and Welfare, Rockville, Md., 1974, pp. 163–171.

Habermann, Edward T. "Orthopedic Aspects of the Lower Extremities." In Rossman, I. (ed.). *Clinical Geriatrics.* Lippincott, Philadelphia, 1971, pp. 309–325.

Hahn, B. H. "Arthritis, Bursitis, and Bone Disease." In Steinberg, F. U. (ed.), *Cowdry's, The Care of the Geriatric Patient,* 5th ed. Mosby, St. Louis, 1976, pp. 11–34.

Henderson, E. D. "Putting the Pieces Together." *Geriatrics,* 31(3):46–47, March 1976.

Howell, T. H. *A Student's Guide to Geriatrics.* Staples, London, 1970, pp. 135–150.

Johnson, K. A. "When Total Knee Arthroplasty is Indicated." *Geriatrics,* 31(3):71–75, March 1976.

Larson, C. B., and Gould, M. L. *Calderwood's Orthopedic Nursing,* 7th ed. Mosby, St. Louis, 1970.

Loxley, A. K. "The Emotional Toll of Crippling Deformity." *American Journal of Nursing,* 72:1839–40, October 1972.

Lutwak, L. "Metabolic Disorders of the Skeleton in Aging." In Chinn, A. B. (ed.), *Working with Older People,* Vol. IV. U.S. Dept. of Health, Education, and Welfare, Rockville, Md., 1974, pp. 172–179.

Marmor, L. "Surgery for Osteoarthritis." *Geriatrics,* 27:89–95, February 1972.

Moidel, Harriet C., Giblin, Elizabeth C., and Wagner, Berniece M. (eds.). *Nursing Care of the Patient with Medical-Surgical Disorders,* 2nd ed. McGraw-Hill, New York, 1976.

Shafer, Kathleen N., et al. *Medical-Surgical Nursing,* 5th ed. Mosby, St. Louis, 1971.

Shoemaker, R. R. "Total Knee Replacement." *Nursing Clinics of North America,* 8:117–125, March 1973.

Sorka, C. "Combating Osteoporosis." *American Journal of Nursing,* 73:1193–1197, July 1973.

Spencer, H., Baladad, J., and Lewin, I. "The Skeletal System." In Rossman, I. (ed.), *Clinical Geriatrics.* Lippincott, Philadelphia, 1971, pp. 289–300.

Stauffer, R. U. "Total Ankle Joint Replacement as an Alternative to Arthrodesis." *Geriatrics,* 31(3):79–85, March 1976.

Thewlis, M. W. *The Care of the Aged,* 6th ed. Mosby, St. Louis, 1954, pp. 599–642.
Trueta, J. *Studies of the Development and Decay of the Human Frame.* Saunders, Philadelphia, 1968.

CHAPTER 14:
Hematologic Problems
Beland, Irene L. *Clinical Nursing: Pathophysiological and Psychosocial Approaches,* 3rd ed. Macmillan, New York, 1975.
Brunner, Lillian S., and Suddarth, Doris S. *Textbook of Medical-Surgical Nursing,* 3rd ed. Lippincott, Philadelphia, 1975.
——*The Lippincott Manual of Nursing Practice.* Lippincott, Philadelphia, 1974.
Clifford, G. O. "Hematologic Problems in the Elderly." In Rossman, I. (ed.), *Clinical Geriatrics.* Lippincott, Philadelphia, 1971, pp. 253–266.
Craytor, J. K. "Talking with Persons Who Have Cancer." *American Journal of Nursing,* 69:744–748, April 1969.
Hugos, R. "Living with Leukemia." *American Journal of Nursing,* 72:2185–2188, December 1972.
Maekawa, T. "Hematologic Diseases." In Steinberg, F. U. (ed.). *Cowdry's, The Care of the Geriatric Patient,* 5th ed. Mosby, St. Louis, 1976, pp. 152–166.
Moidel, Harriet C., Giblin, Elizabeth C., and Wagner, Berniece M. (eds.). *Nursing Care of the Patient with Medical-Surgical Disorders,* 2nd ed. McGraw-Hill, New York, 1976.
Shafer, Kathleen N., et al. *Medical-Surgical Nursing,* 5th ed. Mosby, St. Louis, 1971.
Wilson, P. "Iron-Deficiency Anemia." *American Journal of Nursing,* 72:502–504, March 1972.

CHAPTER 15:
Gastrointestinal Problems
Amberg, J. R., and Zboralske, F. F. "Gallstones After Seventy." *Geriatrics,*

Bargen, J. Arnold. "Gastroenterologic Disorders." In Cowdry, E. V., and Steinberg, F. U., *The Care of the Geriatric Patient.* Mosby, St. Louis, 1971, pp. 80–104.
Becker, G. H., Meyer, J., and Necheles, H. "Fat Absorption in Young and Old Age." *Gastroenterology,* 14:80–92, January 1950.
Beland, Irene L. *Clinical Nursing: Pathophysiological and Psychosocial Approaches,* 3rd ed. Macmillan, New York, 1975.
Berman, P. M., and Kirsner, J. B. "Gastrointestinal Problems." In Steinberg, F. U. (ed.), *Cowdry's The Care of the Geriatric Patient,* 5th ed. Mosby, St. Louis, 1976, pp. 93–118.
Bertolini, A. M. *Gerontologic Metabolism.* Thomas, Springfield, Ill. 1969.
Bhaskar, S. N. "Oral Lesions in the Aged Population." *Geriatrics,* 23:137–149, October 1968.
Brunner, Lillian S., and Suddarth, Doris S. *Textbook of Medical-Surgical Nursing,* 3rd ed. Lippincott, Philadelphia, 1975.
——*The Lippincott Manual of Nursing Practice.* Lippincott, Philadelphia, 1974.
Davidoff, A., Winkler, S., and Lee, M. *Dentistry for the Special Patient: The Aged, Chronically Ill and Handicapped.* Saunders, Philadelphia, 1972.

Elfenbaum, A. "Dentistry for the Elderly in Health and Illness." In Chinn, A. B. (ed.), *Working with Older People,* Vol. IV. U.S. Dept. of Health, Education, and Welfare, Rockville, Md., 1974, pp. 337–358.

————— "Newer Problems of Older Patients—an Introduction to Geriatric Dentistry. In *Dental Clinics of North America.* Saunders, Philadelphia, 1968.

Greenwood, A. H. "Dental Care for the Elderly Poses Special Problems." *Geriatrics,* 31(5):103, May 1976.

McGinty, M. D. "Hiatal Hernia." *Hospital Medicine,* 7:133–143, April 1971.

Moidel, Harriet C., Giblin, Elizabeth C., and Wagner, Berniece M. (eds.). *Nursing Care of the Patient with Medical-Surgical Disorders,* 2nd ed. McGraw-Hill, New York, 1976.

Painter, Neil S. "Diverticular Disease of the Colon: A Bane of the Elderly." *Geriatrics,* 31(2):53–58, February 1976.

Rowe, Nathaniel H. "Dental Surgery." In Steinberg, F. U. (ed), *Cowdry's, The Care of the Geriatric Patient,* 5th ed. Mosby, St. Louis, 1974, pp. 300–309.

Salter, R. H. "Some Aspects of Diverticular Disease of the Colon." *Age and Aging.* 2:225–229, November 1973.

Shafer, Kathleen N., et al. *Medical-Surgical Nursing,* 5th ed. Mosby, St. Louis, 1971.

Silverman, S. I. *Principles and Practices of Dental Care for the Chronically Ill, Handicapped and the Aged.* Symposium, New York University, May 1975.

Sklear, Manuel. "Gastrointestinal Diseases in the Aged." In: Chinn, A. B., *Working with Older People,* Vol. IV. U.S. Dept. of Health, Education, and Welfare, Rockville, Md., 1974, pp. 124–131.

Straus, Bernard. "Disorders of the Digestive System." In Rossman, Isadore, *Clinical Geriatrics,* Lippincott, Philadelphia, 1971, pp. 183–202.

Unger, James L., and McGregor, Douglas H. "When Esophageal Carcinoma Is Obscured by Other Factors." *Geriatrics,* 31(2):53–58, February 1976.

CHAPTER 16:
Genitourinary Problems

Alvarez, W. C. "Will a Prostate Operation Produce Impotence?" *Geriatrics,* 20:996, 1965.

Beland, Irene L. *Clinical Nursing: Pathophysiological and Psychosocial Approaches,* 3rd ed. Macmillan, New York, 1975.

Birnbaum, S. J. "Geriatric Gynecology." In Chinn, A. B. (ed.), *Working with Older People,* Vol. IV. U.S. Dept. of Health, Education, and Welfare, Rockville, Md., 1974, pp. 149–155.

Bowles, W. T. "Urologic Surgery." In Steinberg, F. U. (ed.), *Cowdry's, The Care of the Geriatric Patient,* 5th ed. Mosby, St. Louis, 1976, pp. 275–283.

Brocklehurst, J. C. "The Urinary Tract." In Rossman, Isadore (ed.), *Clinical Geriatrics.* Lippincott, Philadelphia, 1971, pp. 219–228.

————— Dillane, J. B., Griffiths, L., and Fry, J. "The Prevalence and Symptomatology of Urinary Infection in An Aged Population." *Gerontologica Clinica,* 10:242, 1968.

Brunner, Lillian S., and Suddarth, Doris S. *Textbook of Medical-Surgical Nursing,* 3rd ed. Lippincott, Philadelphia, 1975.

————— *The Lippincott Manual of Nursing Practice.* Lippincott, Philadelphia, 1974.

Clark, C. L. "Catheter Care in the Home." *American Journal of Nursing,* 72:922–924, May 1972.

Delehanty, L., and Stravino, V. "Achieving Bladder Control." *American Journal of Nursing,* 70:312–316, February 1970.

Gibbs, G. E. "Perineal Care of the Incapacitated Patient." *American Journal of Nursing,* 69:124–125, January 1969.

Grabstald, H. "Management of Tumors of the G.U. Tract in the Geriatric Patient." *Journal of the American Geriatrics Society,* 14:95, 1966.

Jaffe, J. W. "Common Lower Urinary Tract Problems in Older Persons." In Chinn, A. B. (ed.), *Working with Older People,* Vol. IV. U.S. Dept. of Health, Education, and Welfare, Rockville, Md., 1974, pp. 141–148.

Jeffcoate, T. N. A. *Principles of Gynecology,* 3rd ed. Prentice-Hall (Appleton), Englewood Cliffs, N.J., 1967.

Kahn, A. I., and Snapper, I. "Medical Renal Diseases in the Aged." In Chinn, A. B. (ed.), *Working with Older People,* Vol. IV. U.S. Dept. of Health, Education, and Welfare, Rockville, Md., 1974, pp. 131–140.

Keuhnelian, J. G., and Saunders, V. E. *Urologic Nursing.* Lippincott, Philadelphia, 1971.

Lapides, J., and Zierdt, D. "Renal Function with Aging." *Journal of the American Medical Assoc.,* 201:778, 1967.

Moidel, Harriet C., Giblin, Elizabeth C., and Wagner, Berniece M. (eds.). *Nursing Care of the Patient with Medical-Surgical Disorders,* 2nd ed. McGraw-Hill, New York, 1976.

Owen, M. L. "Special Care for the Patient Who Has Had a Breast Biopsy or Mastectomy." *Nursing Clinics of North America,* 7:373–382, June 1972.

Rossman, Isadore. "The Anatomy of Aging." In Rossman, Isadore (ed.), *Clinical Geriatrics.* Lippincott, Philadelphia, 1971, p. 9.

Shafer, Kathleen N., et al. *Medical-Surgical Nursing,* 5th ed. Mosby, St. Louis, 1971.

Winter, C. C., and Barker, M. R. *Nursing Care of Patients with Urologic Diseases.* Mosby, St. Louis, 1972.

Wright, V. Cecil. "Carcinoma of the Vulva." *Journal of the American Geriatrics Society,* 14(5):232-235, May 1976.

CHAPTER 17:
Neurological Problems

Beland, Irene L. *Clinical Nursing: Pathophysiological and Psychosocial Approaches,* 3rd ed. Macmillan, New York, 1975.

Brunner, Lillian S., and Suddarth, Doris S. *Textbook of Medical-Surgical Nursing,* 3rd ed. Lippincott, Philadelphia, 1975.

———— *The Lippincott Manual of Nursing Practice.* Lippincott, Philadelphia, 1974.

Carini, E., and Owens, G. *Neurological and Neurosurgical Nursing.* Mosby, St. Louis, 1970.

Carter, A. B. "The Neurologic Aspects of Aging." In Rossman, I. (ed.), *Clinical Geriatrics.* Lippincott, Philadelphia, 1971, pp. 123–141.

Cooney, L. M. and Solitaire, G. B. "Primary Intracranial Tumors in the Elderly." *Geriatrics,* 27:94–104, January 1972.

Dayhoff, N. "Soft or Hard Devices to Position Hands?" *American Journal of Nursing,* 75(7):1142–1144, July 1975.

Dervitz, H. L. and Zislis, J. M. "A Medical Perspective of Physical Therapy and Stroke Rehabilitation." *Geriatrics,* 25:123–132, June 1970.

Dolan, M. B. "Autumn Months, Autumn Years." *American Journal of Nursing,* 75(7):1145–1147, July 1975.

Hardin. W. B. "Neurologic Aspects." In Steinberg, F. U. (ed.), *Cowdry's, The Care of the Geriatric Patient,* 5th ed. Mosby, St. Louis, 1976, pp. 364–379.

Hull, J. T. "The Prevalence and Incidence of Parkinson's Disease." *Geriatrics,* 25:128–133, May 1970.

Jacobansky, A. M. "Stroke." *American Journal of Nursing,* 72:1260–1263, July 1972.

Locke, S. "Cerebrovascular Disorders in Later Life." In Chinn, A. B. (ed.), *Working With Older People: A Guide to Practice,* Vol. IV. U.S. Dept. of Health, Education, and Welfare, Rockville, Md., 1974, pp. 50–59.

——— "Neurological Disorders of the Elderly." In Chinn, A. B. (ed.), *Working With Older People: A Guide to Practice,* Vol. IV. U.S. Dept. of Health, Education, and Welfare, Rockville, Md., 1974, pp. 45–49.

Moidel, Harriet C., Giblin, Elizabeth C., and Wagner, Berniece M. (eds.), *Nursing Care of the Patient with Medical-Surgical Disorders,* 2nd ed. McGraw-Hill, New York, 1976.

Shafer, Kathleen N., et al. *Medical-Surgical Nursing,* 5th ed. Mosby, St. Louis, 1971.

Skelly, M. "Aphasic Patients Talk Back." *American Journal of Nursing,* 75(7):1140–1141, July 1975.

CHAPTER 18:
Dermatological Problems

Barrett, D., and Klibanski. A. "Collagenase Debridement." *American Journal of*

Beland, Irene L. *Clinical Nursing: Pathophysiological and Psychosocial Approaches,* 3rd ed. Macmillan, New York 1975.

Blass, M. A. "Improvised Cushions." *American Journal of Nursing,* 70(12):2605, December 1970.

Brunner, Lillian S., and Suddarth, Doris S. *Textbook of Medical-Surgical Nursing,* 3rd ed. Lippincott, Philadelphia, 1975.

——— *The Lippincott Manual of Nursing Practice.* Lippincott, Philadelphia, 1974.

Conrad, A. H. "Dermatologic Disorders." In Steinberg, F. U. (ed.), *Cowdry's, The Care of the Geriatric Patient,* 5th ed. Mosby, St. Louis, 1976, pp. 178–190.

Lang, C., and McGrath, A. "Gelfoam for Decubitus Ulcers." American Journal of Nursing, 74(3):460–461, March 1974.

Moidel, Harriet C., Giblin, Elizabeth C., and Wagner, Berniece M. (eds.), *Nursing Care of the Patient with Medical-Surgical Disorders,* 2nd ed. McGraw-Hill, New York, 1976.

Pfaudler, M. "Flotation, Displacement and Decubitus Ulcers." *American Journal of Nursing,* 68(11):2351–2355, November 1968.

Shafer, Kathleen N., et al. *Medical-Surgical Nursing,* 5th ed. Mosby, St. Louis, 1971.

Tindall, J. P. "Geriatric Dermatology." In Chinn, A. B. (ed.), *Working with Older People: A Guide to Practice,* Vol. IV. U.S. Dept. of Health, Education, and Welfare, Rockville, Md., 1974, pp. 3–27.

Van Ort, S. R., and Gerber, R. M. "Topical Application of Insulin in the Treatment of Decubitus Ulcers: A Pilot Study." *Nursing Research,* 25(1):9–12, January–February 1976.

Vasile, J., and Chaitin, H. "Prognostic Factors in Decubitus Ulcers of the Aged." *Geriatrics,* 27:126–129, April 1972.

Wallace, G., and Hayter, J. "Karaya for Chronic Skin Ulcers." *American Journal of Nursing,* 74(6):1094–1098, June 1974.

Weinstein, L. D., and Davidson, B. A. "Fluid-Support Mattress and Seat for the

Prevention and Treatment of Decubitus Ulcers." *Lancet,* 2:625–626, September 25, 1965.

Young, A. W. "Skin Diseases." In Rossman, I. (ed.), *Clinical Geriatrics.* Lippincott, Philadelphia, 1971, pp. 203–218.

CHAPTER 19:
Sensory Deficits

Amburgey, P.I. "Environmental Aids for the Aged Patient." *American Journal of Nursing,* 66:2017–2018, September 1966.

American Foundation for the Blind. *An Introduction to Working with the Aging Person Who Is Visually Handicapped.* New York, 1972.

Brunside, I. M. "Clocks and Calendars." *American Journal of Nursing,* 70:117–119, January 1970.

———"Touching Is Talking." *American Journal of Nursing.* 73:2060–2063, December 1973.

Chodil, J., and Williams, B. "The Concept of Sensory Deprivation." *Nursing Clinics of North America,* 1970. 5:453, Sept, 1970.

Cockerill, E. E. "Reflections on My Nursing Care." *American Journal of Nursing,* 65:83–85, May 1965.

Condl, E. D. "Ophthalmic Nursing: The Gentle Touch." *Nursing Clinics of North America,* 5:467–476, September 1970.

Davis, H., and Silverman, S. R. *Hearing and Deafness.* Holt, Rinehart and Winston, New York, 1970.

Downs, F. S. "Bedrest and Sensory Disturbances." *American Journal of Nursing,* 74:434–438, March 1974.

Gordon, D. M. "Eye Problems of the Aged." In Chinn, A. B. (ed.), *Working with Older People,* Vol. IV. U.S. Department of Health, Education, and Welfare, Rockville, Md., 1974. pp. 28–37.

Kornzweig, A. L. "The Eye in Old Age." In Rossman, I. (ed.), *Clinical Geriatrics.* Lippincott, Philadelphia, 1971, pp. 229–246.

Nilo, E. R. "Needs of the Hearing Impaired." *American Journal of Nursing,* 69:114–116, January 1969.

Ohno, M. J. "The Eye-Patched Patient." *American Journal of Nursing,* 71:271–274, February 1971.

Reuben, R. "Aging and Hearing." In Rossman, I. (ed.), *Clinical Geriatrics.* Lippincott, Philadelphia, 1971, pp. 247–252.

Rummerfield, P. S., and Rummerfield, M. J. "Noise Induced Hearing Loss." *Occupational Health Nurse,* 17:23–24, November, 1969.

Saunders, W. H., et al. *Nursing Care in Eye, Ear, Nose and Throat Disorders,* 2nd ed. Mosby, St. Louis, 1968.

Seamon, F. W. "Nursing Care of Glaucoma Patients." *Nursing Clinics of North America,* 5:489–496, September 1970.

Senturia, B. H., and Prince, L. L. "Otolaryngological Problems in the Geriatric Patient." In Chinn, A. B. (ed.), *Working With Older People,* Vol. IV. U.S. Department of Health, Education, and Welfare, Rockville, Md., 1974, pp. 38–44.

Worrell, J. D. "Nursing Implications in the Care of the Patient Experiencing Sensory Deprivation." In Kintzel, K. C. (ed.), *Advanced Concepts in Clinical Nursing,* Lippincott, Philadelphia, 1971.

CHAPTER 20:
Surgical Care

Alexander, S. "Surgical Risk in the Patient with Arteriosclerotic Heart Disease." *Surgical Clinics of North America,* 48:513, 1968.

Dodd, R. B. "Anesthesia." In Steinberg, F. U. (ed.), *Cowdry's, The Care of the Geriatric Patient,* 5th ed. Mosby, St. Louis, 1976, pp. 247–257.

Duncalf, D., and Kepes, E. R. "Geriatric Anesthesia." In Rossman, I. (ed.), *Clinical Geriatrics.* Lippincott, Philadelphia, 1971, pp. 421–438.

Glenn, F. "Surgical Principles for the Aged Patient." In Chinn, A. B. (ed.), *Working with Older People,* Vol. IV. U.S. Dept. of Health, Education, and Welfare, Rockville, Md., 1974, pp. 250–266.

—— Moore, S. W., and Beal, J. (eds.). *Surgery in the Aged.* McGraw-Hill, New York, 1960.

Mason, J. H., Gau, F. C., and Byrne, M. P. "General Surgery." In Steinberg, F. U. (ed.), *Cowdry's, The Care of the Geriatric Patient,* 5th ed. Mosby, St. Louis, 1976, pp. 217–246.

Powers, J. H. (ed.). *Surgery of the Aged and Debilitated Patient.* Saunders, Philadelphia, 1968.

Schein, C. J., and Dardik, H. "A Selective Approach to Surgical Problems in the Aged." In Rossman, I. (ed.), *Clinical Geriatrics.* Lippincott, Philadelphia, 1971, pp. 405–420.

CHAPTER 21:
Mental Health and Illness in Old Age

Blank, M. L. "Raising the Age Barrier to Psychotherapy." *Geriatrics,* 29(11):141–148, November 1974.

Botwinick, J. *Aging and Behavior.* Springer, New York, 1973, pp. 25–27, 54–59, 60–66, and 309.

Braceland, F. J. "Predicting the Future of Mental Health Care." *Geriatrics,* 29(11):178–186, November 1974.

Brown, B. S. "How Do Mental Health and Aging Affect Each Other? New Center Will Encourage Search for Answers." *Geriatrics,* 31(2):40–44, February 1976.

Buell, D. "Psychiatrists Pay New Heed to Mental Problems of Aged." *National Observer,* January 25, 1975, p. 17.

Burnside, I. M. "Group Work Among the Aged." *Nursing Outlook,* 17(6):68–71, June 1969.

—— (ed.). *Psychosocial Nursing Care of the Aged.* McGraw-Hill, New York, 1973.

Busse, E., and Pfeiffer, E. *Mental Illness in Later Life.* American Psychiatric Association, Washington, D.C., 1973.

Butler, R. N. "Clinical Psychiatry in Late Life." In Rossman, I. (ed.), *Clinical Geriatrics.* Lippincott, Philadelphia, 1971, pp. 439–460.

—— "Mental Health and Aging: Life Cycle Perspectives." *Geriatrics,* 29(11):59–60, November 1974.

—— "Psychiatry and the Elderly: An Overview." *American Journal of Psychiatry,* 132(9):893–900, September 1975.

—— *Why Survive? Being Old in America.* Harper & Row, New York, 1975, pp. 225–259.

—— and Lewis, M. I. *Aging and Mental Health.* Mosby, St. Louis, 1973.

Casady, M. "If You're Active and Savvy at 30, You'll Be Warm and Witty at 70." *Psychology Today,* 9(6):138, November 1970.

Gage, F. "Suicide in the Aged." *American Journal of Nursing,* 71(11):2153–2155, November 1971.

Garetz, F. K. "Breaking the Dangerous Cycle of Depression and Faulty Nutrition." *Geriatrics,* 31(6):73–75, June 1976.

Garnick, S. "Psychological Study in the Management of the Geriatric Patient." In Chinn, A. B. (ed.), *Working With Older People: A Guide To Practice,* Vol. IV. U.S. Dept. of Health, Education, and Welfare, Rockville, Md., 1974, pp. 321–336.

Gordon, S. K. "The Phenomenon of Depression in Old Age." *Gerontologist,* 13(1):100–105, Spring 1973.

Hall, J. E., and Weaver, B. R. *Nursing of Families in Crisis.* Lippincott, Philadelphia, 1974.

Harrison, C. "The Institutionally Deprived Elderly." *Nursing Clinics of North America,* 3:697–707, December 1968.

Hoogerbeets, J. D., and LaWall, J. "Changing Concepts of Psychiatric Problems in the Aged." *Geriatrics,* 30(8):83–87, August 1975.

Kahn, R. L. "The Mental Health System and the Future Aged." *Gerontologist,* 15(1):24–31, February 1975.

Kastenbaum, R., and Mishara, B. L. "Premature Death and Self-injurious Behavior in Old Age." *Geriatrics,* 26(7):70–81, July 1971.

——— "... Gone Tomorrow." *Geriatrics,* 29(11):127–134, November 1974.

Kern, R. A. "Emotional Problems in Relation to Aging and Old Age." *Geriatrics,* 26(6):83–93, June 1971.

Libow, L. B. "Pseudo-senility: Acute and Reversible Organic Brain Syndromes." *Journal of American Geriatrics Society,* 21:112–120, March 1973.

Looney, D. S. "Senility Is Also a State of Mind." *National Observer,* March 31, 1973, p. 1.

Neugarten, B. L. (ed.). *Middle Age and Aging.* Univ. of Chicago Press, 1968.

Parker, B., Deibler, S., Feldshub, B., Frosch, W., Laureano, E., and Sillen, J. "Finding Medical Reasons for Psychiatric Behavior." *Geriatrics,* 31(6):87–91, June 1976.

Patterson, R. C., Abrahams, R., and Baker, F. "Preventing Self-Destructive Behavior." *Geriatrics,* 29(11):115–121, November 1974.

Post, Felix. *The Clinical Psychiatry of Late Life.* Pergamon Press, London, 1965.

Raskind, M. A., Alvarez, C., Pietrzyk, M., Westerlund, K., and Herlin, S. "Helping the Elderly Psychiatric Patient in Crisis." *Geriatrics,* 31(6):51–56, June 1976.

Yelom, I., and Terrazas, F. "Group Therapy for Psychotic Elderly Patients." *American Journal of Nursing,* 68:1690–1694, 1968.

CHAPTER 22:
Geriatric Pharmacology

Ayd, F. J. "Tranquilizers and the Ambulatory Geriatric Patient." *Journal of the American Geriatrics Society,* 8:908, 1960.

Bellville, J. W., Forrest, W. H., Jr., Miller, E., and Brown, B. W., Jr. "Influence of Age on Pain Relief from Analgesics." *Journal of the American Medical Assoc.,* 217:1835–1841, 1971.

Bender, A. D. "Pharmacologic Aspects of Aging: A Survey of the Effect of Increasing Age on Drug Activity in Adults." *Journal of the American Geriatrics Society,* 12:114, 1964.

——— "Gerontological Basis for Modifications in Drug Activity with Age." *Journal Pharm. Science,* 54:1225, 1965.

——— "The Effect of Increasing Age on the Distribution of Peripheral Blood Flow in Man." *Journal of the American Geriatrics Society,* 13:192, 1965.

——— "Pharmacologic Aspects of Aging: Additional Literature." *Journal of the American Geriatrics Society,* 15(1):68–74, 1967.

Calloway, N. O., and Merrill, R. S. "The Aging Adult Liver, I: Bromsulphalein and Bilirubin Clearances." *Journal of the American Geriatrics Society,* 13:594, 1965.

Davis, L. D., Lawton, A. H., Prouty, R., and Chow, B. F. "The Absorption of Oral Vitamin B-12 in an Aged Population." *Journal of Gerontology,* 20:169, 1965.

Davison, W. "Drug Hazards in the Elderly." *Gerontologica Clinica,* 7:257, 1965.

"Drugs and the Elderly Mind." *Lancet,* 2:126, 1972.

Fikry, M. E., and Aboul-Wafa, M. H. "Intestinal Absorption in the Old." *Gerontologica Clinica,* 7:171, 1965.

Freeman, J. T. *Clinical Principles and Drugs in the Aging.* Thomas, Springfield, Ill., 1963.

——— "Drug Therapy in Aging Patients." *Geriatrics,* 18:174, 1963.

Friedman, S. A., Raizner, A. E., Rosen, H., Solomon, N. A., and Sy, W. "Functional Defects in the Aging Kidney." *Annals of Internal Medicine,* 74:41–45, 1972.

Halford, F. D., and Mithoefer, J. C. "The Effect of Morphine and Respiration in the Aged." *Surgical Clinics of North America,* 40:907, 1960.

Hamilton, L. D. "The Aged Brain and the Phenothiazines." *Geriatrics,* 21:131, 1966.

Herrmann, G. R. "Digitoxicity in the Aged: Recognition, Frequency and Management." *Geriatrics,* 21:109, 1966.

Hurley, J. D. "Cancer Chemotherapy." *Journal of the American Geriatrics Society,* 10:1058, 1962.

Hurwitz, U. "Predisposing Factors in Adverse Reactions to Drugs." *British Medical Journal,* 1:536–539, 1969.

Kayne, R. C., Cheung, A., and McCarron, M. M. *Monitoring of Drug Therapy of Long Care Patients.* Presented at the Second Annual Scientific Session, Western Division, American Geriatrics Society, Los Angeles, 1973.

Keyes, J. W. "Problems in Drug Management of Cardiovascular Disorders in Geriatric Patients." *Journal of the American Geriatrics Society,* 13:118, 1965.

Lamy, P. O., and Kitler, M. E. "Drugs and the Geriatric Patient." *Journal of the American Geriatrics Society,* 19:23, 1971.

Lely, A. H., and Van Enter, C. H. J. "Non-Cardiac Symptoms of Digitalis Intoxication." *American Heart Journal,* 83:149–152, 1972.

Nicholson, W. J. "Medicine in Old Age: Disturbances of the Special Senses and Other Functions." *British Medical Journal,* 1:33–35, 1974.

Olson, E. V., Johnson, B. J., Thompson, L. F., McCarthy, J. A., Edmonds, R. E., Schroeder, L. M., and Wade, M. "The Hazards of Immobility." *American Journal of Nursing,* 67:781–796, 1967.

Pfeiffer, E. "Use of Drugs which Influence Behavior in the Elderly: Promises, Pitfalls and Perspectives." In Davis, R. H. (ed.), *Drugs and the Elderly.* Andries Gerontology Center, Univ. of South California, Los Angeles, 1973, pp. 43–44.

Rubb, T. U. "Use of Drugs in the Older Age Groups." *Pharmaceutical Journal,* 1:507, 1961.

Schwid, S. A., and **Gifford, R. W.** "The Use and Abuse of Antihypertensive Drugs in the Aged." *Geriatrics, 122:172, 1967.*
Smith, W. N., and **Melmon, K. L.** "Drug Choice in Disease." In Melmon, K. L., and Morrelli, H. F. (eds.), *Clinical Pharmacology: Basic Principles in Therapeutics.* Macmillan, New York, 1972, p. 5.
Stewart, R. B., and **Cluff, L. E.** "A Review of Medication Errors and Compliances in Ambulant Patients." *Clinical Pharmacology and Therapeutics,* 13:463–468, 1972.

CHAPTER 23:
Sexuality

Armstrong, E. B. "The Possibility of Sexual Happiness in Old Age." In Beigel, H. G. (ed.), *Advances in Sex Research.* Harper & Row, New York, 1963.
Bengtson, V. L. "Sex in Nursing Homes." *Medical Aspects of Human Sexuality,* 9:21, 1975.
Botwinick, J. "Drives, Expectancies and Emotions." In Birren, J. E. (ed.), *Handbook of Aging and the Individual.* Univ. of Chicago Press, 1960.
——— *Aging and Behavior.* Springer, New York, 1973, pp. 35–49.
Calleja, M. A. "Homosexual Behavior in Older Men." *Sexology,* August 1967, pp. 46–48.
Cameron, P., and **Biber, H.** "Sexual Thought Throughout the Life Span." *Gerontologist,* 13:144–147, Summer 1973.
Christenson, C., and **Gagnon, J. H.** "Sexual Behavior in a Group of Older Women." *Journal of Gerontology,* 20:351–356, 1965.
Comfort, Alex. *The Joy of Sex.* Simon & Schuster, New York, 1972.
——— "Sexuality in Old Age." *Journal of the American Geriatrics Society,* 22(10):440–442, October 1974.
Daly, M. J. "Sexual Attitudes in Menopausal and Postmenopausal Women." *Medical Aspects of Human Sexuality,* May 1968, pp. 48–53.
Davis, M. E. "Estrogen and the Aging Process." In *Year Book of Obstetrics and Gynecology,* 1964–1965. Year Book Medical Publishers, Chicago, 1965.
Finkel, A. L. "The Relationship of Sexual Habits to Benign Prostatic Hypertrophy." *Medical Aspects of Human Sexuality,* October 1967, pp. 24–25.
——— "Sex After Prostectomy." *Medical Aspects of Human Sexuality.* March 1968, pp. 40–41.
——— "Sexual Function During Advancing Age." In Rossman, I. (ed.), *Clinical Geriatrics.* Lippincott, Philadelphia, 1971.
——— **Moyers, T. G., Tobenkin, M. I.,** and **Karg, S. J.** "Sexual Potency in Aging Males: Frequency of Coitus Among Clinic Patients." *Journal of the American Medical Assoc.,* 170:1391–1393, 1959.
Freeman, J. T. "Sexual Capacities in the Aging Male." *Geriatrics.* 16:37–43, 1961.
Goldfarb, A. F., **Daly, M. J., Lieberman, D.,** and **Reed, D. M.** "Sex and the Menopause." *Medical Aspects of Human Sexuality,* November 1970, pp. 64–89.
Jacobson, L. "Illness and Human Sexuality." *Nursing Outlook,* 22(1):50–53, January 1974.
Kent, S. "Continued Sexual Activity Depends on Health and the Availability of a Partner." *Geriatrics,* 30(11):142–144, November 1975.
Lewis, M. I., and **Butler, R. N.** "Neglected by Women's Lib." *National Observer,* June 29, 1972, p. 20.

Lobsenz, N. M. "Sex and the Senior Citizen." *The New York Times Magazine,* January 20, 1974, pp. 8–28.

Newman, G., and Nichols, C. R. "Sexual Activities and Attitudes in Older Persons." *Journal of American Medical Assoc.,* 173:33–35, 1960.

Pfeiffer, E. "Sexuality in the Aging Individual." *Journal of the American Geriatrics Society.* 22(11):481–484, November 1974.

Rubin, H. H., and Newman, B. W. *Active Sex After Sixty.* Arco, New York, 1969.

"Sex Behavior of Older Women." *Sexology,* June 1966, p. 734.

Sontag, S. T. "The Double Standard of Aging." *Saturday Review,* September 1972, pp. 29–38.

Verwoerdt, A., Pfeiffer, E., and Wang, H. S. "Sexual Behavior in Senescence." *Geriatrics,* 24:137–154, February 1969.

Weinberg, J. "Sexuality in Later Life." *Medical Aspects of Human Sexuality,* April 1971, pp. 216–227.

Whiskin, F. E. "The Geriatric Sex Offender." *Medical Aspects of Human Sexuality.* April 1970, pp. 125–129.

CHAPTER 24:
The Dying Process

Allen, B. "Until Death Ensues." *Nursing Clinics of North America,* 7(2):303–308, June 1972.

Becker, Ernest. *The Denial of Death.* Free Press, New York, 1973.

Black, P. McL. "Focusing on Some of the Ethical Problems Associated with Death and Dying." *Geriatrics,* 31(1):138–141, January, 1976.

Cameron, P., et al. "Consciousness of Death Across the Life Span." *Journal of Gerontology,* 28(1):92–95, January 1973.

Davis, Richard H. (ed.). *Dealing with Death.* Andrus Gerontology Center, Univ. of Southern California, Los Angeles, 1973.

Elner, R. "Dying in the U.S.A." *International Journal of Nursing Studies,* 10(3):171–184, August 1973.

Fuchs, Beverly. "On Death and Dying." Unpublished paper presented to Osler Nursing Staff, Johns Hopkins Hospital, Baltimore, November 1976.

Kastenbam, Robert, and Aisenberg, Ruth. *The Psychology of Death.* Springer, New York, 1972.

Klass, D., and Gordon, A. "Goals in Teaching About Death." *The Maryland Teacher,* 23(3):8–9, 22-24, Spring 1976.

Kutscher, A., and Goldberg, M. (eds.). *Caring for the Dying Patient and His Family.* Health Sciences, New York, 1973.

Maguire, Daniel C. *Death By Choice.* Doubleday, New York, 1974.

Mitford, J. *The American Way of Death.* Simon & Schuster, New York, 1963.

Quint, J. C. *The Nurse and the Dying Patient.* Macmillan, New York, 1967.

Schoenberg, B., et al. (eds.). *Psychosocial Aspects of Terminal Care.* Columbia Univ. Press, New York, 1972.

Schultz, R. "Meeting the Three Major Needs of the Dying Patient." *Geriatrics,* 31(6):132–137, June 1976.

Shneidman, E. S. (ed.). *Death: Current Perspectives.* Aronson Jason, New York 1976.

Simms, L. M. "Dignified Death: A Right Not A Privilege." *Journal of Gerontological Nursing,* 1(5):21–25, November–December 1975.

Weisman, A. D. *On Dying and Denying.* Behavior Publications, New York, 1972.

Williams, R. *To Live and To Die: When, Why and How.* Springer-Verlag, New York, 1974.

CHAPTER 25:
Services for the Aged

Beverley, V. E. "Helping Your Patient Choose and Adjust to a Nursing Home." *Geriatrics,* 31(5):115–126, May 1976.

——— "Matching Facilities to the Patients Needs." *Geriatrics,* 31(4):100–110, April 1976.

Hammovitch, M. B., and Peterson, J. E. "Housing Needs and Satisfactions of the Elderly." *Gerontologist,* 9:30–32, 1969.

Lang, J., et al. (eds.). *Designing for Human Behavior.* Dowden, Hutchinson and Ross, Stroudsburg, Pa., 1974.

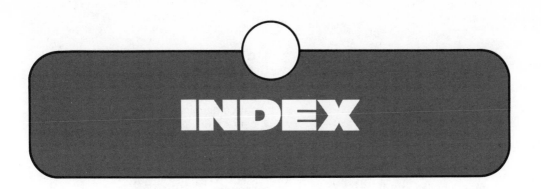

INDEX